The Changing Face of Medicine

A VOLUME IN THE SERIES

The Culture and Politics of Health Care Work

Edited by Suzanne Gordon *and* Sioban Nelson

The Changing Face of Medicine

WOMEN DOCTORS AND THE EVOLUTION OF HEALTH CARE IN AMERICA

Ann K. Boulis
Jerry A. Jacobs

ILR Press
an imprint of
Cornell University Press   ITHACA AND LONDON

First published 2008 by Cornell University Press

Printed in the United States of America

Library of Congress Cataloging-in-Publication Data

Boulis, Ann K., 1968–
   The changing face of medicine : women doctors and the evolution of health care in America / Ann K. Boulis, Jerry A. Jacobs.
      p. cm. — (The culture and politics of health care work)
   Includes bibliographical references and index.
   ISBN 978-0-8014-4446-3 (cloth : alk. paper)
  1. Women physicians—United States. 2. Medical care—United States. I. Jacobs, Jerry A., 1955–. II. Title. III. Series.
   R692.B675 2008
   610.82—dc22   2008019828

Cornell University Press strives to use environmentally responsible suppliers and materials to the fullest extent possible in the publishing of its books. Such materials include vegetable-based, low-VOC inks and acid-free papers that are recycled, totally chlorine-free, or partly composed of nonwood fibers. For further information, visit our website at www.cornellpress.cornell.edu.

Cloth printing   10 9 8 7 6 5 4 3 2 1

*This book is dedicated
to our daughters,
Sophia and Renie Harris
and
Elizabeth and
Madeleine Jacobs*

Contents

Acknowledgments

This project has had a long gestation, and consequently we have accumulated many debts along the way. The research presented here has been funded by research grants from the Josiah H. Macy Foundation and the Robert Wood Johnson Foundation, and a National Academy of Education Post-Doctoral Fellowship for Ann Boulis funded by the Lyle M. Spencer Foundation.

We are grateful to Dr. June Osborn, president of the Macy Foundation, and Dr. Cathy DeAngelis, editor of the *Journal of the American Medical Association*, who played a central role in organizing the Macy Foundation Conference in 2006 where the issues addressed in this book were discussed (Hager 2007). At Cornell University Press, Fran Benson has been very encouraging since the first outline of this project was put together some years ago. Sioban Nelson read several drafts of the manuscript and offered very thoughtful and detailed advice.

We wish to acknowledge the valuable research assistance provided by Arielle Kuperberg, Terry Labov, Daniella Main, and Kristin Turney. Ruth Schwartz Cowan, Jason Schnittker, and Chloe Bird organized seminars and professional panels that gave us the opportunity to present some of our findings. Charles Bosk met with us shortly after the inception of this project and has provided collegial advice as we brought this study to fruition.

We acknowledge the Association of American Medical Colleges (AAMC) for sharing its data on entering and graduating students. The conclusions presented here are our own and do not reflect those of the AAMC. Similarly, we thank Linda Sax and William S. Korn at the UCLA Higher Education

Research Institute for generously providing tabulations of their unique data on American college freshmen.

We have benefited from lengthy discussions with Dr. Stephanie Abbuhl and Dr. Judith Long regarding many issues examined here, especially about the role of women in academic medicine. Special thanks to Gus Harris and to Renee and Matt Boulis for their support throughout this project.

The Changing Face of Medicine

1

Introduction

Betty Friedan was very proud of her daughter the doctor. Friedan's 1963 book *The Feminine Mystique* helped to spark the second wave of the women's movement during the 1960s, and Friedan went on to help establish the National Organization for Women. Her daughter, Emily, entered Harvard Medical School in 1978, just as the number of young women in medical school classes began its rapid ascent.

Encouraging one's daughter to pursue a career in medicine is no longer an unusual idea restricted to feminist leaders who happen to be Jewish. In fact, Americans are now more likely to report that they feel comfortable recommending a career in medicine for a young woman than for a young man. The Gallup Organization has polled Americans on this subject periodically since the Second World War (see Figure 1.1). In 1950 more than one quarter of those sampled reported that they would recommend a career in medicine for a young man, but only 2 percent would do so for a young woman (Saad 2005).[1] The question was not asked again about young women until 1985. By this time the number of respondents who volunteered medicine as a career for young men had declined to fewer than 10 percent, but the level of support for young women physicians had grown to nearly the same level. Since 1998 the proportion who would recommend a career in medicine to a young woman has exceeded that for young men.

A career in medicine is now the top recommendation for young women, surpassing the most prominent alternatives—nursing, teaching, computers, and business—by a wide margin. Moreover, the overall level of endorsement for careers in medicine has rebounded from its lows during the 1980s. We think Betty, who passed away in 2006, would be pleased to know of this trend.

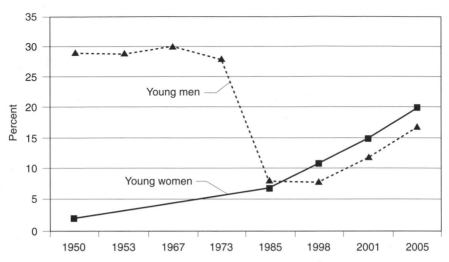

Figure 1.1. Trends in Advice to Young Men and Women. *Source:* Gallup Organization, Saad 2005.

For Friedan, the women's movement was principally about opening up avenues of opportunity for daughters which had previously been reserved for sons. Whereas feminist politics in recent years have centered on debates about abortion, contraception, and gay marriage and parenting, it may be useful to remember that expanding new career possibilities for young women was central to the original agenda. From this vantage point, the burgeoning numbers of women entering the medical profession surely constitutes a success story. Female physicians are not simply a symbol of women's accomplishments; they also constitute a significant fraction of the highest-earning women in the United States. In 2000 they represented nearly one in ten women who earned more than $100,000.[2]

Since the 1970s, women have made significant progress in the U.S. medical profession. Most notably, between 1970 and 2005 women's share of seats in medical schools increased from 11 percent to 48.9 percent (AAMC 2006). During the same period, women's numerical representation among practicing physicians increased nearly ninefold, from 25,000 in 1970 to 225,000 in 2002. In this book we examine whether women's entry into medicine represents a success for feminism or if the story is more complex than the term "success" might suggest. We first document why and how women's representation among physicians in the United States has grown so dramatically since 1970. We then assess the place that women currently occupy in the medical profession and examine how they came to occupy this place. And finally, we consider the impact of this demographic transformation on the provision of health care services. Specifically, we address four questions: (1) How can the feminization of medicine in the United States best be explained? (2) How and why do the career locations and experiences of male and female physicians differ? (3) How are the family lives of physicians changing as the need to balance work and family becomes more salient? and (4) What effect has the feminization of U.S. medicine had on the daily practice of medicine and on the medical profession?

Has the entry of women into the profession resulted from a decline in the status of medicine? In other words, does women's entry represent a turning point in the status of the medical profession? Has the entry of women led to a further deterioration in the status of the profession, impacting the women themselves as well as their male counterparts? Have women become full and equal members of the profession, or have they become ghettoized in a small set of low-paying, low-status specialties? Once they don their white coats, have women begun to change the way medicine is being practiced? Finally, are women bringing a heritage of nurturance and caring to the science of medicine, or do male and female physicians trained in the same procedures make the same diagnoses and deliver the same expert care in essentially interchangeable ways? Will women change the nature of the medical profession and its social position?

Our study follows women (and men) as they enter the medical profession. We chart the pathways that men and women traverse as they become doctors. By comparing these processes for different generations of physicians during a period of rapid change, we are able to better understand how women entered this most prominent of professions and, once there, where they land.

Are gender differences in medicine the result of the choices made by individual women, or do gendered institutions also play an important role? The bulk of research to date highlights the role of individual choice and underplays the effects of institutional arrangements and social pressures. By tracing changes over time, we are better positioned to assess the evolution of choices and constraints that women have faced.

When patients come into a family practice setting, or find themselves in an emergency room or specialist's office, does it matter if the physician is a woman or a man? Will the nature of the encounter be different? Will female physicians be consistently more collegial, more caring, and more attuned to psychosocial issues? Will diagnoses, referrals, procedures, and prescriptions be the same regardless of the physician's gender? Are there gender differences that pertain across the board, or are differences in practice restricted to a limited set of ambiguous conditions or to distinct parings of physicians and patients?

And what will happen to the structure of the profession when women physicians are as numerous as men? Will the increasing number of women physicians change the focus of medical research or influence the leadership style of organized medicine? Will this dramatic demographic change cause all physicians, regardless of gender, to employ a more collaborative approach with other health care providers? Will the presence of women lead to the creation of more family-friendly supports within the profession?

In endeavoring to answer these questions, we draw on a wide array of data sources. Since most sources of data have both strengths and weaknesses, our approach is to cast a wide net in order to gather as much information as possible on the evolution of gender and medicine. Our analysis of the processes of recruitment into the profession takes advantage of multiple longitudinal data sources, including a series of national surveys of college students' career plans which span the 1970s, 1980s, and 1990s and data from the Association of American Medical Colleges (AAMC) surveys of prospective and matriculating medical students before and after graduating from medical school. In order to understand the career experiences of physicians, we analyzed data from 1996 and 2004 on physicians' attitudes and practices from the Community Tracking Study, a nationally representative longitudinal sample of doctors. Our examination of changes in the family lives of physicians draws on data from the 1980, 1990, and 2000 U.S. censuses.

We supplement these rich and varied quantitative sources with dozens of in-depth interviews with female physicians at all stages of the career cycle. We also posted questions on-line at the MomMD and the Student Doctor Network Web sites, and we monitored scores of postings that followed. Both sites include frequent discussions of gender issues in medicine. These data sources are described in more detail in the Appendix.

Perspectives on Gender and Medicine

We draw on three main perspectives on gender and work to inform our answers to the four questions delineated earlier. The first perspective, which we refer to as personal choice, suggests that gender differences in the workforce stem primarily from differences in the choices that men and women make as they pursue education and paid employment. In other words, gender differences in the status of male and female physicians reflect preferences and values that women bring with them into the medical profession (Hinze et al. 1997; Grant et al. 1990). More specifically, this viewpoint asserts that women physicians choose to work fewer hours than men and gravitate toward primary care roles because they give higher priority to the care of their families.

The personal choice perspective also emphasizes the relationship between personal values and gender differences in career choice. The crux of this perspective is best articulated by Carol Gilligan in her book *In a Different Voice* (1982). Gilligan holds that women are generally less competitive and status conscious and more sensitive, caring, and concerned about others' feelings than are men. In the context of medicine, the "different voice" thesis predicts that women will be more interested in close relationships with their patients and less interested in high earnings than their male counterparts. Advocates of the different voice perspective suggest that the tendency for female physicians to spend more time with patients (Dorschner 2003; Ross 2003; Fang et al. 2004) stems primarily from women's desire to know and care for their patients rather than simply treating their specific medical conditions. They also believe that it is the caring nature of women medical students which leads to their disproportionate interest in serving underprivileged patients (Crandall et al. 1993).

The second perspective, which we refer to as the institutional discrimination thesis, suggests that specific industry and organizational characteristics and the behaviors of other key groups in the health services workforce are responsible for many of the disparities between male and female physicians. One of the most common theories in the discrimination perspective is the "structural difference" view (Kanter 1977). This theory holds that differences between men and women workers reflect gender differences in status and power in the organization or the profession. In the medical context it suggests that observed gender differences in practice or status stem from women's weaker organizational or professional position. Advocates of the structural discrimination perspective see the tendency for women to spend more time with patients very differently from those who believe that women are inherently more caring. These analysts maintain that the propensity for women physicians to spend relatively more time with patients results from the greater needs of women physicians' patients and the tendency for women physicians to work as employees. In fact, research shows that a large portion of the time differential among primary care physicians stems from the fact that women physicians see more women patients who often need time-consuming pelvic exams (Franks and Bertakis 2003). In a similar light, researchers have shown that women physicians are more likely to be employees than are their male counterparts, and physicians in such settings spend more time in each patient visit (Kikano et al. 1998). Finally, the structural discrimination perspective offers an explanation of why women physicians are actually less likely to provide charity care even though studies suggest that as graduating medical students, women are more amenable than men to providing such care (Cunningham et al. 1999; Crandall et al. 1993). The evidence suggests that physicians who work as employees spend less time offering their services for free; consequently, women's concentration in positions as employees, typically in hospital settings, accounts for their lower rate of charity care.

A closely related phenomenon involves the social expectations or behaviors of physicians' colleagues and patients. At one extreme, women might encounter more harassment and less mentoring support. At the other, gender-linked behaviors might also be more subtle but the effects no less important. For example, assumptions regarding patients' preferences might cause men to assign breast surgeries to their female colleagues in a general surgery practice (Cassell 1998; McMurray et al. 2000). In a similar light, the expectation that women are good communicators might cause patients with emotional problems to seek them out, and this process of sorting may explain why female physicians see more patients with complex social problems (McMurray et al. 2000).

The third perspective that motivates our analysis focuses on social change. One of the more prominent theories maintains that increases in the representation of women in an occupation are related to declines in the status of the field. The underlying idea here is that women constitute a surplus labor force, and that they enter professions only when more desirable workers—namely, men—are no longer interested.

The dramatic influx of women into medicine and other occupations has prompted social scientists to investigate demographic changes in the labor force (Reskin and Roos 1990; Strober 1984; Cohn 1985). This research examines changes in the status of women workers that accompany their entry into an occupation such as medicine. In particular, Reskin and Roos (1990) suggest that women's entry into male-dominated occupations tends to occur in a similar fashion regardless of the specific profession. A shortage of male employees prompts employers to recruit women. The shortage of men is typically due to a decline in the status of the occupation. In some cases the impetus for the initial departure of men from an occupation is a technological shift that lowers skill levels and earnings in the field. Reskin and Roos also find that, in general, women's entry into male-dominated fields does not result in true integration. Rather, women cluster in the least desirable niches of male-dominated occupations—niches with lower pay, fewer required skills, less autonomy, and limited promotion opportunities.

Another aspect of social change involves generational shifts among women physicians. From this perspective, the first groups of women to enter medicine in the late 1960s and 1970s represented "pioneers" who blazed uncharted paths in a male-dominated terrain. Consequently, these "trailblazers" faced different expectations and challenges than did the "settlers"—those women who followed in their footsteps. The first small, elite group had few role models, and were committed to proving that women could succeed. They also felt so privileged to enter the profession that they tolerated unequal treatment. Empowered by their growing numbers and increasing attention to women's professional issues in the broader labor force, many among the generation of women physicians who entered medicine during the 1990s and beyond seek a fulfilling family life along with the satisfactions of engaging professional work. At the same time, it may be that work expectations are shifting for male physicians as well, as they are increasingly likely to find themselves in dual-career families.

We challenge the assumptions of many of these perspectives along the path to developing a new understanding of women's representation in medicine. Our thesis is that the medical profession reflects and exemplifies broader changes in women's roles in American culture and society. Women's status has changed as a result of political developments (specifically the women's movement); social and cultural changes in education, work, and family life; and the economic forces buffeting American society.

Women's entry into medicine reflects broader accomplishments in the labor force and the professions as well as the unique institutional changes occurring in the U.S. health care system. Our research situates the medical profession in the context of the evolution of women's position in American society. Women's achievements in medicine, however, continue to fall short of complete equality in a number of important areas, as is the case with women in the broader labor market. Careers in medicine are especially demanding in terms of training, working time, and professional commitment, and thus the dilemmas of balancing and integrating work and family life are especially salient among physicians. The economic, technical, and organizational landscape of medicine has rapidly evolved since the 1970s with the rise of managed care and other pressures to rein in the costs of medical care. These forces have limited the extent to which women could remake the medical profession in their own image. Nevertheless, we expect that the influence of women physicians on the medical landscape will continue to grow as they make inroads throughout the profession and in positions of professional leadership.

Relative to other occupational and professional choices for women, medicine ranks high in terms of financial rewards and personal satisfaction. Thus women's successes in the field of medicine are not principally due to a sharp decline in the desirability of careers in the medical profession, as medicine remains at the top of the occupational status hierarchy. At the same time, medicine is a highly stratified and internally differentiated profession, and the inequality within the profession compounds the difficulties women face in pursuing complete equality. Indeed, there are indications of increasing inequality among physicians. Marked disparities by gender remain in specialty areas, ownership and employee status, faculty representation, and leadership positions. Discrimination persists in some stages of the medical career, in some specialties, and in terms of women's access to positions of leadership. But women also face the challenges posed by institutional arrangements which are at least as salient as the lingering resistance and sexist attitudes of some male physicians. Women over the last generation or so have entered a profession designed for the male breadwinner with a stay-at-home spouse. Intense time demands and continuing professional commitments, with few opportunities to leave and reenter, dominate the lives of physicians during their twenties and well into their thirties, spanning most of the childbearing years. Very few women physicians have stay-at-home husbands who provide the kind of support that stay-at-home wives provided an earlier generation of men.

The evidence we have compiled is largely inconsistent with the notion of a "post-pioneer" pattern of female physicians' career choices. We find that women doctors are not dropping out of the labor force, nor are they more likely to marry and have children today than did previous generations. Moreover, the gender gap in work habits and earnings is quickly closing for childless male and female physicians. We also show that women physicians are more similar to other women today in terms of marriage and motherhood than was the case a generation ago. Women physicians face enduring challenges in combining work which are similar in kind, though perhaps more extensive in nature, than those faced by other employed women.

The values that women bring with them to medicine differ from those of their male counterparts. Careers in medicine offer not only financial rewards but also the personal satisfaction of helping others in their times of greatest need. Thus medicine has become a more socially attractive professional option for scientifically oriented women than other technical fields such as engineering. Although evidence indicates that women medical students are more altruistic in their professional goals than are their male classmates, this particular gender gap is not as sizable as one might assume but amounts to only a few percentage points, and changes in the intentions of male and female physicians over time dwarf differences between the two genders. Moreover, the values and preferences of entering medical students are not sufficient to explain subsequent behavior. Ultimately, the structure of the environment in which physicians work and the expectations of peers and patients influence physician behaviors as much as or more than the abstract ideals that physicians hold during and immediately after their training.

Women physicians do interact with their patients in subtly different ways than their male peers, but gender differences in diagnosis and treatment are not extensive. Differences in practice patterns are most evident in areas involving patients' personal privacy and sexually sensitive conditions. As far as the structure of the profession is concerned, women are just beginning to have an impact on the profession and the way medicine in practiced, and more change is likely as their representation continues to grow.

This book is a case study of one profession that plays a key role in the health care sector, which now represents about one seventh of the U.S. economy. It examines the most dramatic demographic change in this sector in the last century. But the issues we raise are likely to be of interest more broadly for what they say about the changing roles of women in contemporary society. Women's entry into medicine is taken as dramatic evidence that the barriers to opportunity for women are rapidly falling in

America. Does the experience of female physicians to date bear out this optimistic view? An alternative view is that gender roles remain deeply entrenched in our institutions and culture. Specifically, the gender division of household labor continues to constrain the choices of all women (Moen 2003). The trade-offs between work and family may be clearest in the most demanding professions, such as law and medicine, which require a high degree of professional devotion (Blair-Loy 2003).

Our study builds on the fine histories of women in medicine written by Walsh (1977), Morantz-Sanchez (1985), and More (1999). The analysis presented here focuses on the period since 1970, thus complementing the important studies of Bowman and colleagues (2002) and Bickel (2000). Lorber (1984) examined the experiences of the generation of women who pioneered the transformation of the profession. With the benefit of additional decades of perspective, we are in a position to examine whether the role of gender in medicine is changing.

Women's Entry into Medicine

Since the 1970s the face of students at American medical schools has changed markedly, with women rapidly approaching 50 percent of entering medical students. While women's arrival has been widely noted, few studies have directly confronted the question of how and why this change is occurring. The next two chapters of the book are devoted to trying to explain this trend. Is women's entry a reflection of the plummeting status of the medical profession, or are the reasons more varied and complex? We examine several interrelated aspects of professional status, including earnings, autonomy, and prestige, as well as the political clout of the American Medical Association. We consider specific historical developments, such as changes in government reimbursement policies and the ebb and flow of concerns over malpractice insurance premiums. We pay considerable attention to the interest levels in the profession exhibited by young men. As we review the 1970s, the 1980s, and the 1990s in detail, we do not assume that the same factors play the same roles in each decade. The series of challenges to the status of the profession is the central concern of chapter 2.

In chapter 3 we set the feminization of medicine in the broader context of changing gender roles in society at large. We examine factors that influence the degree of preparation for careers in medicine, including the extent of women's education, the rates at which young women take math and science courses in high school, and the number of women graduating from college with degrees in biology.

We find that women have entered medicine not so much because of the flight of men but rather because many barriers to access have eroded. The timing of women's entry, as well as the ups and downs of men's applications to medical school, does not map onto the timing of challenges to the authority, status, and earnings of the profession. In many ways, women's entry into medicine is in line with the broader patterns of women's growing share of the labor market, leadership, and power as a whole. Women earn an increasing proportion of college degrees, and they have pursued historically male-dominated academic tracks in increasing numbers, and these changes are beginning to influence our society. Women's entry into the medical profession reflects and exemplifies these trends.

Changes in women's roles are not confined to the United States, nor is the feminization of medicine a uniquely American phenomenon. Our review of the trends in physician employment patterns in developed countries shows an increased representation of women in all of the thirty-five countries examined. Indeed in many of these countries women's share of the profession exceeds that in the United States. In conjunction with this analysis, we discuss the role that foreign-born physicians have played in the feminization of medicine in the United States. Much of our story, however, is uniquely American. The organization and financing of health care differs sharply from that in many other countries, and the evolution of medicine in the United States has followed a distinctive trajectory (Riska 2001). In short, the evolution of gender and medicine sketched in this book is inextricably linked to the distinctively American features of our medical system. Further research will be required to detail fully which elements of our story resonate in other countries.

Careers in Medicine

Next we turn to women's careers in the profession. There are many aspects of the opportunity structure to examine. Traditional indices include earnings, specialties, and access to leadership positions. We are also interested in a number of nontraditional measures of career success, such as the ability to combine work and family. To the extent possible, we address these questions historically, examining how the various gender gaps have evolved as women's representation in the medical profession has increased.

We start in chapter 4 by describing the gendered landscape of the medical profession. We examine the distribution of women by specialty, employee and ownership status, involvement with research, faculty appointments, and leadership positions. We map the connection between these positions in the profession onto earnings disparities among physicians.

Chapter 5 turns to a more detailed consideration of gender and medical specialties. We explore the historical basis of specialty practice in order to understand better how the connection between specialties and gender came to take its current form. We also examine the process of sorting into specialties that occurs during medical school. Do the values and preferences women and men bring into the profession explain their choice of specialties? What role do experiences during medical school play in subsequent career choices? We also examine careers in academic medicine. In this area we seek to resolve an apparent paradox: women express more interest in pursuing academic careers but end up being underrepresented in this segment of the profession. We seek to pin down the role that medical school experiences play in this process. The emergence of the clinical educator track provides a new context for women's entry into academic medicine.

Women continue to occupy a disadvantaged place both in medicine and in the broader professional labor market. This disadvantage stems from lingering discrimination in the workplace, and from the persistence of organizational arrangements that fail to accommodate the needs of parents in a labor force dominated by members of dual-career families (Jacobs and Gerson 2004). Those who suggest that gender differences in physicians' status stem from the tendency for women to choose "controllable" lifestyles and less procedure-focused specialties have not adequately acknowledged how social forces such as male chauvinistic faculty, colleagues, and patients circumscribe the opportunities of women and men physicians. The "choice" explanation simply ignores how social factors have contributed to the structure of medical education and medical work.

In chapter 6 we examine motherhood and marriage. Here we further explore the contrast between the pioneers and the settlers. Are women physicians able to combine work and family? Do they marry at the same rates as women in the general population and to the same degree as their male counterparts? Are women physicians "opting out" of careers in order to spend time with their children? We report surprising evidence regarding the growing length of workweeks for both men and women in medicine, and find little evidence of an increase in part-time employment. We then examine the nature of physicians' families. We find that the status of women has been improving in the families of both male and female physicians. Finally, we examine changing patterns of marriages in which both partners are physicians. The evidence suggests that, despite broadly similar investments in education and training, marriages between two physicians remain far from equal.

Gender Differences in Practice Patterns

Having explored how women entered medicine and their experiences as physicians, we turn to the question of the consequences for medical care. Does it matter in terms of treatment if physicians are men or women? Now that women constitute a major and growing portion of the American medical workforce, it is essential that we ascertain whether significant gender differences in practice patterns exist. Identifying the existence and etiology of such differences will help to ensure that all patients of the U.S. health care system receive the highest-quality care possible and will also help to provide the most equitable work environment for health care providers regardless of gender. Although much research has been done on gender differences in practice, the research is not complete.

The standard view of the relationship between gender and the provision of medical services is that the sex of a physician does not affect the provision of care to patients. Because physicians are carefully screened and rigorously trained, patients can count on physicians to diagnose, treat, and refer patients as medically indicated regardless of whether they wear pants or skirts under their medical garb. Although they note that there are some sex differences, some researchers, such as Mattila-Lindy and colleagues (1998), conclude that socialization into the medical profession makes physicians' practices more alike and diminishes gender differences. While there is no reason to suspect that either male or female physicians provide systematically inadequate care, a variety of perspectives suggest that gender differences in practice styles may exist. One possibility, in keeping with the "different voice" perspective, is that women provide more nurturing care because they are more interested in the satisfaction of their patients.

Another possibility, motivated by the discrimination perspective, is that gender differences in practice stem from the lower status accorded to women in terms of their social roles and organizational positions. For example, the reluctance of nurses to support female physicians might force female doctors to perform a higher portion of routine procedures themselves (Gjerberg and Kjølsrød 2001; Wear and Knight-McNulty 2004; Zelek and Philips 2003).[3]

Similarly, it could be that the gender stereotypes of patients contribute to gender differences in practice (Street 2002). The social change perspective would focus on changes across generations of women physicians and the extent to which the growing representation of women is changing the practice of medicine.

In addition to these perspectives, we examine a fourth possibility: that gender differences are most likely to emerge in the treatment of specific sex-linked diseases, especially, though not exclusively, those involving personal privacy (Bouchard and Renaud 1997; Britt et al. 1996; Ivins and Kent 1993; Fang et al. 2004; Lurie et al. 1997). For example, a female patient might be more reluctant to raise an issue of vaginal itching with a male physician, while a male patient might feel less comfortable raising potential concerns about a prostate condition with a female doctor. At the same time, physicians might be uncomfortable in exploring certain conditions or performing certain procedures with patients of the opposite sex (Lurie et al. 1998).

In chapter 7 we assess these issues and find evidence that women physicians on average do approach patients differently, employing a more collegial approach to the doctor-patient relationship and prioritizing psychosocial issues more than their male colleagues. Research on physician communication, however, highlights similarities between men and women as well. Thus researchers on doctor-patient interactions frequently suggest that physicians of both genders can improve their communication skills.

We present an analysis of vignettes from the Community Tracking Study (CTS) physician survey, which includes physicians' reactions to a series of model patients with presentations designed to suggest multiple appropriate treatment plans. The results reveal a gender effect for sexually sensitive conditions even after differences in practice environment are acknowledged.

With respect to the daily practice of medicine, the similarities between men and women outweigh the differences. Gender matters far more with respect to time spent with patients and communication styles than it does with respect to diagnoses or even treatment regimes. The gender of physician and patient can be of greater significance in areas of personal, especially sexual, privacy.

Chapter 8 examines the question whether medicine is becoming a family-friendly profession. We find that many physicians are working as many hours as ever. We examine the historical roots of the medical culture of long workweeks and find that despite this culture, many physicians express an interest in working less. Given the prevalence of this interest in reduced hours or part-time work, we explore the availability of part-time opportunities and consider the barriers that inhibit more physicians from taking advantage of these choices. We conclude this discussion by examining how physicians handle the demands of family life in the context of extensive professional commitments.

In the final chapter of the book we take stock of the argument and evidence, and discuss the prospects, for further gender integration of medicine in the coming years. Will women emerge as a new majority of physicians? Will they help to foster a more caring, patient-centered medical care system, or will physicians increasingly leave primary care to physicians' assistants and other medical care practitioners? We also discuss the prospects for women's leadership in medicine and the impact women have had on research on women's health.

In this book we examine how women entered medicine, how they are faring in the rapidly evolving medical system, how they are managing to integrate and balance work and family, how they practice medicine on a day-to-day basis, and how they are changing the system of medical care in the United States. These large themes are interconnected in many ways, and the answers to each of these questions echo throughout the other analyses.

Although individual choices play a significant role in determining women's place in medicine, they cannot explain the origins and implications of this profound demographic change. In contrast to much of the available literature, we repeatedly find that the entry of women into medicine, their place in the profession, and their influence on medical practice stem from broad changes occurring throughout American society, from lingering traditional attitudes and arrangements and from independent structural changes in the profession.

The medical profession has been undergoing many fundamental changes in recent decades. In some ways the pace of change regarding gender roles has been slower than other developments, and slower in the United States than has been the case in a number of other countries. As women increasingly become a critical mass in the profession, especially in some specialty areas, they are increasingly poised to make a profound difference in how the medical profession operates. Thus the biggest changes with respect to gender and medicine may lie ahead.

2

Feminization of an Evolving Profession

Over the past several decades health policy researchers and social scientists have debated the status and prestige of the medical profession. While there is nearly universal agreement that medicine enjoyed a uniquely privileged place in our society during the 1950s and 1960s, in the 1970s some policymakers and social researchers began to observe and forecast declines in the earnings, autonomy, control, and prestige of physicians in the United States (McKinlay 1977; Haug 1973). Although the voices predicting that the sky is about to fall on modern medicine have grown in number over time, until recently they have been matched by more optimistic observers who maintain that political and economic pressures have done relatively little to challenge the dominant position of medicine in American society (Mechanic 1991; Freidson 1994). Regardless of the debate over the status of medicine as a profession, however, it is clear that the work experiences of the average physician have changed dramatically since the early 1970s. Most notably, today, physicians at all levels of the profession have significantly less capacity to set prices for their services and to determine their earnings. They are also increasingly likely to face expectations regarding treatment patterns and resource use from both the government and private insurers (Culbertson and Lee 1996; Kelly and Toepp 1994), and they are significantly more likely to face a demanding and critical patient population (Mechanic 2003).

As suggested previously, social researchers (Riska 2001) and physicians (Ross 2003; Levinson and Lurie 2004; Hall 2004) have questioned the implication of women's growing presence in the medical profession. A commonly voiced concern is that increases in the representation of women in the profession will inevitably lead to declines in the status, autonomy, and earnings of all physicians. This concern is based on the assumption that there is an inverse relationship between the status of the medical professional and women's representation in it. For example, Riska (2001) points out that women's representation in medicine was relatively high in the Soviet Union, although the status of the profession was quite low compared with that in Western countries. In contrast, over the course of the late nineteenth and most of the twentieth centuries, medicine in the United States had a relatively privileged status, while women practitioners were scarce. Riska places the Scandinavian case in an intermediate position, with more women doctors but lower status for physicians than in the United States.

While much has been said about both the alleged decline in dominance of the medical profession and the increasing representation of women in medicine, few efforts have been made to assess the relationship between these two trends systematically. In this chapter we begin this assessment by comparing reforms in the structure of medicine and gender differences in interest in the medical profession in the United States over time. We suggest that although the interest and presence of women in the medical profession has grown dramatically since the 1970s, there is little reason to believe that women's entry into medicine was prompted by declines in the status and autonomy of the profession. Instead, our account is a multifaceted one that emphasizes different contributing events and processes occurring during each of the last three decades.

The increasing representation of women among medical students during the 1970s resulted from the confluence of three largely independent trends: the removal of barriers to women's entry into medical education, the sharp expansion in the capacity of medical schools, and the end of the military draft for young men. While challenges to the status of the profession had already begun during this decade, the authority and daily practice patterns of physicians remained resilient.

The 1980s are the period that most closely fits the "male flight" explanation, as male applications to medical school fell substantially. But even at this point there are many discrepancies. Physicians' incomes grew briskly during the decade, and the managed care phenomenon had not yet made significant inroads. Also, the "male flight" argument does not predict and cannot explain the limited growth in female applications during this era, especially in light of the dramatic rise in the numbers of female college graduates and biology majors.

The events of the 1990s clearly depart from the "male flight" thesis. During this decade both male and female applications to medical schools rose sharply, even though some of the most serious challenges to professional autonomy and authority were experienced during this time. Women's representation over the 1990s grew despite sharp increases in the number of men interested in pursuing medical careers.

We begin our discussion with a more detailed review of sociological approaches to the feminization of occupations. The historical analysis is divided into three sections, each of which focuses on a different decade of the thirty-year period in which women's entry into medicine was most pronounced. In each section we ask three distinct questions: (1) Which developments altered the structure of medicine? (2) What were the implications of these changes for the status of the medical profession? and (3) How did these transformations affect women's entry into the profession? We track how the interest of young men and women in medical careers has varied as American medicine has evolved. The analysis in this chapter draws on data pertaining to applications to medical schools, physician incomes, and public esteem for the medical profession in order to pinpoint the times when declines in the status of medicine were most pronounced. We present our own synthesis of trends in the status of the medical profession, drawing on a number of previous studies in this area, including Starr (1982), Stevens (1989), and Freidson (2001), among others.

The Feminization of Occupations

The dramatic influx of women into medicine and other occupations has prompted social scientists to investigate the processes of occupational segregation and integration (Reskin and Roos 1990; Strober 1984; Cohn 1985). This research examines changes in the status of women that accompany their entry into an occupation such as medicine.

Reskin and Roos (1990) present the most comprehensive analysis of women's entry into male-dominated fields. They examine fourteen cases in which women made significant inroads into occupations previously dominated by men. Eleven of these cases are presented in their book *Job Queues, Gender Queues*. The commonality that Reskin and Roos posit is that a shortage of male employees prompts employers to recruit women. The shortage of men is typically due to a decline in the status of the occupation. In some cases the impetus for the initial departure of men from an occupation is a technological shift that lowers skill levels and earnings in the field. For example, the advent of computer technology transformed typesetting from a highly skilled manual field to a much cleaner but less skill-intensive keyboarding occupation. Accompanying this shift was a decline in union strength, which contributed to the rapid switch from a predominantly male to a predominantly female occupation. Some currently employed men left, but more important, young men seeking careers avoided this field.

In this account the status of the field declines first. In response, some male incumbents leave, and few new male recruits are to be found. The subsequent recruitment of women simply confirms and crystallizes the debased status of the occupation. Feminization of a field is thus seen as the *result* of a decline in status rather than its initial cause.[1]

This theory holds that employers generally prefer men, and allow women in only when there is a shortage of available men. Faced with such a shortage, employers (or, in the case of the professions, professional gatekeepers) must seek alternative streams of personnel, and thus actively begin to recruit women. The very presence of growing numbers of women itself, however, signals an imminent decline in the status of the profession. This further deters men from entering the field, thus hastening the day when an occupation previously staffed by men becomes a feminine preserve (England et al. 2007). In short, the typical sequence of events is that there is an initial decline in the status of a field, precipitated by some external event, such as a challenge to the authority of the profession, which leads employers or gatekeepers to recruit women, which in turn further contributes to the decline in status of the field.

The implication of this perspective is that women's advances into the professions represent less than meets the eye. While optimists cite the prevalence of women in fields previously dominated by men, Reskin and Roos maintain that such advances rarely represent true equality or full integration. Moreover, they suggest that occupations are unlikely to maintain a balanced gender profile over any significant period of time. Rather the fields are likely to undergo a gender reversal, starting as male fields, then passing through a brief transition period before becoming female fields. Feminization thus involves a tipping point process just like residential segregation, in which the racial composition of neighborhoods can rapidly switch from predominantly white to predominantly black. This approach has been applied to such instances of occupational feminization as teaching in the nineteenth century (Preston 1995) and banking, as in the case of bank tellers during the 1950s (Strober and Arnold 1987) and bank branch managers during the 1970s (Bird 1990), although Wright and Jacobs (1994) suggest that the case of computer programmers during the 1980s is not fully consistent with this approach.

Does this perspective illuminate the influx of women into medicine? As we have seen, the level of interest that men express in a field is a key element of this theory. Consequently, the number of male and female applicants to medical schools is of central interest.[2]

Figure 2.1 presents trends in male and female applications to U.S. medical schools between 1961 and 2004. The number of men who applied to medical schools did in fact decline from 1975 through 1990. Male applications rebounded sharply during the 1990s, however, a period when women's applications also showed their sharpest increases. The pattern of applications thus suggests that a somewhat more complex discussion of women's entry into the profession may be in order.

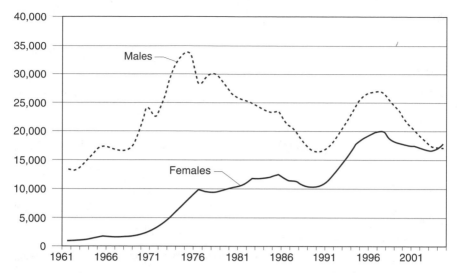

Figure 2.1. Medical School Applications, by Gender, 1961–2004. *Source:* AAMC.

Trends in the number of newly minted MDs is another way of looking at the male flight thesis. Figure 2.2 tracks this indicator over time for men and women. Increases are evident for both men and women though the mid-1980s. Thus the entry of women into medicine in substantial numbers coincided with a notable increase in the number of men for more than a decade. Since the 1980s the number of new male MDs has declined, in part because the overall number of new physicians produced has stabilized at just over 15,000 per year, and because women are making up an increasing share of these new graduates. Even through 2004 the number of new male physicians continued to exceed 8,000, a level first reached in 1971. In other words the number of male physicians has continued to grow despite women's impressive gains. This can be seen most clearly in Figure 2.3, which displays the number of practicing male and female physicians. The number of male physicians more than doubled between 1970 and 2004, increasing from 300,000 to nearly 650,000, even as the number of female physicians rose from 25,401 to 235,627. Therefore a central problem with the male flight thesis is that men did not flee from the profession. The growth in the number of women physicians during this period did not preclude an increase in the number of male physicians.

After 1985, however, women's growing relative presence among newly minted domestic MDs was matched by declines in male medical graduates, given the fixed number of seats in medical schools (see Figure 2.2 for details). In fact, between 1985 and 2003 annual MDs awarded to women increased by 2,004 individuals while annual MDs awarded to men decreased by

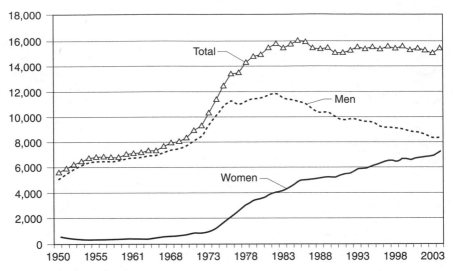

Figure 2.2. New MD Degrees by Gender, 1950–2004. *Source:* NCES, Digest of Education Statistics.

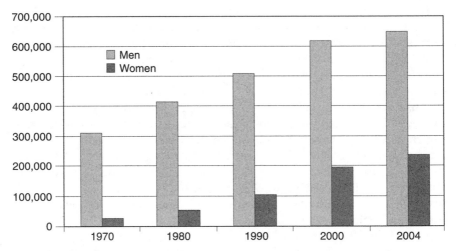

Figure 2.3. Practicing Physicians, by Gender, 1970–2004. *Source:* AMA Masterfile.

2,689 individuals. Thus trends after 1985 are significantly different from trends prior to this point. Women's entry into medicine before 1985 did not reduce the number of men's seats in medical schools, while growth in the number of female MD recipients after 1985 involved an absolute decline in new male medical graduates.

We examine the 1970s, the 1980s, and the 1990s in detail in order to compare the developments in the status of the field with trends in the number of men and women seeking to pursue careers in medicine.

The 1970s

Structural Challenges

The 1970s brought the first major external challenges to the prestige, the autonomy, and the political and corporate power of American physicians. Assaults on the medical profession initially came from four distinct directions. First, business and government became increasingly concerned about rising health care expenditures during the late 1960s and, as a result, sought greater control of their health care costs during the 1970s. These initial increases in costs were sparked largely by the passage of Medicare legislation. Physicians quickly realized that requests for higher reimbursement from Medicare would be honored, and this led to a spiral of increasing costs. Furthermore, unlike the medical advances of the immediate postwar era, advances in medicine in the 1960s and 1970s, which generally prolonged the lives of the chronically ill rather than preventing or curing acute illness, significantly raised the cost of care. Finally, dramatic increases in the cost of hospital stays, including increases in the relative wages of hospital employees, raised overall health care costs (Starr 1982; Aaron 1991).

Second, a series of judicial decisions in the late 1970s challenged the privileged legal status of medicine, thereby limiting the control of organized medicine and other professional organizations over professional work and increasing competition among individual professionals. Court rulings seriously restricted the ability of medical organizations to promote unified behaviors among their constituents and to lobby effectively. Beginning in the 1970s, legal decisions prevented the AMA and state medical societies from making hospital appointments contingent on medical society membership. These rulings also prevented professional organizations from punishing physicians who either accepted salaried positions or actively advertised their services. And most notably, in 1977 the Supreme Court ruled that medical societies were no longer exempt from antitrust regulations, thereby reducing organized medicine's privileged status and acknowledging the business aspects of medicine (Field 1988). Third, the burgeoning movement for patients' rights, such as the right of informed consent and the right to refuse care, entailed demands for greater equality between physicians and patients. And fourth, the early 1970s saw the first major crisis in the cost of physicians' malpractice insurance.

The Status of Medicine

By the end of the 1970s, evidence of the declining status of medicine was growing. Legislative attempts by the AMA to stop federal efforts to control costs were largely unsuccessful. Legal challenges by the AMA successfully slowed the implementation of these reforms but did not eliminate them. By the late 1970s much of this cost-controlling legislation was in the process of being implemented (Starr 1982).

Similarly, although most of the efforts by patients' rights activists were short-lived, at least two had long-term implications. First, in 1973 the American Hospital Association addressed concerns of public groups by adopting a Patients' Bill of Rights, which included the right to informed consent and the right to refuse treatment. Although this reform was couched as an act of goodwill, it came in the midst of international efforts to promote the rights of subjects of medical research, and was probably offered in an effort to prevent government intervention. Shortly before this measure, courts had ruled that patients could sue if their physicians did not fully disclose the risks of a procedure (Starr 1982).

Ironically, given the need for a coherent, coordinated response to unprecedented challenges to the status of medicine, the strength of the AMA declined substantially during the 1970s. Declines were directly attributable to the legal reforms that limited the power of the AMA and to the increasing specialization of physicians in the United States. AMA membership began dropping in the 1960s but continued declining during the 1970s. At the same time, membership in medical specialty societies grew, and these organizations took on greater political power. Nevertheless, increasing divisions within the medical community inevitably weakened its capacity to influence the political process.

Although there is considerable evidence to indicate a decline in the status of the medical profession during the 1970s, when viewed in a large enough historical context, and in comparison to trends in other prestigious occupations, the ultimate implications of structural reforms during the 1970s appear limited. Most notably, at the end of the 1970s physicians still retained most of the control over their profession and practice that they had had a decade earlier. Public membership in health maintenance organizations remained low. In 1980 only 9 million Americans participated in some form of managed care (Luft 1987). The low penetration of managed care implies that oversight of physicians stemmed almost entirely from governmental reforms. And the persistent increases in hospital costs during the late 1970s and early 1980s suggest that the ultimate implications of the legislative reforms of the 1970s were limited. In particular, hospital costs increased at six times the rate of inflation in the early 1980s (Stevens 1989).

Physicians also enjoyed more public confidence than many other institutions or professions in 1980, in spite of a slight decline in public esteem.

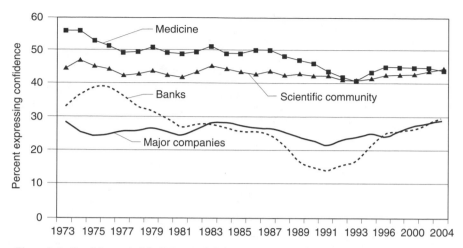

Figure 2.4. Confidence in Medicine and Other Institutions, 1973–2004. *Source:* General Social Survey.

Figure 2.4 presents data on confidence in the medical profession throughout the 1970s, 1980s, and 1990s. The graph indicates the percentage of respondents to the nationally representative General Social Survey who expressed a strong degree of confidence in particular public institutions. It demonstrates that in 1980, 7.2 percent more respondents indicated that they had a great deal of confidence in medicine than was the case for the scientific community. Similarly, 20.6 percent more respondents indicated that they had a great deal of confidence in medicine than U.S. banks and financial institutions.

Furthermore, although adjusted median physician income declined during the 1970s, the magnitude of this decline was limited, especially in light of the experiences of those in other elite occupations. Figure 2.5 documents trends in inflation-adjusted median income for physicians over time. It indicates that income declined 14 percent for men and 2 percent for women. Data from the 1970 and 1980 5 percent U.S. Census samples, however, suggest that adjusted median income for female and male lawyers declined 37 and 25 percent, respectively. And median income for postsecondary schoolteachers declined 24 and 20 percent, respectively. Thus the slight decline in median physician income appears even more insignificant in light of the trends occurring in other prominent professional fields.

In addition, the difference between the median income of physicians and the median income of other prestigious professionals remained robust throughout the 1970s. During this period the median income for male physicians was consistently 50 percent more than the median income of male lawyers, and 200 percent more than the median income of male college faculty.

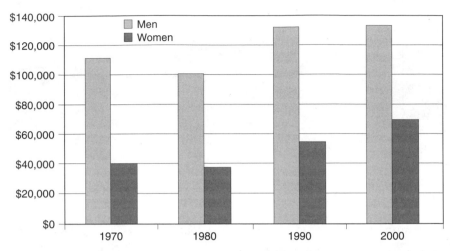

Figure 2.5. Median Income of Physicians, by Gender, 1970–2000. *Source:* U.S. Decennial Censuses.

Along with the setbacks discussed earlier, organized medicine had some successes during the 1970s. Although doctors were unable to stymie efforts to control costs, they did respond rapidly and effectively to the decade's malpractice crisis, by encouraging physicians to organize public demonstrations to focus attention on the implications of malpractice problems for patient access and to demand relief from lawsuits. In fact physicians' reactions to the crisis were readily acknowledged by both the government and the private sector. Reforms were adopted relatively quickly, and the crisis was short-lived (Sage 2004).

Relatedly, statistics on practice organization indicate that physicians were able to adapt well to the evolution in their work environment. During the 1970s the trend away from solo practice slowly began to take shape. In particular, between 1975 and 1983 the proportion of physicians in solo practice declined 5.3 percent from 54.2 to 48.9 percent. At the same time, the proportion of physicians in practices of five or more increased 5.9 percent from 16.8 to 22.7 percent. Physicians also began to alter the legal organization of their practices. In particular, between 1975 and 1983 there was a significant trend away from sole proprietorships and partnerships toward physician-owned professional corporations. The proportion of physicians who worked in professional corporations increased from 31 to 54 percent during this period (Center for Health Policy Research 1983). The trend away from solo practice served to insulate physicians from the potentially devastating effects of lawsuits and began to position them to succeed in an increasingly technology-intensive industry. Physicians in group practices are better able to maintain expensive technology in their offices. They can also provide more comprehensive care and ultimately earn more. Although the tendency to incorporate advanced significantly, in 1980 physicians were still largely independent of for-profit corporations. Finally, much of the gain in the numbers of employee physicians during the 1970s was the result of temporary increases in employee status among younger doctors rather than a major alteration in the standard physician career.

In sum, although medicine endured several assaults during the 1970s, these reforms ultimately had limited implications for the status of the profession overall. Using the characteristics of a profession offered by Leicht and Fennel (2001), we find that the status of medicine as a profession was not significantly affected by the reforms of the 1970s. First, in 1980 medicine was still founded on a theoretically driven knowledge base. In fact that base grew considerably during the 1970s. Second, the long period of training required to obtain membership in the medical profession was maintained and even expanded as a result of reforms in the graduate medical education system. Third, as discussed earlier, at the end of the 1970s the majority of the American population still had great confidence in not only their physicians but also the institution of medicine. Fourth, in 1980 physicians still had a great deal of autonomy over their work. Most notably, as mentioned earlier, they faced relatively limited oversight from the insurance industry or government.

Yet a few key trends of the 1970s, including the growing number of physicians, the increasing specialization of physicians, and the significant changes in the legal status of organized medicine set the stage for further challenges to the profession. Each of these developments resurfaces as the evolution of medicine proceeds.

The Interest of Women and Men in Medicine

In light of the general strength of medicine during the 1970s, how can we make sense of trends in medical school application? There is little reason to believe that the initial surge in female applicants during the early 1970s stemmed from declines in the status of medicine. The initial growth occurred too early in the decade for this to be true.

Instead, evidence indicates that this trend stemmed largely from the women's movement. In the late 1960s and early 1970s, activists from the feminist and civil rights movements were working collaboratively, lobbying Congress and suing public institutions to address discrimination against women and minorities, including those applying to medical school. And these efforts were largely successful for women. In 1972 Title IX of the Higher Education Act was passed, which banned discriminatory policies in admissions and salaries in any school receiving federal funds. This legislation reversed exceptions in Title XII, the landmark civil rights legislation of 1964, which permitted medical schools to continue discriminating actively and openly (More 1999).

Women's response to the new law was immediate and overwhelming. Between 1970 and 1974, two years after passage of Title IX, the number of women applicants to medical school more than tripled, increasing from 2,289 in 1969–70 to 7,201 in 1973–74, as can be seen from Figure 2.1. And the increase in applications translated into significant growth in the number of female medical students. Between 1970–71 and 1979–80, the representation of women among accepted medical students expanded precipitously from 12.3 to 28 percent (see More 1999, 219).

The implications of this trend are best understood in light of the dramatic growth in medical school capacity. Concerns about a relative neglect of ambulatory care and regional shortages of physicians prompted federal efforts to increase overall medical school enrollments and the population of physicians practicing primary care. In particular, in 1971, at the behest of President Nixon, and on the advice of the Carnegie Commission on Higher Education, Congress introduced capitation grants to medical schools. This reform caused the amount of federal aid to medical schools to be directly tied to the size of their student population (Starr 1982, 397).

The capitation grants created a clear incentive for medical schools to increase enrollments, and they responded quickly. As a result, between 1970 and 1980 the overall annual number of acceptances to U.S. medical schools rose from around 11,509 to 16,886 (More 1999, 219). The legislation of the early 1970s followed related initiatives of the 1960s. With the help of federal funds, between 1960 and 1980, forty-one new medical schools were constructed, half of them between 1961 and 1971. Most of the women entering medical schools in the 1960s and many who entered in the 1970s filled spots that had been recently created (More 1999, 193).

This increase corresponded to significant growth in the total population of female medical students from 3,894 in 1970–71 to 17,248 in 1980–81 (AAMC 2006). During the same period, however, the population of male medical students also grew precipitously from 36,593 to 47,941. Thus it is hard to support the hypothesis that the decline in male applications stemmed from the increase in female applications. In the 1970s women merely occupied a significant minority of the additional medical school spots. They did not drive men from the field.

So if the decline in male interest in medicine was not driven by the increase in female interest, what propelled the trend in male medical school applications? When this trend is placed in its historical context, an alternative explanation becomes clear. While the decline in male applications during the 1970s is unmistakable, it appears to be matched by a corresponding increase in male applications during the late 1960s. In fact, Figure 2.1 demonstrates that in 1980, male applications to U.S. medical schools were still significantly greater in number than they had been at their previous low point of 1966. In this context, it is the excessively high level of male medical school applications in the early 1970s, rather than the declining level of applications in the latter half of the decade, which appears anomalous and in need of explanation. And there is an obvious explanation for this peak. Much of the increase during the late 1960s may have represented efforts to avoid the draft for the Vietnam War, so it seems only reasonable that the elimination of the draft in 1973 would contribute to a decline in the number of men endeavoring to study medicine.

Thus the historical trends do not confirm the hypothesis that the large influx of women into medicine during the 1970s drove male applications down. We further maintain that there is little evidence to support the idea that the initial growth in female interest in medicine stemmed from a decline in status. There was simply not enough time between the first assaults on the profession and the increase in female applications to establish a cause and effect. Instead, the evidence suggests that the growing number of women medical school applicants and medical students was a product of the political activism of the women's movement and the dramatic increase in medical school capacity. And trends suggest that the decline in male applications during the later 1970s reflected the end of a draft-induced elevation in male interest in the profession rather than any rise in the number of female physicians.

The 1980s

Structural Reform

While the first major independent assaults on the status of medicine came during the 1970s, the reforms of the 1980s were significantly more pronounced. Most notably, between 1980 and 1991 enrollment in managed care exploded. In the first half of the decade, enrollment more than tripled, climbing from 9 million, a relatively small proportion of insured employees, to 31 million, or about 36 percent of all insured employees (Miller et al. 1993, 3). The bulk of this growth, from 9 to 28 million, occurred between 1980 and 1986 (Luft 1987, xvii). Furthermore, although enrollment in managed care still involved only a minority of the population in 1990, by that time most of those with fee-for-service-style insurance had plans that included some degree of oversight and cost control. In 1987, 41 percent of enrollees in traditional health insurance were subject to utilization management. That share rose to 95 percent by 1990 (Miller and Conko 2001).

While enrollment in managed care skyrocketed, the federal government adopted a series of reforms designed to control health care costs. The most powerful of these was the adoption of prospective payment to hospitals in 1983. Before that time Medicare paid hospitals according to their costs. After prospective payment, hospitals were paid a preset rate for each admission which depended on a patient's diagnosis. Diagnoses were arranged into 467 diagnosis-related groups, or DRGs.[3] The goal of prospective payment was to empower the government to be a more careful purchaser of Medicare services.

But prospective payment was by no means the only federal effort to reign in health care spending. In 1986 Congress created the Physician Payment Review Commission (PPRC). Three years later the PPRC issued recommendations for a physician payment scale called the Resource Based Relative Value Scale, or RBRVS. This system for reimbursing physicians was adopted almost in its entirety in 1989 but was not implemented until 1992. Together the growth of managed care and the adoption of federal efforts to control costs set the stage for significant curtailments of physicians' economic and clinical autonomy, and provided political momentum for efforts to rationalize, bureaucratize, and potentially de-skill medical practice through health outcomes research and practice guidelines. In particular, in 1989 Congress increased funding for outcomes research and began funding a significant effort to develop clinical practice guidelines for the treatment of common ailments affecting the Medicare population (Culbertson and Lee 1996).

Although the health workforce was not a major focus of reforms during the 1980s, at least two government policies were adopted which affected the future character of the medical profession. First, the addition of new medical schools and the expansion of the size of existing medical schools during the 1970s began to generate concerns about a surplus of physicians.

Until 1980 the supply of domestic physicians in training was growing. After 1985 it stabilized, largely because funding for medical education was capped. It should be noted, however, that capping growth in medical education does not immediately cap growth in domestically trained physicians because of existing momentum: those already in the training system have to work their way through it. Furthermore, if the number of physicians retiring every year is smaller than the number of those starting to practice, the total population will continue to grow. This has been the case for domestically trained physicians because the bulk of additional physicians have not aged out of the working population.

As early as 1980 the Graduate Medical Education National Advisory Committee concluded that the nation faced a potentially serious surplus of physicians if steps were not taken to limit the number of positions in U.S. medical schools and to restrict immigration of international medical graduates. The specter of an impending physician surplus prompted Congress to end general federal support to American medical schools for undergraduate medical education (Blumenthal 2004). This action not only served to curtail growth in the number of domestically trained physicians but also prompted significant increases in the cost of medical education for aspiring physicians. According to a 2003 report by the AMA, between 1983 and 2003 medical student debt increased at a rate of approximately 1 percent more per annum than inflation. This overall trend led to a 173 percent increase in mean student debt to $104,000 as of October 2003 (American Medical Association Task Force 2003). Ultimately this policy stopped the growth in the number of domestic medical students but did not stop the growth in either the total population of physicians working in the United States or the number of physicians in training.

The second major workforce reform involved reimbursing hospitals specifically for the number of graduate physicians they trained. Because of the limit on domestic medical students, this reform encouraged growth in the number of foreign medical graduates in the United States. Ironically, this provision nearly negated efforts to control physician supply in its entirety. The total number of physicians in training continued to grow throughout the 1980s as a result of the increasing representation of foreign-trained physicians.

Although most of the assaults on physicians' work during the 1980s came primarily from public and private forces concerned with controlling health care costs, grass-roots feminist efforts and homosexual-related health efforts surrounding the breast cancer movement and the outbreak of the AIDS epidemic during this period had significant effects on the course of public investment in medical research and in the way medical research funds are distributed. These efforts not only challenged the dominance of elite physicians in research but also pressured physicians in patient care to adopt more collaborative styles of service (Bix 1997).

The Status of Medicine

At the end of the 1980s there was ample reason to believe that the status of medicine was teetering. As described earlier, a series of federal laws had been passed which dramatically restricted physicians' economic and, to a lesser extent, clinical discretion. They also increased public surveillance of medical behavior and attempted to restrict physicians' earnings. Furthermore, as in the 1970s, the efforts of organized medicine to stymie or protest reforms were largely unsuccessful.

Not surprisingly, physicians did not react positively to many of the reforms and challenges of the 1980s. The adoption of prospective payment and the growth of managed care both within formal managed care organizations and within fee-for-service-style insurance inevitably caused discontent. The 1980s saw the rise of opinion pieces and editorials lamenting the decline of physician autonomy, control, and satisfaction (Stoeckle 1988; Tarlov 1983; Weinstein 1988; Burnside 1989), but relatively little systematic analysis of trends in the status of individual physicians was conducted during this period. The few surveys that were administered did suggest that physician satisfaction was declining (Rubin 1988).

Nevertheless, the reactions of individual physicians to overall trends in health care demonstrated their resilience as individuals and the stability of the profession. Individual physicians reacted promptly and effectively to the initial cost control reforms of the 1980s. Despite these reforms, Medicare costs for physician services continued to rise dramatically owing to the provision of significantly more services for each Medicare beneficiary and increases in physician fees. It should be noted that increases in the quantity of services during this period were not merely the result of strategic behavior on the part of physicians. The 1980s brought a dramatic expansion in the availability of effective but costly medical technologies, especially in the treatment of heart disease (Aaron 1991). Together, these trends suggest that physician income from Medicare increased during the 1980s.

Data on physicians' earnings from the 1980 and 1990 U.S. Census samples suggest that it was not just income from Medicare that was expanding during the 1980s. As can be seen in Figure 2.5, inflation-adjusted income for employed male and female physicians increased significantly during the 1980s. In particular, adjusted female earnings increased 37 percent, and adjusted male earnings increased 15 percent.

Nor does it appear that physicians achieved these gains by putting in longer work weeks. Data from the 1980 and 1990 census samples suggest that the median workweek for employed male physicians remained constant at fifty hours during the 1980s, while the median hours worked for employed female physicians increased 12.5 percent from forty to forty-five a week.[4]

In addition to sustaining significant income growth, physicians of the 1980s were generally able to maintain traditional practice structures. In spite of the growth of managed care, the bulk of physicians were able to retain small group or solo practices until the very end of the decade. Prior research suggests that before 1988 there were only small declines in the prevalence of solo practice and modest increases in the extent of physician employee arrangements. In fact the rate of working as a solo practitioner declined only 2 percentage points between 1983 and 1988 (more significant declines in solo practice occurred in the 1970s), and the tendency to work as an employee increased only 3.7 percentage points between 1983 and 1986 (Marder et al. 1988; Kletke et al. 1996). As in the 1970s, much of the increase in doctors working as employees occurred among very young physicians, many of whom had negotiated a temporary employee status as a way of "buying into" a previously established practice. Although the trend toward employee status and group practice accelerated after 1987, the rate of increase was relatively slow until the 1990s (Kletke et al. 1996).

Furthermore, in spite of dramatic increases in cost and the rise of managed care, public esteem for medicine as an institution remained relatively high and constant until the end of the decade. In particular, Figure 2.4 suggests that the proportion of the public expressing a great deal of confidence in medicine was roughly 50 percent between 1977 and 1987. The relative esteem for medicine is especially pronounced when compared to the downward trends in confidence in banks and financial institutions. Between 1977 and 1987 the level of strong confidence in banks and financial institutions declined 11.4 percentage points.

How can we reconcile the persisting confidence in medicine shown in Figure 2.4 with the sharp decline during the 1980s in the number of Americans who would recommend a career in medicine to a young man? We believe that the confidence data are a more reliable barometer of the standing of the field than are the Gallup data on recommending a career. The Gallup survey asked respondents to volunteer the name of an occupation or profession they would recommend. This means that many highly regarded professions such as judge, college professor, and even rocket scientist do not appear on the list at all. The fact that "computers" was the leading field recommended for a young man during the 1980s does not mean that this occupation had displaced medicine from its perch at the top of the occupational prestige hierarchy. Certainly the pay, autonomy, and authority of computer programmers or even computer systems analysts do not compare with those of the medical profession. The public visibility of the computer industry as a career no doubt reflects the rapid growth and high visibility of personal computers (during the 1980s) and the Internet (during the 1990s).

Finally, although the AMA was not able to stem the tide of cost control or battle managed care effectively, it did continue to have some political success. As in the 1970s, AMA efforts to secure reforms to malpractice were remarkably successful in the late 1980s. Although the U.S. medical profession was arguably at its wealthiest stage, physicians successfully obtained tort reform in most states that had not previously enacted it. Given the stability of public esteem for medicine and the positive earnings growth of physicians, most social scientists believed that the dominant status of medicine was not significantly influenced by the reforms of the 1980s. Most notably, in a special edition of the *Millbank Quarterly* in 1988 several authors suggested that although medicine had experienced significant turbulence during this period, the evidence was still not sufficient for them to conclude that physicians were deprofessionalizing (Wolinsky 1988; Light and Levine 1988). Many of the reforms of the 1980s had dramatic implications for individual physicians, but their ultimate effect did not materialize until the next decade. The primary reform, DRG reimbursement of hospitals, which was adopted early enough in the decade to alter the structure of medical practice, focused on medical institutions and thus had only an indirect influence on individual physicians.

The Interest of Women and Men in Medicine

If the "male flight" thesis applies to any period, it is the late 1980s. Male applications to medical school fell after more than a decade of challenges to the status of the medical profession. A closer examination suggests, however, that even during the late 1980s, the thesis does not account for all of the relevant facts.

As in the 1970s, there were significant challenges to the status of the medical profession, but the profession weathered these assaults well, especially in terms of the rise in income of physicians. Similarly, declines in the status of the profession do not correlate with trends in female applications to medical school. If women were entering medicine because of declines in status, then an increase in female applicants in the final years of the 1980s would be evident. There was, however, actually a slight decline during these years, which roughly matches a slight increase during the first half of the decade.

Furthermore, during these final years of the decade male and female applications begin to ebb and flow at roughly similar rates. In other words, the curves of male and female applications begin increasingly to resemble each other. Thus women's entry into the profession does not respond to male exit: the two genders began to respond similarly to external factors.

So if the drop in male interest in medicine is not explained by male flight in response to status decline, why did the number of men applying to medical school decline while the percentage of women applying increased slightly during the first half of the decade and declined slightly during the second half? The drop in male applications during the 1980s was due in large part to the stagnation in the number of men receiving bachelor's degrees, the relative stability after the Vietnam War in male interest in medicine, and declines in the percentage of men pursuing biology as a college major. By 1990 only 4 percent of male undergraduates obtained their degrees in biology, down from 7 percent in 1978 (National Center for Education Statistics 2004). There were corresponding increases in the number of men pursuing degrees in business and computer science during this period.

A final factor may have contributed to the decline in male applications during the 1980s. As we will see in chapter 3, between the late 1960s and the late 1980s undergraduate students on America's campuses became much more committed to materialistic values and much less committed to pursuing altruistic endeavors. Medicine has long been seen as a desirable profession in terms of the opportunities it affords to serve others as well as its financial rewards. A general reduction in the emphasis placed on altruistic career goals may have contributed to undercutting one of the main attractions of a medical career and contributed to a decline in applications to medical school. That is, male students may have been less attracted to medicine because during the 1980s the values associated with medicine became relatively less important, and because alternative pathways to high income such as business and computer science beckoned. In this atmosphere it is not surprising that students began taking the path of least resistance toward high earnings, thereby avoiding the intense period of training associated with medicine and the mounting costs of medical education that began during this period. Thus we suggest that the popularity of medicine ultimately declined for both genders during this period because of changing norms.

The 1990s

Structural Evolution

While legislation passed during the 1980s had dramatic implications, its immediate effects on individual physicians and the overall health care system were modest in effect. In spite of concerted efforts to control health care costs during the 1980s, they rose consistently throughout the decade. Employers saw persistent increases in health insurance rates as a major problem and focused their attention on cutting these costs in order to maintain competitiveness in an increasingly global economy. This trend translated into efforts to eliminate health insurance entirely for low-wage jobs and to increase cost sharing for workers with higher wages. Consequently, low-wage jobs were increasingly outsourced to companies that did not offer health care coverage, and employee costs for health insurance were increased among the white-collar population. The share of employers paying the full cost of family policies fell from 46 percent in 1983 to 24 percent in 1993. And, as discussed earlier, employers also began offering managed care (Cutler and Gruber 2001). Together these trends led to significant increases in the percentage of the population without insurance and to increasing anxiety regarding medical care coverage and expenses among the middle class.

The onset of the 1990s brought the first major effort by the federal government to reform health care in twenty years. The Clinton health plan represented the first attempt to effect large-scale systemic restructuring in U.S. health care since the early 1970s. Although it received significant initial support, the proposal floundered as a result of political missteps and well-financed opposition to government intervention on the part of the insurance industry.

After the failure of the Clinton plan, federal-level attempts to reform health care during the 1990s were either unsuccessful or very incremental and generally insignificant in the everyday sense for the medical practitioner. (The one possible exception to this trend is the 1996 HIPPA legislation—the Health Insurance Portability and Accountability Act—which dramatically increased the bureaucratic responsibilities of physicians but did not infringe on clinical discretion.) The medical care environment of the 1990s was shaped more by the implementation of 1980s-era reforms rather than the passage of new legislation. The first reform, which took effect in 1992, was the Resource Based Relative Value Scale, the preset system for reimbursing physicians, which placed increasing value on primary care and decreasing value on surgical and invasive specialty services. The second major reform involved an increasing emphasis on clinical guidelines through the establishment of the Agency for Health Care Policy Research. Ultimately, both of these reforms limited the autonomy of individual physicians. While the RBRVS restricted the capacity of physicians to set prices for their services, the movement toward clinical guidelines pressured physicians to change their clinical practice.

As physicians faced the prospect of increasing federal restrictions on their economic and clinical autonomy, the evolution of private health insurance continued. In spite of tremendous growth during the 1980s, in 1991 still only a minority of the population had some official form of managed care. (As suggested earlier, many enrolled in traditional insurance were managed in some way by the early 1990s.) But the speed of managed care growth accelerated dramatically in the 1990s. By 1996 only 27 percent of those with employer-sponsored insurance persisted in traditional fee-for-service-style plans (Phelps 2003, chap. 11). Between 1990 and 1995 the number of Americans enrolled in health maintenance organizations grew from 36.5 million to 58.2 million. And by 1999 only 8 percent of persons with employer-sponsored health insurance had traditional indemnity insurance (Dudley and Luft 2001). Thus by the end of the 1990s the penetration of managed care in the American health care system was nearly comprehensive.

While managed care became increasingly pervasive, the character of this system evolved as the decade progressed. At the start of the decade, consumers and physicians had little influence over the aggressive cost control techniques employed by many managed care companies. Struggling to contain health care costs, health plans introduced restrictions on consumer access and provider behavior, such as limiting the choice of out-of-network physicians and requiring referrals by a gatekeeper to see a specialist.

Both patients and providers reacted negatively to many of the efforts by managed care to control insurance costs during the first half of the 1990s. As the economy improved, coalitions of patients and providers began to lobby for more protections. In 1994 the AMA drafted its version of a Patient Bill of Rights and began pressuring Congress to adopt reforms on behalf of patients and physicians. Although efforts at the federal level were stymied, many states responded to concerns about patients' rights in relation to managed care. In the second half of the decade, many states passed incremental legislation providing protection against managed care companies (Reed and Trude 2002). Between 1996 and 1998 nearly six hundred bills regulating managed care organizations were introduced in statehouses across the country, and at least some provisions were enacted in every state (Marsteller and Bovbjerg 1999). By 1999, forty-eight states had bans on gag clauses preventing physicians from telling patients that certain procedures were not covered by their insurance, forty-two states had laws requiring insurers to cover at least a forty-eight-hour hospital stay for mothers after an uncomplicated vaginal birth, and thirty-eight states had emergency care services mandates (American Academy of Family Practice 2000).

The successful passage of state protection occurred in the midst of significant negative press for managed care. In a systematic review of the nation's leading newspapers' coverage of managed care during 1995, Bernard and Shulkin (1998) found that only 8 percent of articles presented a positive image of managed care, while two thirds of all coverage was highly unfavorable.

Together the success of state-level reforms and the significant negative press prompted many managed care companies to soften their approach to cost control. Most notably, managed care organizations started relaxing the requirement that enrollees get a referral to see a specialist and started developing more PPO (preferred provider organization) style plans with greater overall flexibility for beneficiaries. Evidence reveals a growth in enrollment in PPOs at the expense of more traditional managed care (Gabel et al. 2002).

Although the bulk of the backlash against managed care focused on patients' rights, physicians also benefited from reform. During the latter part of the 1990s, the nature of physicians' relationships with managed care improved.

Data from the Community Tracking Study physician survey indicates that between 1997 and 2001 there was a modest increase in the proportion of practice revenue from managed care contracts but a significant decrease in plans' use of capitation or fixed monthly payments, and there was a decline in the use of direct financial incentives to influence physicians' clinical decision making (Strunk and Reschovsky 2002).

The Status of Medicine

The growing presence of managed care and the strength of the RBRVS have posed a significant problem for many individual physicians and for the status of the profession overall. In particular, physicians generally believe that managed care has had negative effects on numerous facets of medical practice (Warren et al. 1999). There is a negative relationship between the portion of a physician's revenues that come from managed care and his or her professional satisfaction (Stoddard et al. 2001). Given the steady growth of managed care, surveys administered during the 1990s revealed increasing discontent among practicing physicians. In particular, the 1995 Commonwealth Fund Survey of more than 1,700 practicing physicians indicated that approximately 40 percent reported that they were spending less time with patients and had less ability to make good decisions for their patients than they had had three years earlier (Adams 2002). And research suggests that there has been a long-term decline in physicians' satisfaction with a variety of work-related factors. In a comparison of physician surveys from 1986 and 1997, Murray and colleagues (2001) demonstrated that in 1997 fewer than two thirds of survey respondents were satisfied with most areas of their practice, and fewer than half were satisfied with the time they were able to give individual patients, leisure time, or incentives for high quality. The authors also show that these responses indicated significant declines in satisfaction in these three areas. Murray and her colleagues also note that in 1986 about 75 percent of respondents indicated that they were satisfied or very satisfied with their earnings. By 1997 that estimate had fallen to 55 percent. Evidence indicates that trends in the U.S. health care system have been especially difficult for older physicians (Hueston 1998). In particular, research has revealed a positive association between the likelihood of retirement and HMO penetration (Wozniak 2001).

Mounting physician dissatisfaction was no secret during the 1990s. Throughout this period the general discontent of physicians had been appearing in the popular press all over the country (Hobson 2005; Jenkins 1997; Batz 1998; Toner 1999). And many of those articles highlight the relationship between managed care and physicians' concerns (Kilborn 1998; Kowalczyk 2004). The growth of managed care not only influenced physicians' satisfaction but also affected the organization of their practices. In the first half of the 1990s there was a dramatic increase in the frequency with which physicians worked as employees rather than full or partial owners of a practice. Although the prevalence of primary care employee physicians grew only 3 percent between 1983 and 1989, by 1995 this figure increased by 22 percent (Buchbinder et al. 2001). Research on trends in practice organization between 1983 and 1994 indicates that although the trend was most pronounced for primary care providers, the frequency with which all physicians worked as employees increased dramatically in the early 1990s. Most physicians with employee status work in hospital settings rather than in HMOs (Kletke et al. 1996).

The tremendous growth in managed care and the adoption of the RBRVS contributed to relatively stagnant physician incomes. Data from the 1990 and 2000 5 percent census samples indicate that adjusted median physician income for males declined around 2 percent and adjusted median income for female increased around 7 percent (see Figure 2.5). Data from the Community Tracking Study physician data and from the AMA socioeconomic statistics indicate that while physician income grew during the early 1990s, it declined by 5 percent in the latter half of the decade. This decline is especially remarkable when compared to trends for other professions. According to data from the Bureau of Labor Statistics, the adjusted wages of workers in professional, specialty, and technical occupations grew 3.5 percent between 1995 and 1999 (Reed and Ginsburg 2003). There is also some direct evidence linking managed care to the stagnation in physician incomes. For example, a survey by Ernst and Young of New York City found that doctors in practices that receive more than 50 percent of their gross revenues from managed care contracts earned an average of $116,600 in 1995, down from $137,900 in 1994. The same study indicated, conversely, that physicians in practices receiving less than 50 percent of their income from managed care organizations had an income increase from $108,000 to $115,000 on average across specialties (Conrad 1998).

In addition to significant challenges to autonomy and income, physicians in the 1990s also had to confront declining public esteem. Between 1990 and 2000 the proportion of General Social Survey respondents who had a great deal of confidence in the medical profession declined by 5.3 percentage points. The downward trend in public confidence has continued into the twenty-first century. Surveys by Harris Interactive in 1998 and 2004 indicate that although medicine was consistently rated higher on a prestige scale than any of the other twenty-two professions in the survey, confidence in physicians fell by 9 percentage points during this period (Harris Interactive 2004). Although declines in overall confidence in medicine are small, they are notable, and there is evidence that they coexist with a potentially stronger trend toward consumerism among patients. Research also suggests that although general public confidence in medicine remains relatively high, over time, the public has adopted more negative sentiments toward the profession (Pescosolido et al. 2001). By the mid-1980s as many as two fifths of persons studied were behaving to some extent in a consumerist manner when interacting with physicians. And a more recent Community Tracking Study (2000–2001) found that 38 percent of those surveyed had "looked for or obtained information about a personal health concern" from a source other than their physician. Those with college education or higher were most likely to seek independent information and use the Internet (Mechanic 2003, 941–46).

The Interest of Women and Men in Medicine

In light of the general decline of medicine during the 1990s, how should the trends in medical school applications be understood? The male flight perspective would predict significant declines in applications from men and a corresponding increase in applications from women as a result of the deterioration in the status of the profession. But the actual pattern during this period represents a rather different picture. From 1990 through the early years of the twenty-first century, trends in male and female applications moved in concert. During the first half of the 1990s there were dramatic increases in both male and female applications, despite the challenges facing the profession, but the rate of growth in female applications was slightly higher than the corresponding rate for men. Then in 1996 both male and female applications began to decline, though the rate of decline for female applications was slower than for male applications.

There is a relatively straightforward alternative explanation for the trends during the 1990s: instead of being driven by male flight, the dramatic increases in medical school applications during the early 1990s stemmed from the faltering economy. After the stock market crash in 1987, opportunities in business become significantly less lucrative and less plentiful, and the average salaries of other prestigious occupations began to falter. In contrast, the salaries of physicians remained strong throughout the 1980s (Schwartz and Mendelson 1990) and even continued improving in the early 1990s, while the incomes of other professionals lagged behind the cost of living (Reed and Ginsburg 2003).

The decline in applications to medical school during the latter half of the 1990s also seems to be directly tied to the economy. As the economy boomed and the Internet bubble expanded, the potential earnings of other professions outside of medicine improved significantly, even as the general work environment for physicians remained stressed. As suggested earlier, there was some evidence of a backlash against managed care, and some concessions were made to physicians during this period. Nevertheless, the concessions did not fully account for the continuing growth of managed care, and during the latter half of the decade physicians' median income declined, while the income of other professionals grew (Reed and Ginsburg 2003; Center for Health Policy Research 2003).

The attractiveness of medicine for women may also derive in part from the evolution of the profession. In the early 1990s the implementation of the RBRVS caused the relative earnings of primary care physicians to increase. Since women are disproportionately represented in these fields, their earnings relative to those of their male colleagues improved during this period (Center for Health Policy Research 2003). The lesser decline in female applications can also be attributed to the growing female advantage in college completion and in the tendency to major in biology. We discuss these trends in greater detail in chapter 3.

Taken collectively, the evidence presented here indicates that the growing representation of women in American medicine does not stem from declines in the profession's status. While the autonomy and authority of individual physicians have declined, medicine as a whole remains a highly paid and well-regarded profession. And despite all of the developments reviewed here, medical training continues to offer opportunities for service, prestige, and high income. Although the incomes of male physicians have dropped as a whole, a significant minority of this group earn extremely high incomes.

Instead, increases in the number of women medical students and practicing physicians are due to a series of independent social trends in American society and structural developments in U.S. health care. Thus women's presence in medicine is intimately intertwined with the larger society.

More specifically, women's initial entry into medicine occurred primarily because of the successes of the women's movement during the early 1970s and because of the dramatically increased capacity of the country's medical education system. Female medical students during the 1970s largely occupied medical school seats that had been recently created. Their presence did not represent a direct challenge to male dominance in, or male access to, the medical profession.

Women's increasing share of seats in American medical schools during the 1980s was driven primarily by declining male interest in medicine rather than by sustained growth in female interest. In fact, female applications to medical school remained relatively constant during the 1980s. Although medicine suffered many assaults during that decade, it maintained its overall power, prestige, and earning potential. During the 1980s, as was the case in the 1970s, there is little evidence to support the specific linkages posited by the male flight argument. Instead it appears that declines in male applications to medical school stemmed from multiple social forces, including the lack of growth in the number of male recipients of bachelor's degrees, the growing popularity of business majors and the declining interest in biology, and a growing emphasis among college students on materialism. In other words, male applications to medical school declined because business became more popular while the supply of male college graduates remained constant rather than because medicine became less desirable as a career.

Finally, as in the 1970s and 1980s, during the 1990s we fail to find support for the male flight argument. Medicine sustained a significant and lasting decline in status, autonomy, and income during the 1990s, but ironically-interest in medicine among both male and female students increased markedly, especially in the early 1990s. These declines contrast with the potential earnings and work environment offered by other demanding professions. Over time, women's presence in medicine has grown while the profession has sustained an increasing number of assaults on its autonomy and prestige. Nevertheless, the relationship between these trends is weak at best. Since the late 1980s, the ebb and flow of female interest in medicine increasingly mirrors trends among men. Thus the logic of substitution that underlies the male flight thesis has not been operative.

Although it does not appear that women's entry into medicine was driven by declines in the status of the profession, the question remains as to how women's increasing presence in U.S. medicine grew and why the process occurred as it did. In the next chapter we offer an alternative explanation for this profound demographic shift.

Our account focuses on the evolution of women's social roles in concert with the transformation of the medical profession. While external factors consistently tilted toward increased representation of women in the medical profession, developments internal to the profession played a positive role in some cases but in other cases inhibited women's access to, and success in, medicine.

3

Applying for Change

In Chapter 2 we asked whether a decline in the status of the profession precipitated a decline in men's interest in medicine, thus paving the way for women's entry. Despite the many challenges to the profession, physicians remain highly respected and well compensated. There was a drop-off in the number of men's applications to medical school during the 1970s and 1980s, but this was followed by sharp increases during the 1990s. Government efforts to reduce discrimination played an important role in opening doors for women, as did the growth in the size of medical school classes. In this chapter we turn our attention to the social factors that facilitated women's entry.

Much more research has been focused on the experiences of women in the medical profession than explaining why they began to arrive in such large numbers in the first place. The rapid evolution of women's status in American society is an essential component of the explanation for their sustained entry into medicine. In particular, the expansion of educational opportunities for women has helped to create a growing pool of candidates with the background and interest necessary for pursuing a career in medicine. Foreign physicians have also contributed to the feminization of medicine. A complete account of women's entry into medicine thus must include broader currents in American society as well as in other societies around the world, in addition to factors specific to the medical profession.

In this chapter we highlight some of the key demographic trends that contributed to women's entry into the American medical workforce during the last decades of the twentieth century. In particular, growth in the population of female college graduates—and thus in the population of potential physicians—and increases in the tendency of female college students to express interest in medicine contributed to the growing presence of women among practicing physicians. On the negative side of the ledger, higher levels of attrition for women both before and during medical school continue to inhibit women's entry into the medical profession. This suggests that there continue to be more barriers to, and less support for, women's professional career pursuits than is evident for men.

We start by presenting overall trends in the medical workforce, followed by a discussion of the surprising role of foreign physicians in the process of women's entry into medicine. Returning to the U.S. population, we then examine how the premedical pipeline has evolved since the 1970s. Our analysis focuses on women's educational pursuits in high school and in college as well as the interest that college students express in pursuing careers in the medical profession. The chapter concludes with the issue of leaks in the medical pipeline, including an assessment of trends in the attrition rates of male and female students before and during medical school.

Overall Trends in the U.S. Medical Workforce

Figure 3.1 presents data on the percentage of physicians who are women from 1970 (7.6 percent) to 2004 (26.6 percent). The data reveal that women's representation has been growing at an increasing rate—by 4 percentage

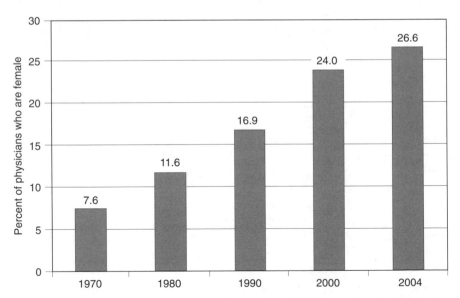

Figure 3.1. Women's Representation in Medicine, 1970–2004. *Source:* American Medical Association.

points during the 1970s, 5 percentage points during the 1980s, and 7 percentage points during the 1990s—to the point where women made up over one quarter of all U.S. physicians by the end of the twentieth century. Thus, while there was a rapid surge of women into medical schools as soon as the doors were opened wide in the early 1970s, women's entry into medicine has been the result of a gradual and sustained evolution that has still not been fully completed. (The trend is even more pronounced for osteopathic physicians.)[1] This overview suggests that both short-term and longer-term changes were essential in increasing women's representation in the profession.

The surge in women's representation in medical schools in the early 1970s in response to expanded opportunities was just the beginning of a longer process of social change. The early successes of women in gaining admission to medical school slowly spawned greater interest and awareness on the part of a new generation of women. Interest in medical school among college freshman women climbed slowly and steadily year after year. In short, it seems quite clear that there was a positive feedback loop between declining discrimination, expanded opportunities, women's early successes, and the continued growth in women's interest in medicine over time. The legacy of the 1972 Title IX legislation described in chapter 2 was not simply an immediate, short-term jump in women's applications. Instead, the full effect of this law continued to accumulate strength and momentum throughout the 1970s, 1980s, and 1990s, and is still being felt today as the number of young women aspiring to careers in medicine continues to grow.

Foreign Physicians

Immigrant or foreign-born physicians have made up a significant minority of the U.S. medical workforce since the end of World War II. As we saw in chapter 2, during the 1980s, payment incentives to hospitals based on the number of residents trained opened the door to more foreign-trained physicians. Data from the U.S. Census samples suggest that the representation of foreign-born physicians has been increasing steadily over time. Between 1970 and 2000, foreign-born physicians increased from 20 to 26 percent of the physician population, even as the number of U.-S.-born physicians was rapidly growing.

The representation of women has been increasing in both the native-born and foreign physician populations. Between 1970 and 2000, women rose from 6 to 25 percent of the U.S.-born population of doctors and from 17 to 31 percent of the foreign-born population. In other words, although women were better represented among foreign-born physicians early on and remain so, U.S.–born women are catching up and passing immigrant women. Data from the Association of American Medical Colleges (AAMC) indicate that in

2000, 46.6 percent of allopathic medical students in the United States were female (AAMC Data Book 2007, Table 3.9). During the same year, 40 percent of foreign-born physicians under age forty were female. As recently as 2000, nearly one third (30 percent) of female physicians in this country were foreign born. Thus overall, immigrant physicians have made a significant contribution to the feminization of the U.S. medical workforce.

Why has women's presence grown so significantly in the population of foreign-born physicians? One important contributing factor is that women are increasingly well represented among physicians in countries around the world, including those that send physicians to the United States.[2] Figure 3.2 displays the proportion of physicians who were female in 2004 in twenty-eight developed countries, drawing on data from the Organization for Economic Cooperation and Development (2007). The United States is far from the top of the list in terms of women's representation; indeed it is closer to the bottom. In several of the eastern European nations, such as Poland and Hungary, women physicians have long been quite common, as these countries followed the Soviet Union's model of feminized but relatively low status medicine. Yet many western European countries surpass the United States as well, including Spain (44 percent female), Sweden (41 percent female), and the Netherlands (38 percent female). The case of the Netherlands is somewhat surprising, since part-time employment rather than full-time professional careers is typical for women there. Since western European countries had relatively few women in medicine in 1970, the relatively high representation of women reflects rapid growth rather than a long-standing historical pattern.

This international evidence suggests that women are well represented among foreign physicians in the United States because the entry of women into the medical profession has not been restricted to this country. These data further suggest that the United States has not been at the forefront, as many other countries have incorporated women into medicine more rapidly than has been the case in the United States.

Another factor contributing to the growing presence of women among immigrant physicians involves the changing racial and ethnic background of foreign-born physicians in the United States. According to data from the U.S. Census, in 1970, 19.4 percent of all immigrant physicians were Asian. By 2000 this number had grown to 45.7 percent. In 1970 Caucasian immigrants made up 60.9 percent of all foreign-born physicians. By 2000 they were only 36.7 percent of the group. At the same time, women have consistently been better represented among foreign-born Asians than among foreign-born Caucasians. In 1970, 25.6 percent of immigrant Asian physicians and 15.6 percent of immigrant white physicians were female. The corresponding numbers in 2000 were 33.6 and 27.7 percent. Thus the increasing relative presence of Asians in the immigrant physician workforce appears to be causing women's presence among immigrant physicians to grow.

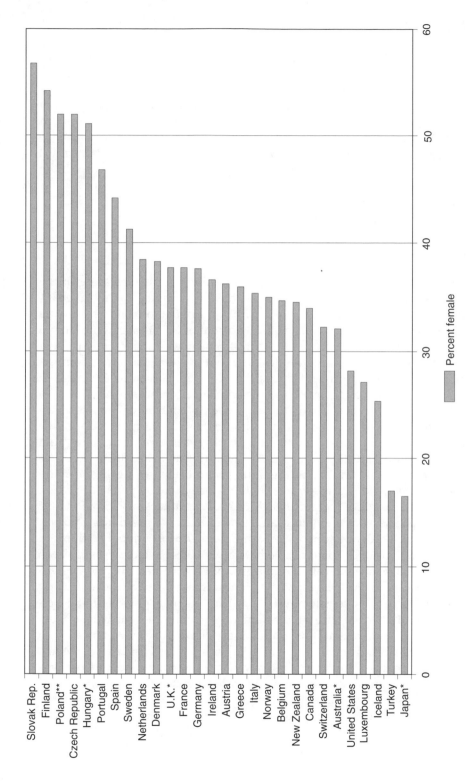

Figure 3.2. Women Physicians in 28 Countries, 2004. *Source:* OECD, 2007.

The leading countries of origin for female foreign-born physicians under age fifty are India (with 21.9 percent), China (8.3 percent), the Philippines (6.5 percent), Pakistan (3.0 percent), and Taiwan (1.8 percent). These five countries account for over 40 percent of foreign-born female physicians in this age group. The high proportion of women among these foreign-born physicians reflects the fact that many women have been training to become physicians in these sending countries. For example, in India over one third (37.5 percent) of those earning medical degrees in 2000 were women (India Central Bureau of Health Intelligence 2005). In China 41.0 percent of physicians and 46.0 percent of new medical graduates were women in 2002 (China Ministry of Health 2004).[3]

Racial and Ethnic Diversity

Census data suggest that racial and ethnic diversity is increasing in the U.S. medical workforce overall. Women have contributed to this diversity, and racial and ethnic groups have in turn contributed to women's growing representation in medicine. In 2000, 78 percent of physicians in the United States were white, 15 percent were Asian, 4 percent were black, and 3 percent Hispanic. The significance of this development can be gleaned from comparing physicians by age group. Of physicians over age fifty in 2000, 81 percent were white; of those age forty and younger, 71 percent were white.[4]

As we have just noted, one of the major factors contributing to this diversity is the presence of substantial numbers of foreign-born physicians. The representation of immigrants in the U.S. physician workforce grew from 20 percent in 1970 to 26 percent in 2000, including an increasing representation of physicians born in Asia. Yet immigration is by no means the entire story. Graduates of U.S. medical schools are also becoming more diverse.

Figure 3.3 displays the percentage of 2004 graduates of U.S. allopathic medical schools by race, ethnicity, and gender. Just over two thirds (68.6 percent) of male graduates were white, compared with just under two thirds of female graduates (63.7 percent). Female physicians have consistently been a more racially and ethnically diverse group. This is especially true for African Americans. In 2004 the representation of African Americans was nearly twice as high among female physicians as among male physicians (8.6 percent versus 4.4 percent). In absolute numbers, African American women were 1.6 times as numerous in this graduating class as African American men (658 versus 404). Women represent a larger share of Hispanic and Asian physicians in this graduating class as well, although the gender disparity is much lower than is the case among African Americans. Women physicians are thus more racially and ethnically diverse than are their male counterparts. To the extent that this diversity represents a strength of American medicine, women deserve their share of the credit.

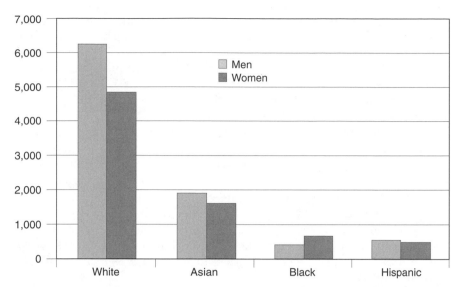

Figure 3.3. Race, Ethnicity, and Gender among 2004 MD Recipients. *Source:* 2004 CTS Survey.

The Evolving Status of Women

We maintain that the growing representation of women in the medical profession is a manifestation of a large-scale, transformation in the academic behavior and professional ambitions of young American women and in Americans' beliefs about women's place in society. In response to the rebirth of the women's movement during the late 1960s, opportunities for women have expanded in a number of important ways.

One key shift in behavior with wide ramifications for society in general and medicine in particular is the steady growth in the number of women obtaining college degrees (Jacobs 1996). In 1960 men outnumbered women in caps and gowns by roughly two to one. By 1982, a mere two decades later, women had completely erased this gap and had attained parity in college completion for the first time. Surprisingly, the growth in women's representation among college graduates did not stop once women had reached parity with men; instead women continued to outpace their male counterparts. By 2004 women were earning 57 percent of bachelor's degrees to men's 43 percent, a female-to-male ratio of nearly 1.4 to 1 (National Center for Education Statistics 2006a; Buchmann and DiPrete 2006).

Through 1975, college graduation rates climbed for both men and women in similar absolute numbers, although the rate of growth was higher for women since they were starting out at a much lower level. In 1975, the year after the military draft for the Vietnam War ended, trends in college graduation for men and women began to diverge. In the ensuing three decades the number of bachelor's degrees awarded to men increased only 14 percent, while the number of bachelor's degrees awarded to women increased 84 percent. This difference ultimately resulted in women's receiving 215,000 more bachelor's degrees than men in the 2003–4 academic year. The expansion in women's representation in college added to the pool of women with the potential to apply to medical school.

These high rates of college completion coincided with more rigorous educational choices dating back to the high school years. Girls in high school are increasingly taking the math and science courses that are necessary prerequisites for college entry. This preparation is particularly useful for the choice of many college majors and careers that require these skills.

By the 1980s, girls had begun to surpass their male counterparts in taking many key math and science courses in high school. According to the National Center for Education Statistics, female high school graduates in 2000 were more likely than their male peers to have taken algebra II, biology, advanced placement or honors biology, and chemistry. Young women have exceeded their male counterparts in taking honors or advanced placement biology courses since 1982, and the gap is growing at a slow but steady pace. Among high school graduates in 2000, 19 percent of women and 14 percent of men had completed AP biology. The same pattern is evident for general high school chemistry. By 1990 women high school graduates had surpassed men in completing chemistry courses. In 2000, 66 percent of female high school graduates had completed a course in chemistry, compared with 58 percent of their male counterparts (Freeman 2004).

These developments are echoed by trends in college majors related to medical careers. Although only about half of the applicants to medical school are biology or life science majors, this group is nonetheless a useful barometer of interest in medical school.[5] Women now surpass men in the share of biology majors, and since there are more women than men receiving college degrees, the pool of women receiving degrees in biology now substantially exceeds that for men. In 2004 over 37,000 women received bachelor's degrees in biology, compared with only 23,000 men (Freeman 2004).

Among high school students, there are areas in math and science where young men maintain an advantage. Male students continue to be more likely than females to take physics. And males are more likely to enroll in both AP physics and AP chemistry. This disparity means that although males are less likely to take AP biology, they take more science AP tests overall. The story is similar for advanced mathematics. Women are catching up to men, but a disparity still exists. The percentage of male graduates who had taken any form of calculus increased from 6 to 12 percent, and the percentage of female graduates who had taken calculus increased from 4 to 11 percent between 1982 and 2000 (National Center for Education Statistics 2004). Yet women take only 47 percent of the AB calculus AP tests and only 44 percent of the BC calculus AP tests.[6] Furthermore, although girls get better grades overall in high school, their performance in selected advanced math and science classes lags slightly behind that of their male peers. For example, in 2002 the average score on AP calculus tests was 3.5 for boys and 3.3 for girls (Freeman 2004).

As in the case of high school enrollment and achievement, gender imbalances across college majors remain. In 2001 women earned 51.3 percent of all social science and history degrees, 59.5 percent of all biology and life science degrees, 41.2 percent of all physical science and science technology degrees, and 19.9 percent of all engineering degrees (National Center for Education Statistics 2004).

The remaining gender gaps in math and the physical sciences contribute to gender differences in performance on the physical science portion of the Medical College Admissions Test (the MCAT). In 2005 the average female MCAT taker scored 0.3 points lower on the verbal section, 1.1 points lower on the physical science section, and 0.7 points lower on the biological science section.

One factor contributing to women's lower performance on the MCAT involves differences in their academic choices during college. Data from the AAMC on MCAT takers in 1998 suggest that students who major in physical sciences such as chemistry and physics score significantly higher on the physical science portion of the MCAT. There are also positive relationships between a student's science MCAT scores and the student's number of credit hours in physics, biochemistry, and organic chemistry (author's analysis of 1998 MCAT premedical questionnaire data). Our summary of these trends in educational patterns is that even though a small gender gap in MCAT scores remains, there is a large and growing pool of young women with the necessary science background to succeed in medical school and in medical practice. As we will see, the remaining differential in MCAT scores has become less important in recent years. Increases in the educational investments of young women both facilitate and reflect their increasing aspirations.

Female college students are becoming not only more numerous but also more ambitious and more interested in graduate education. Surveys of college freshmen conducted annually by the Cooperative Institutional Research Program (CIRP) indicate a sharp increase in women's plans to pursue graduate education. In 1966 only 40.3 percent aspired to graduate degrees (which could include a master's degree in education). By 2001 more than three fourths expressed an interest in pursuing graduate degrees, slightly more than did the men (77.3 percent of the women compared to 73.1 percent of the men). By contrast, in 1966 freshman men were much more likely

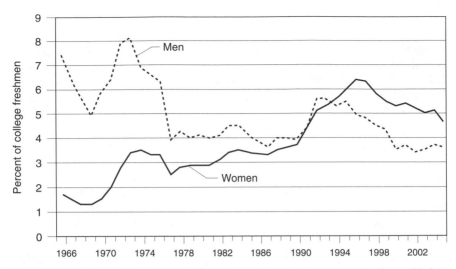

Figure 3.4. Freshman Interest in Medical Careers by Gender, 1966–2004. *Source:* Higher Education Research Institute, UCLA.

than their female peers to aspire to graduate degrees: 58.4 percent versus 40.3 percent (Astin 1998).[7]

Women's interest in medicine has grown as part of this broader trend in the pursuit of graduate education. Figure 3.4 presents trends in the number of U.S. college freshmen reporting medicine as their probable career choice. Interest among female freshman has climbed nearly consistently since the early 1970s, shortly before laws were passed preventing discrimination against female medical school applicants and shortly after a dramatic increase in the number of domestic medical school openings. The rate of increase, however, was fairly modest from the mid-1970s through the early 1990s, until the level of women's interest began to exceed that for men in 1992. Despite a gradual increase among women over men, the overall historical trends in interest in medicine are largely similar for men and women from the late 1970s onward.

Curricular Reform in U.S. Medical Schools

Another factor that may be contributing to growth in the number of women attending U.S. medical schools is the change in priorities of medical school admissions committees and in the nature of academic medical curricula. Medical schools have been incorporating and institutionalizing training in a broad range of topics related to health care which do not involve physical or life sciences. Such subjects include health outcomes research and evidence-based medicine (Barzansky and Etzel 2003), bioethics (Scott 1991;

Miles et al. 1989; Barzansky and Etzel 2003), communication (Kalet et al. 2004), empathy (Kahn et al. 1979), cultural competence (AAMC 2005), and women's health (Henrich 2004), as well as a more general exposure to the humanities (Kennedy 2006).

Medical schools have also been reforming their approach to education to encourage more problem-based learning, more peer collaboration, more self-motivation, more student-level independence, and more computer-assisted learning (Jonas et al. 1991). In the process, many schools have been limiting students' experiences in more competitive environments by limiting grades and providing opportunities for retesting. And administrators have been discouraging the traditional "teach by humiliation" approach, as well as restricting demands for rote memorization.

One of the main manifestations of this trend was the restructuring of the Medical College Admissions Test in the early 1990s so as to broaden the types of knowledge assessed. Shortly thereafter, the percentage of medical school applicants with social science majors increased (Cooper 2003).

But the MCAT is only the first of a series of changes in the evaluation of physicians. Beginning in 2004, students taking step 2 of the National Medical Licensing Exam were required to pass a clinical skills test in which they evaluate ten standardized patients in fifteen-minute intervals. Students receive three scores for the test: assessment of an integrated clinical encounter (based on the checklist from the standardized patients and global ratings of the encounter note), a test of communication skills, and an evaluation of English language skills. Students must pass all three components in order to practice medicine in the United States. This marks the first time since 1964 that medical students have had to pass a clinical skills test, and the first time that communication skills have been highlighted in the evaluation (Santana 2003).

Another manifestation of the increasing salience of social science to modern medicine was the effort by the Institute of Medicine to examine the behavioral and social science curricula in medical school. The resulting document (Institute of Medicine 2004) highlights the need for physicians to understand how social conditions such as poverty and personal behaviors such as smoking influence health and to acknowledge how a physician's background and beliefs can influence patient care.

Advocates of the "different voice" perspective might suggest that the reforms in medical education stem largely from the increasing presence of women in the profession, and that it is women's more altruistic and nurturing demeanor that is driving these reforms. Although we cannot definitively adjudicate this claim, we suggest that the primary impetus for these innovations stems largely from two series of studies, one that documents differences in the care that minority and female patients receive and one that suggests that patient behaviors play a major role in determining health outcomes. These studies resulted in part from the development of health services and health outcomes research as a federal priority. We discuss the role that female leadership played in this and other areas of medicine in chapter 9. Regardless of their origins, however, these reforms increased the attractiveness of medicine to female students.

Why Medicine?

Women in 2004 constituted 46.4 percent of the U.S. labor force. Does the growth of their share in medical school classes simply reflect these broad changes in women's social roles, specifically higher college completion rates and higher labor force participation? While these society-wide trends no doubt play an important role, women have entered some occupations in much greater numbers than others. For example, in 2004 women made up 29 percent of computer professionals, 27 percent of lawyers, 46 percent of biologists, and 50 percent of pharmacists, but only 14 percent of engineers (all figures obtained from Dye 2005). Clearly, factors specific to the medical profession are required to account for the level of and trends in women's representation in medicine.

The altruistic nature of medical work contributes to its appeal to women. Some young adults are attracted to careers that will pay well, others are more interested in helping people, while still others are interested in working with things. This trio—money, people, and things—has long played a prominent role in sociologists' and vocational counselors' lists of salient job attributes (Konrad et al. 2000). Careers in medicine tend to be attractive because they draw people oriented in any and all of these directions. Medicine is a career that offers an unusual combination of high pay and job security. Doctors, however, also derive tremendous satisfaction from being able to help people on a daily basis. And finally, many areas of medicine involve enough gadgets and gizmos to satisfy those with a technical orientation.

The Higher Education Research Institute at UCLA has administered a nationally representative survey of U.S. college freshmen annually for several decades. We were able to obtain special tabulations of these data on the professional priorities of students who indicated a serious interest in medicine as a career and their peers.[8] Specifically, for the years 1978, 1982, 1987, 1992, 1997, and 2002, data were obtained on the importance placed on "being very well off financially" and "helping others who are in need." We compared college freshmen who identified themselves as premedical (those who identified medicine as a "probable career goal") at four-year institutions with their peers at the same institutions. The data on these issues are presented in figures 3.5 and 3.6.

Since the 1970s the expressed desire for financial success has increased among college students across the board. The vestiges of the antimaterialist

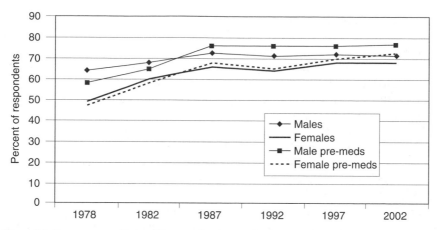

Figure 3.5. Importance of Being "Financially Very Well Off" for College Freshmen by Premed Status and Gender, 1978–2002. *Source:* Higher Education Research Institute, UCLA.

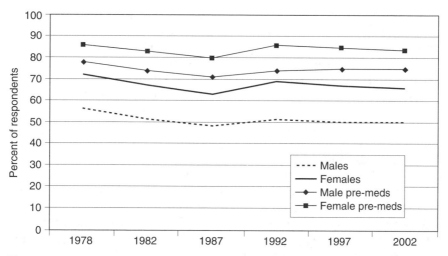

Figure 3.6. Importance of "Helping Others" for College Freshmen by Premed Status and Gender, 1978–2002. *Source:* Higher Education Research Institute, UCLA.

1960s gave way to the full-throttled careerism of the 1980s. The trends in the values of medical students need to be understood against the backdrop of the goals and values of their classmates.

As a group, in 1978 freshman men interested in careers in medicine were actually less likely than their classmates to identify financial success as an "important or very important priority" (58 percent of prospective premeds, versus 64 percent for freshmen overall). By 1987 male premeds had pulled ahead of their peers in regard to their desire for financial success, and by 2002 male premeds had surpassed their classmates by 6 percentage points in the emphasis placed on financial success (77 percent versus 71 percent). This is ironic because it appears that medicine has become increasingly attractive to those who prioritized money as a key factor in their career choices despite the numerous challenges to the profession reviewed in chapter 2.

The pattern is very much the same for women. In 1978 freshman women who aspired to a career in medicine were less likely to cite the importance of financial success than were their peers (47 percent of freshman premedical students versus 56 percent of other students). By 1987 women in general were more likely to respond that financial success was important or very important to them than were their non-premed classmates. By 2002 female freshmen who aspired to careers in medicine had become slightly (72 percent versus 68 percent) more interested in financial success than had been the case twenty-four years earlier and also in comparison with their non-premedical peers.

In addition to the financial attractiveness of the profession, the ability of physicians to help those in need is another important reason why medicine is attractive to women. Relative to fields such as engineering, the altruistic dimension helps to set it apart. Premedical students consistently stand out from other college students in terms of their altruistic orientation over the period examined. Premeds are more likely to say that they would like to help others than are other students. And since the 1970s, as the salience of altruism has declined among college students, the gap in altruistic orientation between those interested in medicine and others has increased.

Figure 3.6 displays trends in the importance of "helping others in need" from the American freshman surveys. In 1978 female premedical students expressed more altruism than their peers. At that time, 86 percent of female premeds cited the importance of helping others in need, versus 72 percent of other female freshmen, for a 14 percentage point "altruism" advantage. The altruism advantage is even more evident for male premedical students, who were 23 percentage points more likely to volunteer that "helping others" was important or very important to them.

In the ensuing two decades, the reported altruism of all groups declined, but this trend was felt less among premedical students than among others. By 2002, 83 percent of female freshman premeds cited the importance of helping others, down from 86 percent in 1978. But because altruism declined even faster among women interested in pursing other careers, the differential in favor of female premeds increased from 14 percentage points in 1978 to 19 percentage points in 2002. The same general pattern held for men as well. Altruism among male freshman premedical students dropped slightly, from 78 percent in 1978 to 75 percent in 2002. The 23 percentage point gap in 1978 grew to a 26 percentage point gap by 2002.

Finally, because women's representation among medical aspirants is increasing, the altruism of the medical aspirant population has remained relatively constant, falling only from 81.1 percent to 79.9 percent between 1978 and 2002. In other words, the priority placed on altruistic motives has been declining for both males and females, but because women are consistently more altruistic than men, the growth in women's representation offsets the overall decline in altruism. Thus throughout this period, an altruistic orientation differentiates those who pursue careers in medicine from those interested in other fields. Women have historically placed a greater emphasis on being able to help others, and this has contributed to the popularity of medicine as a career choice.

Some would no doubt see these data through the lens of the "different voice" perspective mentioned in chapter 1: in other words, women come to medicine for different reasons and with different priorities than do men. While there is no doubt that some women bring a different orientation with them from that of men, the matter is more complex than is conveyed by the "different voice" thesis.

Our first observation is that there is a great deal of overlap in the orientations of young men and women interested in careers in medicine. Both groups value helping others as well as being well off financially. Men and women resemble each other in these respects (as in many others) more than they differ. Second, the extent to which the general culture values altruism varies over time. Thus women premeds in 2002 were more focused on making money than were men premeds in 1978. The extent of interest in helping others is therefore not a fixed attribute of males and females but instead varies over time.

Third, it is important to keep in mind that the values that students bring with them into the profession will be shaped and reshaped during their medical education as well as their early years in the profession. The value accorded a social orientation to medicine, as opposed to technical and other norms, may be altered during the course of medical education and may depend on the specific medical school a student attends. And finally, the ability of physicians to live up to their ideals is shaped by many factors that are increasingly out of their control. Thus while the connection between gender and altruism has contributed to the rising interest of women in medicine, we caution against treating altruism as an unchangeable gender-linked dichotomy.

These results are also inconsistent with the idea that a feminine commitment to caring has begun to pervade the entire profession. The trends to date have indicated just the opposite: the medical profession has not been insulated from the growing emphasis on materialism in American culture and society.

These data point to a generational shift in medicine that is quite different from the ones often discussed in the medical literature. While Bickel and Brown (2005), among others, have suggested a general trend away from traditional notions of pecuniary success, the data suggest that today these traditional values are as strong as, if not stronger than, in previous generations.

The data on goals and values thus do not conform to the expectations of a "post-pioneer generation" perspective. Today's women are not more altruistic than their predecessors. Quite the contrary. A generational shift has increased the emphasis on financial success while slightly tempering the levels of reported altruistic motives. It is not easy to reconcile these data with the thesis that the status of medicine is declining. Not only are those interested in financial success still pursuing careers in medicine, but also the gap between premeds and other students in the emphasis placed on financial goals has grown over time.

One possible reason for the persistent interest of premedical students in money is the development of careers that merge the financial rewards of business and management with medical training. Doctors have become so interested in the business side of medicine that since the 1980s more than forty medical schools have added an optional fifth year of schooling for those who want to earn an M.B.A. degree as well as an MD. Some graduates go directly to Wall Street or into health care management without ever practicing medicine (Uchitelle 2006).

As noted earlier, during the 1980s college students as a group moved away from choosing altruistic careers. This trend likely depressed interest in careers in medicine for both men and women during that period of time. Thus, while altruism plays a role in explaining women's pursuit of medicine rather than other fields, its relative decline also helps to explain the dip in interest in medicine during the 1980s.

How do these results fit with data on the values of prospective medical students? We drew on data from students who took the MCAT exam over the period 1999 to 2004. In this analysis there is unfortunately a shorter time line because of inconsistencies in the way the first-year medical questionnaire asked the question regarding career goals and values. Table 3.1 presents results for eight different reasons for pursuing medicine. Interest in helping people is by far the most common reason cited. It is striking, however, that there is a decline in the popularity of this response for both men and women between 1999 and 2004. This trend echoes a similar pattern found for freshman premedical students. We were also struck by the frequency with which "intellectual challenge" and "interest in research" were mentioned. Income trails far behind. This finding is actually not uncommon when the reasons for specific career choices are elicited in this manner.

The results in Table 3.1 also show striking similarities in the priorities of male and female aspiring medical students and thus discount the possibility that gender differences in essential values are driving differences in the

Table 3.1. Reasons for Pursuing Medicine, by Gender, 1999 and 2004

	1999		2004	
	Men	Women	Men	Women
Interest in helping people	64.63	71.23	51.54	63.60
Intellectual challenge	35.16	34.96	46.60	49.04
Interest in research	16.00	16.43	21.97	23.51
Job security	16.31	16.67	20.09	19.85
Independence	11.34	10.58	16.60	14.45
High income	5.63	4.26	7.79	6.58
Authority	2.85	2.02	4.91	4.72
Status and prestige	3.16	2.02	5.45	3.95

Source: AAMC Premedical Questionnaire.

careers of male and female physicians. Both men and women were most likely to list interest in helping people, intellectual challenge, job security, and research as the most highly motivating aspects of the profession. Thus, the motivations of medical school aspirants have changed over time for both men and women.

Women are slightly more likely to cite altruistic reasons for their career choices, and men are slightly more likely to cite income. This difference is corroborated by previous research documenting similar types of gender differences in motivation for medical students in the United States and abroad (Vaglum et al. 1999; Bickel and Ruffin 1995; Neittaanmaeki et al. 1993). The similarities in the responses of men and women in Table 3.1, however, overshadow the modest differences.

Another potential explanation for disproportionate increases in female interest in medicine is what appears to be a growing perception among young women that medicine offers more secure employment and more opportunities for work-family balance than other technical fields. One female undergraduate biochemistry major we interviewed described the decision this way: "It is harder to hold down a job as a woman who just does research. As a doctor you're always going to have a job. As a researcher, you have to be in lab seven days a week, all day." She was struggling to decide between medical school, graduate school in chemistry, and an MD-Ph.D. program. Although she did not say so directly, she seemed to believe that medicine offers a part-time option that does not exist in science.

Similarly, another recent graduate from residency explained in an interview that although she had majored in chemical engineering in college, she had elected to go to medical school because she thought that there would be more opportunities to work part-time in medicine than in the corporate world.

Although we detect a growing sense among potential medical students that medicine offers part-time opportunities, it remains to be seen whether these expectations will eventually be realized. As we show in chapters 6 and 8, with the exception of general pediatrics and psychiatry, female physicians have relatively low rates of part-time work. Many of the women entering medicine in search of a work-family balance may be surprised by what they find.

Persistence

Do the freshmen who check off medicine as a career goal end up finding their way into medical school? While there is surprisingly little research on persistence with medical aspirations prior to entering medical school, there is substantial evidence that women abandon their interests in science more readily than men (for example, see Sax 1992). And there is some limited evidence that, prior to the 1990s, women who aspired to careers in medicine were less likely to realize their goal than their male counterparts (Fiorentine and Cole 1992; Antony 1998).

Our analysis indicates that gender differences in persistence with medical aspirations remain. Figure 3.7 presents trends in the ratio of male and female medical school applicants to the number of college freshmen expressing interest in medicine four years earlier. It suggests that with the exception of the few years between 1972 and 1976, persistence with medical aspirations has been higher for males than for females, and that the gender difference in persistence has been relatively constant during this period.

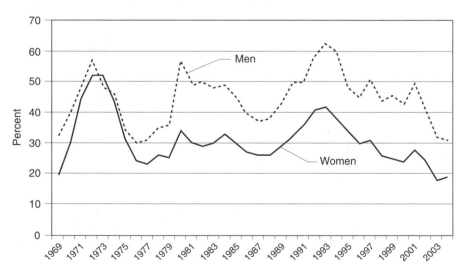

Figure 3.7. Estimated Freshman Medical School Yield, by Gender, 1970–2004. *Source:* NCES and HERI, UCLA data.

This analysis is only a rough approximation because the data utilized do not follow the same individuals over time. Thus some may have switched into medicine, perhaps even after college. Panel data that do follow the same individuals over time, however, also show disproportionate female attrition. To fill the gaps, we examined data from the National Center for Education Statistics' Baccalaureate and Beyond longitudinal survey (B&B), a nationally representative panel study of students completing undergraduate degrees in 1993. These data indicated that the female advantage among college freshmen was thus reversed by graduation. In 1994, one year after college graduation, 4.2 percent of males and 2.3 percent of females intended to become physicians.[9] Of this group, by 2003, a decade after graduation, 55 percent of males and 36 percent of females reported that they were "medical practice professionals." So, attrition during and after college is higher for females than for males.[10]

The limited evidence indicates that the gender differential in attrition from the medical pipeline continues after students matriculate at U.S. medical schools. Data suggest that this attrition has increased steadily since 1973 and that women drop out of medical school at consistently higher rates than men (Fitzpatrick and Wright 1995).[11] In general, however, most students who enter medical school eventually graduate. The gender gap in attrition is just a few points—10.4 percent on average for women versus 6.3 percent for men between 1988 and 1992—but the gap has been consistent over time. Thus the bulk of attrition from medical careers occurs before students begin their studies.

Yet receipt of a Doctor of Medicine degree is necessary but not sufficient to practice medicine. Today students must complete one year by law, and three years in actual practice, of graduate medical education or residency. While relatively little evidence exists about attrition from residencies overall, research indicates that gender affects the odds of attrition from graduate medical education in surgery, and that overall attrition from surgery is significant. For example, average one-year attrition from general surgery residency programs in 2000 was 20.2 percent (Cochran et al. 2002). Other research suggests that female general surgical residents are more likely to drop out than their male colleagues (Bergen et al. 1998). When women leave general surgery residencies, it is more likely for family reasons such as lifestyle considerations or to join a spouse in another geographic location, and when men leave it is most likely to pursue another medical specialty (Bergen et al. 1998).

Similarly, women are more likely than men to drop out of obstetrics-gynecology residency programs (Jancin 2002). This result is surprising in light of evidence suggesting increasing problems facing men in obstetrics (Lyon 2002). And, as in general surgery, men who drop out of obstetrics do so primarily to pursue a different medical specialty. Women, in contrast, quit residency primarily for family reasons, with the two most commonly cited causes being spouse relocation and child care issues (Jancin 2002).

In sum, although women now surpass men in terms of aspiring to medical school (and even equal shares would favor women at this point, since they outnumber men among college graduates), women continue to leak out of the medical pipeline in disproportionate numbers. This leaves roughly similar numbers of men and women entering medical school.

What factors contribute to this small but persistent gap in retention in the premedical pipeline? Performance on standardized tests may contribute to the gender disparity. Women continue to garner slightly lower scores on the science portion of the MCAT tests, and test performance is related to entry into, and persistence in, medical school.[12]

But we suspect that test scores are not the entire story. A significant portion of this attrition and academic difficulty may stem from differences in the socioeconomic backgrounds of female and male medical students. As we have seen, female physicians are more diverse than are their male counterparts. They are more likely to be members of racial and ethnic minority groups, and are also likely to have grown up in families with relatively limited financial resources. Previous research indicates that ethnic minorities and lower-income students experience more difficulty in medicine (Cooter et al. 2004; Fadem 1995). Consequently, women students as a group are more likely to encounter the obstacles associated with lesser access to financial support.

In addition to these greater financial constraints, the incomplete transition in the way American society views women and men, as well as persistent differences in how male and female residents are treated, contribute to the ongoing gender differences in attrition. On the one hand, there has been a dramatic increase in the number of Americans who believe that married women can and should work outside the home. In particular, data from the General Social Survey (GSS) indicate that the acceptability of women's employment outside the home grew steadily between 1974 and 1998 (Bolzendahl and Myers 2004). Most notably, the proportion of male Americans who disapprove of married women's working for pay declined from 37 to 17 percent between 1972 and 1998 (the last year for which data were available regarding these questions). The comparable figures for American women were 32 and 18 percent respectively. These changes reflect the replacement of earlier generations who grew up with different attitudes and expectations by those more accustomed to women's paid employment, and in part reflect attitudes adapted to the new realities (Brooks and Bolzendahl 2004).

On the other hand, many Americans continue to embrace the ideal of a female homemaker and male breadwinner. In 2004 over one third of men (37 percent) and women (35 percent) responding to the General Social Survey reported believing that it is better for the man to work and the woman to tend to the family. Furthermore, throughout the 1990s evidence suggests that many men and women continued to expect a wife to sacrifice her career for her husband even if her career was prestigious (Novack and Novack 1996; Simon and Landis 1989; Wethington et al. 2003). Even if they support the idea of a woman working for pay, they still accept traditional gender norms regarding domestic and financial responsibilities.

In particular, the full incorporation of mothers of young children into the world of paid work continues to evoke ambivalence. In 2004, 36 percent of women and 52 percent of men responding to the GSS agreed that preschool-aged children suffer if their mothers work. Some of the attrition of women from the premedical school pipeline may well reflect this continuing ambivalence regarding women's roles.

A related factor may involve the challenges women physicians face in combining work and family. In other words, it may be the challenging prospect of combining a fulfilling family life with very long workweeks that discourages some women from pursuing careers in medicine. We examine trends in this area in chapter 6 and again in chapter 8. For example, Lovecchio and Dundes (2002) find that women who abandoned medical aspirations were significantly more likely than their male peers to attribute their career switches to the incompatibility of a physician's life with plans to have a family (95 percent of women versus 52 percent of men). To a lesser extent, the authors also found that more women admitted that low grades had been a deciding factor in their revised career plans (76 percent versus 61 percent of men).

But differences in persistence are not merely a result of gendered expectations surrounding family life. Although the evidence is limited, there is reason to believe that male and female students are treated differently at all stages of medical and premedical training. In particular, it appears that female science students get less attention than do their male classmates (Greenfield 1998). This issue is examined in more detail in the context of medical education in chapter 5.

A final factor contributing to the greater attrition of women is the resistance they face from men. One specific manifestation of this is sexual harassment. A representative study released by the American Association of University Women (2006) indicates that sexual harassment is widespread on college campuses and that these experiences are especially detrimental for female students. Since women in medicine are disproportionately members of racial and ethnic minorities, they are likely to face discrimination based in racial and ethnic prejudice as well.

Research indicates that harassment does not stop in college. Women are also more likely than men to experience general and sexual harassment during medical school (Bickel and Ruffin 1995; Nora et al. 1996). Results from the AAMC graduating student questionnaire suggest that roughly one in six female students reported mistreatment of any kind in 2004, compared with one in eight of their male classmates. Two thirds of all mistreatment reported by female students was sexual in nature, while only one third of mistreatment reported by male students was sexual (Yamagata et al. 2006). There is also a qualitative difference between the types of sexual mistreatment that male and female students encounter during medical school. The most frequent type of perceived gender discrimination involves educational inequalities, and male students are more likely to report this type of problem, especially in regard to experiences involving obstetrics-gynecology (Nora et al. 1996). Female students are more likely to report all other types of harassment, including stereotypic comments, sexual overtures, offensive, embarrassing, or sexually explicit comments, and inappropriate touching (Witte et al. 2006).

We have culled through many different data sources and summarized a number of important historical developments in order to bring women's entry into medicine into focus. The entry of women into medicine marched on steadily for three decades, even though the 1970s, the 1980s, and the 1990s differed in many important respects

The first key development that allowed women to enter medicine was the decline in legally sanctioned barriers to their entry. The prohibition in 1972 of sex-based discrimination in higher education opened the doors of medical schools to women. Thus women's entry into medicine is clearly due to a decline in discrimination that resulted from the successful legislative agenda of the women's movement.

The second key development was the expansion of the number of seats in medical schools that occurred during the 1970s. As a result of this development, women began entering medicine during a period of a rapid growth in the medical profession. In short, the story of women's entry into medicine begins with expanding opportunities, in terms of both reduced discrimination and the substantial expansion in the number of seats in medical school classes.

Third, by the early 1970s there was a significant pool of women ready and able to enter medicine. Many women were drawn to medicine because of its humanitarian dimension as well as its scientific interest. The biological sciences had long attracted more women college students than other natural science fields such as geology and physics. As the doors of medical schools opened to them, there were many talented women eager to fill out applications. In this way the early 1970s resembled the 1940s, when women rapidly filled the medical school seats vacated by men who were off at war (Walsh 1977; Morantz-Sanchez 1985). In both cases there was no need for a long period of altered gender role socialization to adjust to these opportunities: there was a pool of women ready to seize the moment and jump at the chance to join the medical profession.

Yet the entry of women into medicine in response to expanded opportunities in the early 1970s was just the beginning of a longer process of social change. The early successes of women in gaining admission to medical school slowly spawned greater interest and awareness on the part of a new generation of women. Interest in medical school among freshman women climbed slowly and steadily year after year. In short, it seems quite clear that there was a positive feedback loop between declining discrimination, expanded opportunities, women's early successes, and the continued growth in women's interest in medicine over time. The legacy of the 1972 Title IX law was not simply a short-term surge in women's applications. Instead the full effect of this law continued to accumulate momentum throughout the 1970s, 1980s, and 1990s, and is still being felt today as the number of young women aspiring to careers in medicine continues to grow.

This positive feedback process was set in a broader context of changes in women's roles. Women's increased participation in higher education expanded the pool of potential applicants to medical school. Not only had women become the majority of college degree recipients by the late 1980s, but also by the 1990s female high school students were graduating more fully prepared to enter premedical studies in college than were their male counterparts. Thus the developments in the 1970s sparked short-term responses on the part of women that generated a secondary series of responses which ultimately played out over a longer period of time. Women's entry into medicine can best be understood as an interactive process of expanding opportunities, which leads to a positive feedback loop, which generates greater interest and better preparation. And we should also keep in mind that roughly one third of women physicians were foreign-born, and thus the developments in medical education in the United States are only part of the story of women's expanded role in U.S. medicine. All of these short-term and long-term changes were still not sufficient, however, to reduce the attrition of women from the premedical pipeline. Women remain disproportionately vulnerable to leaving medicine at all stages of the process, before, during, and after medical school.

In chapter 2 we cast doubt on the commonly cited theory that women's entry into medicine stemmed from declines in the profession. In this chapter we have offered an alternative explanation for this profound demographic transformation. Rather than simply filling a gap left by men, an expanding pool of young women was available as a result of changes in women's roles in contemporary society, especially with respect to changes in educational decisions. The women's movement played a key role in helping to open doors to medical school and, in a broader way, by signaling more generally the importance of a greater acceptance of women in professional roles. Women were also drawn into the profession by the growing need for physicians, especially during the 1970s, and some specific changes in the nature of medical education, especially during the 1990s.

Having described why women entered medicine, we concentrate in the next few chapters on how this process occurred. Our goal is to describe more fully the place that women occupy in medicine in the United States and to explain why women physicians continue to occupy different spheres of medicine from that of their male peers.

4

The Gendered Map of
Contemporary Medicine

Thus far our focus has been on women's entry into the medical profession as a whole. Now we turn to the question of how women are faring once they enter the profession. Substantial gender-based disparities remain within the medical profession. In the following chapters we examine how such differences have changed since women began entering medicine in significant numbers, and what factors are responsible for the persistent gaps between the career experiences of male and female physicians. In contrast to much prior research which emphasizes individual choice, we suggest that a more complete account requires a discussion of structural changes in the profession as well as experiences of discrimination.

This chapter focuses on describing the current state of professional inequality and documenting how that inequality has changed over time. Our analysis addresses gender differentiation in five realms: (1) specialty fields, (2) practice ownership, (3) patient profiles, (4) research and faculty positions, and (5) leadership positions. We conclude by examining how each of these aspects of gender differentiation relates to gender disparities in income.

The pace of gender integration varies significantly across the different realms of the medical profession and across time periods. While data indicate that the gender gaps in practice ownership and earnings have declined steadily over time, our findings with regard to specialization are somewhat less positive. The distribution of female and male physicians across medical specialties is significantly more similar today than it was a generation ago. The pace of gender integration by specialty, however, has slowed in recent years. These patterns are also reflected in the specializations of residents. In the absence of change, women will remain overrepresented in some fields and underrepresented in others for the foreseeable future.

The gap between women physicians' representation in medical research and their presence in the profession overall is larger today than it was a generation ago. Women are better represented among biomedical researchers with Ph.D.s rather than MDs. Although the total number of women physicians in all realms and at all levels of medicine has grown significantly, the presence of women at the upper tiers of the profession lags behind women's overall representation in medicine. Women remain strongly clustered in the lower tiers of the profession. Gender equality remains elusive in medicine, but slow progress is occurring in some areas.

Finally, although there is some evidence that the gender gap in income is decreasing over time, the differential remains significant. Historically, research has attributed much if not all of this gap to gender differences in specialties and work effort. Nevertheless, a small but growing recent literature suggests that a large portion of earnings inequalities cannot be attributed to individual choices. We build on this research with independent analyses of three different nationally representative data sources which reveal a significant unexplained disparity in the earnings of male and female physicians.

Gender Segregation of Medical Specialties

Figure 4.1 documents the percentage of each medical specialty made up by women physicians between 1975 and 2005. Variation in women's presence in the profession is clearly evident from these figures. There is only one specialty—pediatrics—with a majority (53 percent) of female practitioners in 2005. At the other end of the spectrum, there are four specialties with fewer than 6 percent female practitioners: neurological, orthopedic, thoracic, and urological surgery. Although the representation of women increased in all medical specialties between 1975 and 2005, the extent of this increase varied widely, from 4.0 percentage points for thoracic surgery to 34.3 percentage points for obstetrics and gynecology, but by 2005 women were more numerous in all medical fields.

There has been substantial continuity over time in the gendered ranking of individual specialties. Let's define "markedly underrepresented" as a field in which the percentage of women represents less than half of their overall presence in the profession. In 2005 women were markedly underrepresented in ten of thirty-seven specialty fields. In 1975 women were markedly underrepresented in the same ten specialties, plus general surgery and occupational medicine. As Figure 4.1 suggests, the fields with persistent underrepresentation of women include all surgical specialties except obstetrics and gynecology and several procedure-intensive medical fields, including cardiovascular disease and gastroenterology. Thus the specialties

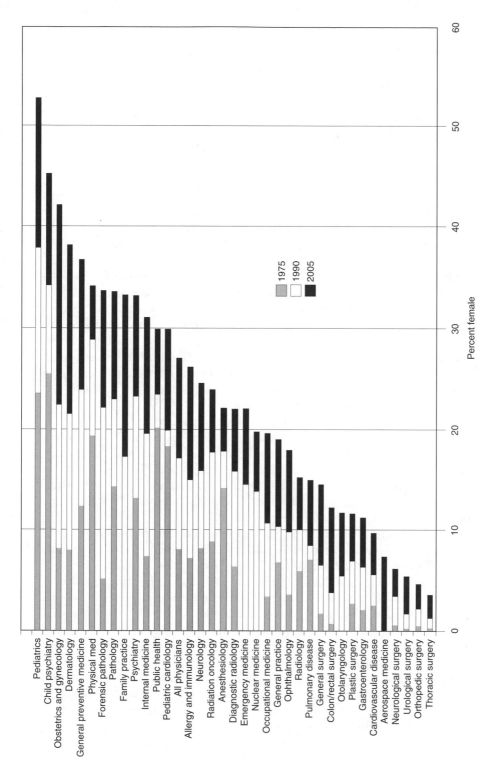

Figure 4.1. Gender Composition of Specialties, 1975–2005. *Source:* American Medical Association, Physician Characteristics and Distribution.

that were male-dominated in the 1970s have remained so, even though in absolute terms there were more women in each of these fields by 2005 than had been the case a generation earlier.

Interestingly, there has been more gender integration in the fields that were disproportionately female in the 1970s. In 1975 women were markedly overrepresented (defined as 50 percent greater representation in a field than in medicine overall) in ten fields, including preventive medicine, psychiatry, anesthesiology, pathology, pediatric cardiology, physical medicine, public health, pediatrics, and child psychiatry. In 2005 women were markedly overrepresented in only three fields: child psychiatry, obstetrics-gynecology, and pediatrics. Thus in terms of specialty, there are relatively few female "ghettos" within the profession. Rather the remaining disparities are more a case of persisting "male bastions" than of emerging "female ghettos."

Although the presence of women in the profession more than tripled between 1975 and 2005, throughout the thirty-year period, women physicians remained consistently underrepresented in about 40 percent of all specialties. At the same time, women remained concentrated in about 60 percent of all specialties, in fields such as pediatrics, child psychiatry, preventive medicine, pathology, and public health. Over time, the fields with fewer women have stayed largely constant. Overall the correlation between women's representation in 1975 and in 2005 is .77 (when calculated across the thirty-seven specialties measured in both years).

Despite this strong pattern of temporal stability, there are specialties that proved to be exceptions. In particular, between 1975 and 2005, internal medicine, forensic pathology, dermatology, and obstetrics and gynecology all feminized more than the medical profession overall. The percentage of women in radiation oncology, diagnostic radiology, and allergy and immunology grew significantly between 1975 and 2005, and all of these fields included relatively few women during the 1970s.

How does gender inequality in 2005 compare to gender inequality at the beginning of women's entry into modern U.S. medicine? To answer this question we calculated the index of dissimilarity across specialties for each year from 1970 through 2005. This index measures the percentage of women or men who would have to change specialty in order for physicians to be distributed equally by gender across specialties. This is a useful measure that can help to reveal the overall trend toward integration or segregation across all of the detailed specialties. Gender segregation by specialty declined between the early 1970s and 2005, although the level has been essentially constant since the late 1980s. In 2005, one quarter of women would have had to change specialties in order to be distributed in the same proportions as men, down from one third in 1970. This index declined to 25 in 1985 and has changed less than one point since that time.[1]

The distribution of men and women across residency programs shows much the same pattern. The overall level of gender segregation for residents closely matches that observed for practicing physicians. Moreover, the trend line remained flat over the most recent ten years for residents, just as it did for practicing physicians. (The index of segregation was 24.4 in 1994 and 24.7 in 2004.) Since we found little forward momentum among either practicing physicians or residents, we can predict that, barring unforeseen developments, current patterns will persist into the future.

Although female physicians continue to pursue distinct medical specialties, their tendency to receive board certification no longer differs significantly from that of their male peers. Data from the AMA Physician Masterfile for 1994 indicate that 67 percent of active female physicians and 73 percent of active male physicians were board certified in at least one specialty. According to the 2004 wave of the Community Tracking Study (CTS) survey of physicians, 86 percent of women and 85 percent of men were board certified in their primary specialty.[2] Thus, at least in the most recent period studied, the slight gender gap in board certification had closed.

Employee and Ownership Status

Gender inequality in medicine is not limited to differences in specialization and board certification. Persistent differences are also evident in the major professional activities of male and female physicians. Data from the AMA Physician Masterfile presented in Figure 4.2 document the percentage of women by major professional activity between 1975 and 2005. The data indicate that in 2005 women remained underrepresented among physician administrators and, since 1990, among physician researchers as well. Women were slightly underrepresented in office-based practice, since they have been consistently overrepresented, relative to their presence in the profession overall, among full-time hospital staff. Because women were disproportionately recent graduates, they were also consistently overrepresented among residents and fellows. Interestingly, evidence increasingly shows that women are more likely than men to enter academic medicine, although they continue to be underrepresented at the highest tiers of the academic medicine hierarchy (Nonnemaker 2000). (We examine the pathways into academic medicine in more detail in chapter 5.)

The clustering of women into specific niches of medicine is not fully portrayed by the data from the AMA Masterfile. Women tend to occupy the lower-status and less well paid patient care positions. U.S. women physicians have also been consistently less likely to have an ownership interest in their practices (Cotter 1986; Collins et al. 1997). Results suggest that the gender gap in ownership is declining, but only because the rate at which male physicians work as employees is increasing. Using data from the American

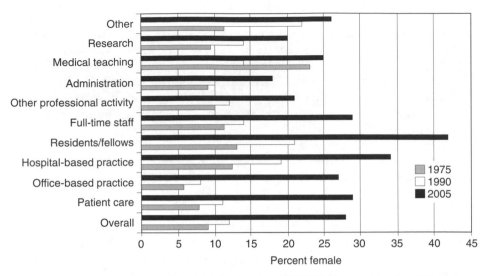

Figure 4.2. Major Professional Activity, by Gender, 1975–2005. *Source:* American Medical Association.

Medical Association, Cotter and colleagues (1986) showed that only 23.5 percent of male physicians were employees in 1985 compared with 45.5 percent of female physicians. Our analysis of the 1996 CTS indicates that 62 percent of female physicians and 38 percent of male physicians had no ownership interest in their physician practice. By the 2004 wave of the CTS, 59 percent of female physicians and 41 percent of male physicians had no ownership interest in their primary physician practice. So between 1985 and 2004 women went from being 1.93 times more likely to work as employees to 1.43 times more likely to work as employees. Unlike the prior era, however, the 1996–2004 period was marked by a significant increase in the percentage of male physician employees and a slight decline in the rate at which women physicians work without an ownership interest.

Patient Attributes and Sources of Compensation

Women physicians see patients from a greater variety of backgrounds than do their male counterparts (see Figure 4.3). Female physicians are more likely than male physicians to see minority patients. Specifically, they are more likely to be in practices where more than one quarter of the patients are black, Hispanic, or Asian. Women physicians see more patients who are on Medicaid than do their male counterparts, but they are less likely to see patients on Medicare. One reason is that Medicaid patients are often children seen by pediatricians, while Medicare patients are typically elderly. After

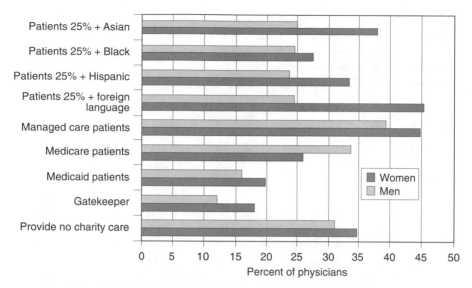

Figure 4.3. Patient Profiles by Gender, 2004. *Source:* 2004 CTS Survey.

the 1997 creation of the State Children's Health Insurance Program (SCHIP) by Congress dramatically improved the access of children to health care, pediatricians saw more poor and minority patients than did physicians in other specialties.[3]

We analyzed the gender gaps in the likelihood of having minority patients. Specialty and practice setting are major factors in influencing the profile of patients a physician sees.[4] Analysis of the 2004 CTS indicates that women physicians are 17 percent more likely than men to have African Americans make up more than 25 percent of their practice. After controlling for the gender gap in personal characteristics such as age and race, we found that the gender gap in the tendency to have more than 25 percent African American patients declined to 7 percent, and after controlling for personal characteristics and specialty, we found that the difference was entirely explained.

Women physicians are also more likely to be in a "gatekeeper" role, which means that patients must receive their permission before seeking specialized services. These differences reflect the specialties that women pursue and the sources of financial reimbursement. Women physicians are more likely than men to practice in managed care settings, although the difference has declined to just a few percentage points.

Women are less likely than their male counterparts to provide charity care. A majority of both male and female physicians provide at least some patient care for free, but this practice is more common for men than for women. This particular finding might seem odd, especially to those who assume that women are more caring than men and less concerned with making money. What this pattern reflects, however, is women's structural location in medicine, since women are more likely to be employees, and employees are less likely to offer their services for free.[5]

Research Positions

Since the early 1990s the representation of women physicians in research positions has declined. Data from the AMA suggest that women's representation improved between 1975 and 1990, but since then these gains have been reversed. According to the AMA, between 1975 and 1990 the number of physicians dedicated to research increased from 7,944 to 16,930, or 113 percent. During the same period, the total number of physicians increased by only 56 percent. And during this time, women also made up a larger percentage of physician researchers than physicians overall.

After 1990, however, the outlook for physician researchers changed dramatically. The overall number of physicians continued to grow, but the total number of physicians dedicated primarily to research declined slightly from 16,930 in 1990 to 14,598 in 2000. In this context of overall decline, the number of female physician researchers fell from 2,856 to 2,700 between 1990 and 2000. Consequently, women's representation in medical research went from parity in 1990 to a 6 percent point deficit in 2000. In other words, in 1990 women were 17 percent of all physicians and 17 percent of medical researchers. By 2000 women were 24 percent of all physicians but only 18 percent of medical researchers. So it has been difficult for women to maintain their representation as the number of medical researchers declined.

Data on research grants corroborate the shift of physicians away from research careers. Between 1978 and 1998 there was no net growth in the number of first-time research grant applications submitted by MDs. From 1994 to 1998 the number of first-time NIH (National Institutes of Health) grant applications submitted by MDs declined by 25 percent. The decline in physician-sponsored research was foreshadowed by declines in medical students' interest in research. During the decade from 1987 to 1997, male and female medical students steadily lost interest in research careers. Guelich and colleagues (2002) report that declines in intent to pursue research careers were steepest at the ten most research-intensive medical schools. The concentration of women in the youngest cohorts may thus in part explain the growing gap between women's presence in medicine overall and women's presence in medical research.

The growing underrepresentation of women among physician researchers needs to be understood in the context of a long-term shift in opportunities for federally funded medical research. In particular, there has been a shift toward research by scientists with Ph.D. degrees and away from research funding for MDs.

Since the late 1960s, Ph.D.s have been applying for NIH funding in far larger numbers than have MDs and have received correspondingly more awards. For example, in 1967, 43 percent of the awarded research project grants went to MDs and MD/Ph.D.s, compared with 53 percent for Ph.D.s. The fraction of awards to MDs fell progressively during the next twenty years to a low of 25 percent in 1987. There was little change in these fractions between 1987 and 1997. Since 1970, the success rates for MDs and Ph.D.s have been virtually identical; that is, MDs have fared as well as Ph.D.s at the hands of NIH study sections and advisory councils when they compete. But physician scientists have become a progressively smaller minority of those seeking and obtaining NIH project support (Rosenberg 1999). Over time, the role of physicians in federally funded medical research has been declining.

There has been growth in women's representation in MD-Ph.D. programs, but even this trend has not kept pace with women's representation in medicine. Prior research indicates that the absolute growth of women in both the NIH-sponsored Medical Scientist Training Program (MSTP) and the Howard Hughes Cloisters Program has been substantial. Between 1980 and 1996 women's representation in the MSTP increased from 16.6 to 29.1 percent (Guelich et al. 2002). Nevertheless, although this growth is significant, it trails women's presence in medical school overall. During the same period women's representation among medical students increased from 25.3 to 41.7 percent (Bickel et al. 2002). Between 1980 and 1996 women's presence in the Howard Hughes–funded Cloisters Program, a program to train medical scientists, increased from 28.7 to 42.1 percent, but this program is much smaller than the NIH-funded MSTP (Guelich et al. 2002).

Participation in a medical scientist training program is not a necessary prerequisite for a career in medical research. Many physicians pursue research without earning a Ph.D. In fact, historically, fewer than one quarter of all physician scientists have participated in medical scientist training, and since enrollment in such training has remained strong, it follows that attrition from medical research is strongest among those without such formal research-related education (Varki and Rosenberg 2002). Nevertheless, students in the medical scientist training programs receive superior mentoring and better formal preparation, and, perhaps most important, accrue less educational debt because of the associated scholarships (Ley and Rosenberg 2002). Therefore they are probably more likely to persist with their research interests than other aspiring physician scientists, at least in part because they are better able to tolerate the relatively reduced salaries that accompany careers in medical research. In any event, the underrepresentation of women in medical scientist training programs contributes to their limited presence in research.

Women's representation among faculty has increased at all ranks between 1994 and 2004 (see Figures 4.4a and b). Overall, women represent 31 percent of clinical science faculty and 28 percent of basic science faculty at medical schools. Their share is lowest among the ranks of full professors, but even here, there were notable increases over the course of the decade from 1994 to 2004. Among the basic sciences, women professors' share grew from 11 to 18 percent while increasing from 8 to 14 percent in the clinical sciences. It is clear from Figures 4.4a and b that women's representation is substantially higher among the nontenured faculty. This pattern will not be fully reflected in the tenured ranks in future years because not all of these faculty members will be promoted, and research indicates that those women who are promoted are promoted more slowly than their male colleagues. This inequality persists even after differences in productivity are acknowledged (Tesch et al, 1995; Wright et al 2003).

Trends in the representation of women among tenured medical school faculty reflects the growth of opportunities in medical schools. Between 1985 and 2004 the number of tenured and tenure-eligible MD clinical faculty increased by 56 percent: from 14,026 in 1985 to 21,921 in 2004. During the same period the number of tenured or tenure-eligible basic science faculty increased from 7,243 to 9,540, or about 31 percent. Thus the growth of women's representation among full professors at U.S. medical schools occurred in the context of overall absolute growth in medical faculty (Bunton and Mallon 2007).

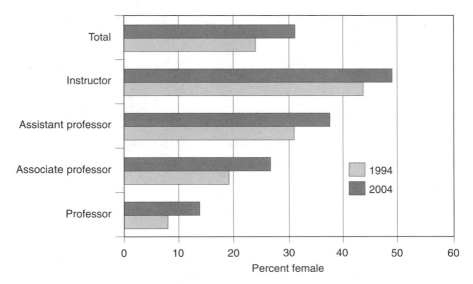

Figure 4.4a. Women's Representation in Medical School Faculty, Clinical Fields, by Rank, 1994–2004. *Source:* American Medical Association.

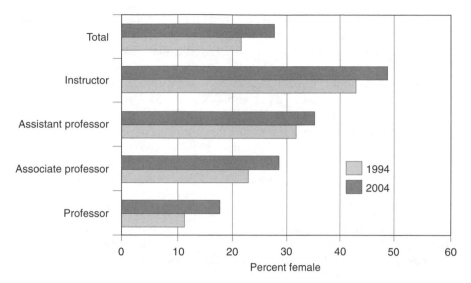

Figure 4.4b. Women's Representation in Medical School Faculty, Basic Sciences, by Rank, 1994–2004. *Source:* American Medical Association.

Although women's presence among physician researchers is declining, women's representation in the population of non-physician biomedical researchers has been growing.

Given the increasing prevalence of Ph.D.s in the community of medical researchers, it is worth briefly considering gender-related trends in this population. Most notably, since the mid-1990s there has been significant growth in the number of biomedical-related life science Ph.D.s, and women account for a sizable portion of this increasing population. Beginning in the 1960s, the number of Ph.D.s awarded annually in the life sciences more than tripled over the next thirty years: 7,696 life science doctorates were awarded by U.S. universities in 1996, compared with 2,095 degrees in 1963. In 1963 fewer than 10 percent of life scientists receiving Ph.D.s were female. By 1996 the fraction was over 40 percent.

Furthermore, women were more likely to be receiving their doctoral degrees from the top universities. Historically the top twenty-six life science graduate programs have awarded over one quarter of all life science Ph.D.s, and these programs award a disproportionate share of Ph.D.s to women (National Research Council 1998). This means that women are well positioned to play central roles in biomedical research.

When the trends in the training backgrounds are compared to trends in the distribution of research funds by gender, the rising role of female Ph.D.s in medical research becomes apparent. Looking at all NIH research grants over the period from 1994 to 2004, we find that the participation of women has increased. In 1994, 20 percent of the awards and 17 percent of the awarded dollars went to female principal investigators. In 2004, 25 percent of the awards and 21 percent of the awarded dollars went to female principal investigators. Finally, the future of research looks bright for women if their representation in postdoctoral fellowship programs is any indication. In 1990 women were 38.3 percent of NIH postdoctoral fellows. In 2005 women were 47.4 percent of NIH postdoctoral fellows.

The funding patterns are reflected in publication of findings. Reviewing trends in six prominent medical journals, Jagsi and colleagues (2006) found that the proportion of articles with women as lead authors increased from 5.9 percent in 1970 to 29.3 percent in 2004. Since women were only 26.6 percent of all physicians in 2004, women physicians are actually overrepresented among lead authors in prominent medical journals. Nevertheless, Jagsi and colleagues emphasize that the distribution of female lead authors is not even across medical journals. The proportion of women lead authors increased most sharply in *Obstetrics and Gynecology* and the *Journal of Pediatrics* and remained low in the *Annals of Surgery*.

Thus the situation of women in biomedical research is somewhat complex and contradictory. Overall there has been progress in women's representation in research, but increasingly this is due to the presence of women with Ph.D.s in the basic sciences rather than MDs.

Women in Positions of Leadership

As with practice ownership and specialization, there have been significant improvements in the number of women physicians in positions of leadership in medicine. In a number of important areas, however, this progress actually trails the growth of women in the profession as a whole. One need only peruse the National Library of Medicine's on-line archive, "Changing the Face of Medicine," to understand the scope of progress that has occurred since the early 1970s. We offer a few highlights from this exhibit.

Women physicians have historically held major leadership positions in governmental health organizations. The National Institutes of Health appointed its first woman institute director, Ruth Kirschstein, in 1972, only a few years after the large-scale growth of U.S. women physicians began. Yet even in public health, the status and power of women physicians has greatly improved. Most notably, in 1990 President George H. W. Bush appointed Dr. Antonia Novello to become the first female surgeon general. The following year he appointed Dr. Bernadine Healy as director of the National Institutes of Health. Since the early 1990s women physicians have maintained a strong presence at the top of many governmental health organizations. President Bill Clinton appointed the second woman, Joycelyn Elders, to be surgeon general in 1993. And in 1994 Dr. Linda Rosenstock was named director of the National Institute for Occupational Safety and Health (NIOSH) in Washington, D.C. A decade later three of the twenty NIH institute directors were women.

Women physicians have also made significant progress in other aspects of medicine. As in government, there is a long history of remarkable female physicians in medical societies, and the recent gains of women have been substantial. The first female president of the Texas Medical Association, Dr. May Owen, was elected in 1960. In 1997 the American Medical Association elected its first female president, Nancy Dickey, and in 2008 Nancy Nielsen followed in her footsteps. The proportion of women in the AMA House of Delegates grew from 5 percent in 1988 to 10 percent in 1994 and 20 percent in 2006.[6]

As expected, women's representation in specialty societies depends on their presence in each field of practice. For example, by 2006, 35 percent of the American Academy of Pediatrics (AAP) chapter presidents were women, 13 percent of committee chairpersons were women, and 34 percent of the AAP section chairpersons were women (AAP Committee on Pediatric Workforce 2006).

There are also signs of growth in the number of female physicians in private administrative positions. According to Barbara Linney of the American College of Physician Executives (ACPE), the total female membership in the ACPE increased from 625 in 1996, when women were 5 percent of members, to 1,125 in 2006, when women were 12 percent of members. Furthermore, a nationally representative survey of physician administrators sponsored by ACPE and conducted by Cejka Search found a 2 percent rise in the number of women physician executives between 2003 and 2005 (Cejka Search 2005).

There has also been significant growth in the number of women leaders within academic medicine. In 2005 women made up 12 of 125, or 9.6 percent, of medical school deans, a considerable increase from the 4.8 percent share they held as recently as 1999 (Magrane et al. 2004). And there are more women among physician administrators as well. Between 1975 and 2000 the number of female physician administrators more than doubled, increasing from 1,020 to 2,310, or 129 percent. The representation of women among physician administrators is also growing. In 2005 women were 18 percent of physician administrators, double the share evident in 1975.

In spite of these trends, however, the number of women in medical leadership has not kept pace with the growth in women physicians overall. As the foregoing discussion indicates, women's presence at the highest levels of AMA leadership, among physician executives, and among public health leaders falls short of women's presence in the medical profession overall (recall that 26 percent of physicians were female in 2004).

Furthermore, the growth in female physician leaders has not been uniform. Mirroring trends in specialization, those women physicians who have pursued administrative careers are more likely to be found in the less prestigious public administration positions. For example, while a national survey of members of the American College of Physician Executives and the Society for Chief Medical Officers conducted in 2000 found that only 7 percent of physician executives were female (Xu et al. 2001), at the same time a survey of the nation's community and migrant health centers found that 41 percent of clinic directors were women (Samuels et al. 1999).[7]

The incomes of female physician administrators reflect their tendency to cluster in the lower tiers of the administrative hierarchy. Research indicates that the incomes of physician executives fall within a huge range. According to the 2005 study by Cejka Search, of the fifteen titles that responded to the 2005 survey, the highest-paid physician executives were medical directors of single-specialty groups, reporting an average yearly income of $340,000, compared to executives working for government-run institutions, who reported incomes of $170,000 (Cejka Search 2005).

The persistent underrepresentation of women among prestigious medical administrators and the clustering of women in public administration is even more understandable when the relatively slow growth of administration is acknowledged. The total number of physician administrators grew from 11,161 in 1975 to 16,210 in 2000, for a 45 percent increase. This compares to a 107 percent increase in the total number of physicians during the same period. Previous research on the professions indicates that administrative positions are prestigious, so competition was probably fierce for these positions (Abbott 1988). Whenever competition is strong, decision makers can maintain social prejudices (Kongar 2006). More recent research on physicians in administration suggests that the corporatization of medicine will lead to increases in the need for physician administrators (Romano 2002; Lyons 2001). If this occurs, we suspect that the representation of women in medical administration will increase significantly, since women's representation in medicine responds to increases in the capacity of the profession.

The clustering of women in less prestigious positions is also evident in organized medicine. On the one hand, in spite of the progress just discussed, women remain relatively underrepresented in the leadership of traditional medical associations. Although the number of female AMA delegates has grown, for example, women's representation in the AMA House of Delegates remains well below the representation of women in the profession overall. Similarly, our earlier discussion demonstrates that even in the American Academy of Pediatrics, the share of women in leadership does not compare to their presence in the specialty.

The skewed distribution of women leaders in organized medicine is echoed in statistics on membership. Women have been consistently underrepresented in the AMA (McDonald 1985), and more recent research suggests that this tendency persists in at least one of the state branches (Williams 1999): although women made up 42 percent of all medical students, they were only 11 percent of the members of the Tennessee Medical Association.

In contrast to medical societies, women are very active in physicians' unions, environmental health organizations, and efforts to promote socialized medicine. For example, there is increasing evidence of women physicians' potential as leaders and administrators in one burgeoning type of physician association—unions. In 1999, women constituted a sizable proportion of physician union membership; 34 percent of the Doctors Council members are female, while only 26 percent of practicing physicians are female. The overrepresentation of women in physicians' unions stems directly from the higher likelihood that women will assume salaried positions and thus be eligible for union membership (Scherzer and Freedman 2000).

Recent literature indicates that women physicians provide highly visible leadership for unions (Scherzer and Freedman 2000). In 2000 the House of Delegates for the Doctors Council, the major physicians' union in the United States, was more than 30 percent female. Similarly, in the same year six of the thirteen members of the executive board of the Council of Interns and Residents were women (Scherzer and Freedman 2000).

Differentiation and Earnings

Given the significant and persistent differences in the positions held by male and female physicians, it is not surprising that significant and persistent gender differences exist in physician earnings. In fact an analysis of the 2000 census suggests that the gender gap in medicine is larger than it is for any other profession: female physicians earn on average 63 percent of what their male colleagues earn (Weinberg 2004).[8]

Until quite recently the debate on the earnings gap in medicine has paralleled the debate on gender differences in other aspects of the profession. Historically, systematic research and the popular press have attributed gender differences in physician earnings to differences in individual choices (Baker 1996; Sasser 2005; Uhlenberg and Cooney 1990), and in particular to differences in how male and female physicians choose their specialties and how they react to marriage and parenting.

Several studies have concluded, however, that even after controlling for work effort, specialty, and other relevant factors, women physicians earn substantially less than their male colleagues. For example, a survey of physicians in hospital positions indicated that women earn less despite similar work schedules and commitments (Hoff 2004). Furthermore, in a nationally representative 1995–96 study of full-time academic medicine faculty, Ash and colleagues (2004) found that female academic physicians earned significantly less than their male counterparts, and that the size of the earnings gap grew over time. The authors discovered that the gap persisted even after professional characteristics were taken into account. Other researchers found that women otolaryngologists earned between and 15 and 20 percent less than their male colleagues even after controlling for professional hours and hours spent in the operating room per week, type of practice, and years since completion of residency (Grandis et al. 2004). A study of family practitioners indicated that both white and black female family physicians earn significantly less than their male peers even after differences in work effort are factored into the analysis (Weeks and Wallace 2006). Data from the Physician Work Life Study, a large, nationally representative survey administered in the mid-1990s, found, even after controlling for age, minority status, specialty, practice type, time in current practice, Medicaid or uninsured status of patients, regional salary variations, ownership status of practice, number of hours worked per week, and proportion of hours spent in hospital-based activities, that female physicians earned about $22,000 less annually than their male colleagues (McMurray et al. 2000).

We supplement the available research in this area with three related analyses. The first takes advantage of the 1996 and 2004 CTS physician surveys to assess how gender difference in professional status relates to the gender gap in earnings. The second uses data from the 1980, 1990, and 2000 censuses to track inequality in earnings in the medical profession. Finally, we draw on data from the Young Physicians Survey in order to examine how marriage and parenting influence incomes in the medical profession.

Table 4.1 presents average earnings estimates from the 2004 CTS by gender and specialty, practice ownership, and practice type. (The income data from this survey pertain to the preceding year, 2003.) Overall, women physicians earned an average of $140,904 and men physicians an average of $199,160 in 2003. Thus women's earnings were 71 percent of their male colleagues.

Several aspects of physicians' practices have distinct influences on the gender gap in earnings. On the one hand, the gap depends greatly on specialization. There is a marked range in average earnings by specialty, with pediatricians earnings the least, $140,716, and surgeons earning the most, $237,514. Thus the concentration of women in pediatrics and other relatively poorly reimbursed fields contributes significantly to the gender gap in earnings.

On the other hand, the estimates presented in Table 4.1 suggest that we cannot entirely attribute the difference to the clustering of women in specific areas. As the table demonstrates, the gender gap in earnings persists even after the data are stratified by specialty. The earnings gap ranges from

Table 4.1. Physicians' Average Income by Gender and Practice Characteristics

	Men	Women	All
Specialty			
Internal Medicine	$158,146	$116,056	$147,944
Family Practice	$157,388	$110,795	$143,710
Pediatrics	$168,596	$111,625	$140,716
Medical Specialties	$211,574	$166,191	$202,532
Surgical Specialties	$243,135	$187,793	$237,514
Psyc	$158,497	$130,034	$148,962
ObG	$218,623	$196,322	$210,822
Total	$199,160	$140,904	
Ownership Status			
	$213,721	$153,741	$202,426
	$178,194	$132,115	$163,085
Medical School, Hospital-Based, and Private Practice			
	$185,888	$131,632	$173,148
	$229,922	$158,905	$215,237
	$198,703	$157,346	$184,153
	$173,410	$118,327	$155,858
	$189,021	$147,703	$177,094

Source: 2004 CTS (note: income data pertain to 2003).

a high in pediatrics, where women earn only 66 percent on average of what men earn, to a low in obstetrics and gynecology, where women earn 89 percent of what men earn.

The gender gap in income also clearly reflects gender differences in ownership. On average, employee physicians or those with no ownership interest in their primary practice earn only 80 percent of what physicians with an ownership interest earn. Thus the overrepresentation of women among employees contributes to the gap between male and female physicians' earnings.

As in the case of specialization, however, gender differences in ownership do not explain the entire gender gap in income. Even stratified by ownership, the income of female employee physicians is on average 72 percent of what male employee physicians earn, and female owners earn an average of 74 percent of what male owners earn.

Differences in male and female earnings also stem from gender differences in practice structure. Table 4.1 shows that average salaries range from a low of $155,858 for physicians based in medical schools to a high of $215,237 for physicians in group practice. Average salaries in HMOs and hospital-based practices fall in the middle. Thus the overrepresentation of women in medical schools and hospital-based practices (11.8 percent of women in the

2004 CTS and 8.5 percent of men in the CTS report a medical school as their primary practice type; 13.7 percent of women and 11.5 percent of men report hospitals as their primary practice type) contributes to the gender gap.

Nevertheless, even after we stratify by practice type, the gender gap in earnings persists. Table 4.1 demonstrates that the gender gap ranges from a high in group practices, where women earn about 68 percent of what men earn, to a low in hospital-based medicine, where women earn about 79 percent of what men earn. The gender gap in earnings in HMOs and medical schools falls in the middle. Women in these types of positions earn about 75 percent of what their male colleagues earn.

We combine these various factors into a single analysis in order to assess their unique contribution to the gender gap in earnings. These results are presented in Appendix Table 1.[9]

Even after controlling for multiple factors including demographic characteristics, specialty, practice ownership, practice structure, and work effort, we find that women physicians continue to earn less than their male colleagues. In 2003 women physicians' annual earnings trailed their male counterparts' by over $21,340. This figure represents the net gap in earnings which persists even after gender differences in specialization and in work effort have been taken into account, the two most common factors affected by women physicians' disproportionate focus on family.

In spite of the persistent gender differences in status, there is some evidence that the gender gap is closing. Based on our parallel analysis of the same CTS sample, the net gender gap in earnings in 1995 was $24,090, which narrowed to $21,340 by 2003. This represents an unexplained differential of 23 percent, down slightly from 28 percent in 1995. So it appears that the gender gap is declining but that the rate of decline is so slow that women will continue to earn significantly less in medicine for the foreseeable future.

Growing Inequality

It is informative to place gender disparities in the context of the overall structure of earnings. Some occupations show a wider disparity in earnings than others. This greater dispersion creates more room for disparities between groups. For example, in some occupations, such as elementary school teaching, earnings tend to be clustered together, and thus there is less room for earnings disparities between groups. There is more disparity in earnings among physicians than is the case among elementary school teachers, and thus there is more opportunity for gender-linked disparities.

Inequality in earnings among physicians has been growing over time. This trend is evident from our analysis of U.S. Census data. Most notably, between 1990 and 2000, the ratio of the ninetieth-percentile earner to the tenth-percentile earner increases from 7.2 to 10.1 for men and from 8.0 to

14.1 for women. The trends between 1980 and 2000 are even more extreme. The ratio of ninetieth-percentile to tenth-percentile earner increases from 4.9 to 10.1 for men and from 7.8 to 14.1 for women.

Growing inequality is also evident among medical specialties. Our analysis of income data from the AMA Socioeconomic Monitoring System suggests that between 1975 and 2000, the ratio of median surgeon income to median physician income increased from 1.20 to 1.37. During the same period, the ratio of median pediatrician income to median physician income declined from 0.84 to 0.71. In other words, the disparity in earnings between the average surgeon and the average pediatrician climbed from 1.43 in 1975 to 1.90 by 2000. This trend implies that while the level of segregation by specialty has remained constant over the last few decades, the financial implications of this segregation have grown.

Growing inequality is typically bad news for the groups at the bottom of the heap. Thus the growth of inequality in the U.S. labor market has presented a challenge to women and minorities, who have to "swim upstream" to overcome this structural change in the labor market (Morris and Western 1999). As noted previously, however, female physicians narrowed the gap in earnings relative to their male counterparts, perhaps in part because of significant absolute growth in the number of women practicing the better-remunerated specialties.

The increase in overall income inequality suggests an increasing bifurcation in the medical profession. Increases in income inequality among physicians stem in part from increasing differences in the earnings of physicians in different medical specialties, and in part from increasing differences in the work effort of physicians.

Explaining Gender Differences in Income and Work

In this section we examine the role of marriage and parenting in contributing to the gender difference in income for physicians. Since the CTS data do not include information on the marriages and families of physicians, we turn to other surveys to address these questions, specifically the 1990 and 1996 Survey of the Practice Patterns of Young Physicians. These data allow us to examine both specialty and family attributes. This analysis indicates a significant unexplained gender difference in earnings regardless of household composition and data source. It also suggests that such differences are most pronounced for physician parents.

In order to identify the percentage of the gender gap attributable to gender differences in specialty and practice environment, we conducted a series of parallel analyses with the Survey of the Practice Patterns of Young Physicians. The analyses focused on employed, non-resident physicians in the 1990 and 1996 versions of this survey. The results are summarized in

Appendix Table 1. Controlling for physician specialty and practice environment explains a substantial additional portion of the gender gap in earnings but does not explain the entire gender gap. (The one exception to this conclusion involves single childless physicians in 1996. We attribute this difference to the small size of this group.)

We find a significant unadjusted gender difference in earnings for physicians in the Survey of Young Physicians. Furthermore, the gender difference remains essentially stable between 1990 and 1996 for physicians in the three marriage and family groups. These data are unique in that they follow the same individuals over time as they grow older.[10] We also find that the gender difference in earnings is most pronounced for married parents. The gender gap in these data is between 1.4 and 2.1 times larger for married parents than for married childless physicians.

The gender gap for parents remains relatively constant over time as these individuals move through their life cycle. For married parents, age and weekly work hours explain 26 percent of the gender difference in 1990 and 23 percent of the gender difference in 1996. We find that controlling for specialty and practice location, in addition to age and work hours, enables us to explain 44.3 percent of the gender gap in 1990 and 38.2 percent of the gender gap in 1996. Thus among married parents, specialty and practice environment explain an additional 18.8 and 15.5 percent of the gender gap in logged earnings. It is important to emphasize that, while specialty and practice location increase our understanding of the gender gap, they do not fully explain it for married parents.

The results presented in this chapter suggest that the significant influx of women into medicine has been accompanied by a modest decline in the gender gap among physicians in some areas along with persisting and even growing gender gaps in others. There was a modest decline in the gender segregation of specialties through 1985, but the level of segregation by specialty has remained constant since then. Women physicians are more likely to see poorer patients, and are more likely to treat members of racial and ethnic minority groups.

While women have made some progress in the ranks of academic faculty, they have fallen behind in leadership positions relative to the overall increase of women in the profession. The situation for women in research is more complex. The representation of women physicians is lagging in research, but that is principally due to the shift in research support toward scientists with Ph.D. degrees. The trends for women Ph.D.s in the biomedical research fields in terms of postdoctoral fellowships, research positions, funding, and publication have been positive. Among physicians, the gender gap in earnings is substantial, and has narrowed only slightly in recent years. The growing degree of inequality within the profession has contributed to the persistence of the gender gap. We find that the usual suspects—specialty, age, work effort, ownership, practice structure, revenue source, and other such factors—contribute to but do not fully explain the gender disparities in earnings. We now turn from this overview of disparities to an appraisal of the causes of these gender differences.

5

Gender, Sorting, and Tracking

In the previous chapter we offered a detailed portrait of women's place in the medical profession. It is clear that women are not distributed equally across all segments of medical work. They continue to cluster disproportionately in the lower tiers of the medical hierarchy. There has been significant absolute growth in the number of women at all levels and in all facets of American medicine. While women's distribution across specialties has become slightly more even, the numbers of women in research and in leadership positions have not kept pace with the growing numbers of women physicians overall.

In this chapter we consider why women physicians continue to occupy a disadvantaged place in the medical profession. The focus here is on professional experiences; the next chapter examines how changes in the personal lives of women physicians have contributed to gender differences in the profession. While the distinctive goals and priorities of female physicians have affected their status, independent structural changes and external social pressures have also played a significant role in creating and maintaining the unique place that female physicians occupy in the profession. As in the case of women's entry into the profession overall, individual choices do not fully explain women's place in U.S. medicine.

Our analysis focuses principally on the allocation of women and men across specialties, as in chapter 4. Practice ownership, research and faculty positions, and access to leadership roles are also considered.

We examine the historical roots of gendered specialization. Given the historical continuities in specialties documented in chapter 4, understanding the historical foundations of these choices will help us understand the current landscape. In a number of cases, specialties do not really match the gender stereotypes often held about these fields. Specialties have also changed over time with respect to such key issues as the growth of employment opportunities and changes in work schedules. We discuss the relative contributions of individual preferences and gendered experiences during medical school, as well as patients' desires and expectations. Historical material, survey data on medical students, and qualitative interviews with women physicians at various stages of their careers help to shed light on these issues.

Like segregation by specialty, women's place in medical research is something we attribute largely, but not entirely, to discriminatory pressures and independent structural change. Women in medical school have fewer research experiences than men and receive less research-related mentoring. And women are concentrated in specialties with fewer research opportunities. Furthermore, over time, the role played by physicians in medical research appears to be declining relative to that of researchers with doctoral degrees in the biomedical sciences.

The status of women physicians in leadership and administration can also be traced to independent structural changes. In particular, the appointment of several women leaders during the 1990s resulted from the independent grass-roots effort to promote research on women's health. In a similar light, the limited growth of medical administration positions and the slow turnover in these positions also contributed to the relatively slow increase in the number of female physician administrators. Finally, much of the gender gap in academic leadership reflects the results of discrimination, although gender differences in aspirations may also contribute. We suggest that similar processes may influence women's access to positions in medical administration as well.

The Historical Roots of Gendered Specialties

Why did women physicians initially cluster in distinct specialties, and why has that gender segregation by specialty persisted? Given that the gendered nature of specialties tends to remain stable over time, digging into the historical causes of these differences should be informative.

As we noted earlier, much of the available research suggests that the persistence of gender differences in specialization is primarily attributable to gender differences in priorities and interests. More specifically, research during the 1990s suggests that the disproportionate tendency for women to seek out fields offering controllable lifestyles explains much if not most of the persistent gender segregation by specialty within medicine (Redman et al. 1994; Xu et al. 1995; McFarland and Rhoades 1998; Baxter et al. 1996). Researchers have also found a relationship between gender differences in the motivation to study medicine and gender differences in specialization. The idea here is that women gravitate toward primary care because of their disproportionate interest in helping people and their relative lack of interest in financial remuneration and medical technology (Schubot et al. 1996).

While women and men have distinct priorities surrounding work and family, and such priorities do influence career choices, these personal choices do not fully account for the large and persistent gender differences in medical specialization. In fact, they may well play a smaller role than is commonly believed.

One of the major limitations with the work and family explanation of gender segregation in medicine is that it does not explain gender differences in specialization during the initial phases of women's entry into medicine. In the 1970s these differences in specialization could not have stemmed primarily from differences in the desire for a controllable lifestyle, since the differences in work schedules across specialties then were quite modest. Table 5.1 documents the average time spent in patient care for physicians by specialty in selected years from 1974 to 2001. We see, for example, that in 1974 surgeons worked only two hours more per week than pediatricians (46.3 and 44.2 hours, respectively). This small difference is unlikely to explain the concentration of women in pediatrics and men in surgery.

Psychiatry (37.3 hours) is the obvious outlier in Table 5.1, but this only adds support for our argument. If the disproportionate desire for controllable work schedules drove the specialty choices of female physicians of this era, then psychiatry would have been the most female-dominated field in the mid-1970s. Data presented in chapter 4, however, show that in 1975, 23.4 percent of pediatricians were female, as opposed to only 13.1 percent of psychiatrists. So psychiatry, the field with the most controllable hours, was

Table 5.1. Length of Workweek by Specialty, 1974–2001 (Mean Number of Hours in Patient Care Activities)

Speciality	1974	1978	1984	1999	2001
GP/FP	45.5	49	53.5	50.6	50.7
IM	46.2	49.2	53.1	54.2	56.2
Surgery	46.3	48.9	51.3	55.6	55.9
Peds	44.2	46.1	50.7	49.5	49.4
ObG	48.1	51.6	54.1	59	55.7
Radiology	41.4	41.9	50.5	56.2	59.3
Psyc	37.3	41	44.6	42.3	44
Anesthesia	44.7	47.2	54.4	53.5	58.7
All MD	44.5	47.5	51	51.6	52.8

Note: Ophthalmologists were removed from 1999 surgery estimate.
Source: AMA Socioeconomic Monitoring System.

significantly less female-dominated than pediatrics in the initial phase of women's entry into medicine.

Table 5.1 reveals that over time the range in work effort across specialties has been expanding. Doctors in all specialties are putting in longer work-weeks than they did in the 1970s, with the overall time spent in patient care increasing by more than eight hours per week. Pediatricians in 2001 worked 49.4 hours per week on average but still trailed surgeons by more than six hours per week. Thus the link between specialty and work schedules has grown over time, and the requirements of the most demanding specialties have increased.

It should be noted that the gender gap in the workweek was larger in the 1970s than it is today. Specifically, women worked 42.4 hours on average, compared to 51.7 hours for men. Nevertheless, we question the link between the gender gap in working time and specialty choice during this era because the difference in demands across specialties was quite modest. Since the evidence does not support this reasoning, there must be alternative explanations for the gender gap during the initial stages of women's entry into medicine.

We suggest that gender differences in specialty choice during the 1970s resulted primarily from: (1) gender stereotypes among faculty and students, (2) women students' attempts to avoid conflict and harassment and to seek out social support, (3) biases in the process by which residency candidates were selected, (4) gender differences in academic experiences, (5) differences in the growth rate of particular medical specialties, and (6) a historical legacy of women physicians specializing in the care of children as a way of combating overt prejudice in other aspects of the profession. In other words, the initial clustering of women physicians into distinct specialties occurred primarily as a result of discrimination or its sequelae and secondarily from the different facets of medicine that most attract male and female students.

Research conducted during the 1970s often suggested that both students and faculty had preconceived notions about the fit of personalities and the demands of certain medical specialties (Ducker 1978; Fishman and Zimet 1972). For example, surgeons were thought to be aggressive and unemotional, and pediatricians were thought to be empathetic and collegial (Lorber 1984, 32).

It was also suggested that women physicians were especially likely to have characteristics that made certain specialties, such as pediatrics and psychiatry, particularly appropriate for them. Like all stereotypes, these gendered assumptions emphasized certain attributes of medical specialties and deemphasized others with a different gender valence. There were, and still are, valid arguments for supporting and for discouraging women in all medical specialties. For example, although some physicians might argue that women do not have the physical stamina to do surgery, others offer the counterargument that women have greater and more precise manual dexterity because their hands are usually smaller (O'Connell 2001, 37) and because they are disproportionately exposed to needlework activities as children. During an interview, one very accomplished female surgeon recounted proudly how she had made a quilt out of her son's sports jerseys, and then added, "It was easy. I've always been good at sewing."

Although it is hard to quantify the subtle social pressures experienced by women in the initial phases of integration, current research has shown that students generally enter medical school without a firm commitment to a specific field. Research has repeatedly shown that most students select their specialty during medical school. Many enter without a clear specialty preference, and most who do enter with a preference ultimately change it (Kassebaum and Szenas 1995; Babbott et al. 1988). Further, together the association between role models and specialty choice (Wright et al. 1997) and evidence that male medical students are more likely to encounter encouragement to pursue a career in surgery (Mayer et al., 2001; Dresler et al., 1996) suggest that medical school experiences play a significant role in determining students' specialty choice and segregating students by gender.

Even students who signal interest in a specific field normally demonstrate a willingness to alter their preferences. Research during the 1980s found that the most frequently cited difficulties in choosing a specialty experienced by first-, second-, and third-year medical students included lack of specialty information, equal appeal of several specialties, diverse interests, lack of decisional support, unknown interests, and unidentified personal abilities (Savickas et al. 1986). Under conditions of uncertainty, people tend to rely disproportionately on preconceived stereotypes (Balsa et al. 2003) and to be more receptive to and less critical of external advice. Thus both women and men medical students of the 1970s were probably very vulnerable to social pressures to pursue gender-appropriate careers.

Prior studies suggest that gendered stereotypes surrounding the various medical specialties exerted a powerful force on women in the initial wave of integration (Lorber 1984, 32). Frances Conley summarizes this phenomenon in her book *Walking Out on the Boys:* "The message heard by us women was that only a certain few disciplines were open to us and that we should not expect a built-in support system. Dedicated career counselors steadfastly maneuvered us into pediatrics, psychiatry, pathology, general internal medicine and family practice. My female classmates all complied" (Conley 1998, 24).

Some survey research from the 1970s and early 1980s also demonstrates a disconnect between the preferences of women students and their ultimate specialty choices which does not match trends among men. One study showed that only a slightly greater percentage of women preferred pediatrics compared to men but over twice as many women entered pediatrics.

Almost the same percentage of men who preferred family practice chose it, but women chose this specialty nearly twice as often as they expressed interest in it (Matteson and Smith 1977). These differences corroborate Dr. Conley's interpretation of her experiences during medical school. Something guided the women medical students disproportionately into primary care. That "something" was probably the gendered ideas of faculty and counselors.

But women medical students often encountered more than the subtle pressures associated with stereotypes. Historical reports indicate that gender discrimination and sexual harassment of women medical trainees was common in the 1970s (Walsh 1977). And more recent surveys suggest that it has remained very frequent. For example, a 1997 study of senior medical students at fourteen medical schools indicates that 83 percent of women and 41 percent of men experienced sexual harassment or gender discrimination during their undergraduate medical education (Nora et al. 2002). If this harassment were evenly distributed across the profession, then its presence would not influence specialty choice. But research suggests a different reality. This study and others have consistently indicated a specialty hierarchy surrounding harassment of female physicians and medical trainees. In particular, general surgery is associated with higher levels of harassment than other specialties (Nora et al. 2002; Frank et al. 1998). And survey research indicates that exposure to gender discrimination and sexual harassment during undergraduate education may influence some medical students' choice of specialty and, to a lesser degree, ranking of residency programs (Stratton et al. 2005).

It is hard to know with certainty what students mean when they say that they have experienced gender discrimination or sexual harassment. Research in this area suggests that such experiences take fundamentally different forms for men and women students. Men primarily complain about being denied access to hands-on educational experiences during pediatrics and obstetrics and gynecology clerkships. For women, they are more likely to involve sexual overtures, offensive or sexually explicit remarks, or inappropriate touching (Witte et al. 2006). A female physician we interviewed who graduated in 1989 reflects on her experiences:

> I really didn't have a clue. I think I was immature. I was mature for the average 20-year-old but too immature to be in medical school. So a lot of shit I took not getting that I should have spoken up. But it really didn't feel safe. There weren't a lot of channels so it wasn't at all uncommon to have your boob grabbed in surgery.... The men got abused too. It was just, I felt, more humiliating as a woman because there was more sexual stuff. They used to line you up at the beginning of the ortho rotation and give you each a humiliating nickname and refer to you by that name during the rotation.... My name was chesty.

It should be noted that the existing research on the relationship between academic experiences and specialty choice is very limited. Our research on Thomas Jefferson University medical school students indicates that gender segregation increases during medical school, a pattern not evident in one Australian study (Redman et al. 1994). A more recent study based on a multi-school survey indicates, however, that exposure to gender discrimination and sexual harassment during undergraduate education may influence some American medical students' choice of specialty (Stratton et al. 2005).

It is not simply personal experience with sexual harassment that affects the choices of female medical students. Women students who are considering a specialty are usually in the process of completing their clinical rotations, so they are often able to witness the types of treatment that adult female attending physicians in specific fields must confront. The following comment posted on the Student Doctor Web site illustrates this idea:

> First off, let me just say that this is only my experience. Older men are often not PC. It is pretty common for them to make sexual comments directed toward the younger women. I was following a female urologist around and she was constantly being pestered by the older men. After one of the exams, one guy said to the woman "after that exam I feel like we should go outside and have a smoke." In the same day another guy asked her if she wanted to join him for a bath and said they should exchange numbers. Of course, both of the men were joking but the lady was as red as a beet. So, if a woman cannot let a constant barrage of comments like that roll off her shoulder, it [urology] probably isn't the right field to go into. (posted July 15, 2006, by "flip a coin")

Research from the Women Physicians Health Study indicates that sexual harassment is not confined to medical trainees. Practicing physicians routinely experience such treatment, and it is most common in the male-dominated fields (Frank et al. 1998).

A second indirect manifestation of harassment involves disparaging treatment of racial and ethnic minorities. In this instance, minority women would endure the harassment directly, but all women could view the behavior and interpret it as evidence of a hostile work environment. One woman surgeon who trained during the 1980s recalled how an attending brushed against her inappropriately when she was a resident performing surgery. The attending then commented that it was the first time he had touched a Puerto Rican without getting AIDS. Although this particular woman was clearly the target of the offensive comment, it is probable that other students witnessed the harassment and potentially used this evidence when electing a specialty.

Research during the 1970s suggests that gendered social pressures and overt sexual harassment were not the only explanations for the initial clustering of women in certain specialties. Researchers of the era also hypothesized that segregation developed because of women physicians' need for acceptance. It was thought that women students chose fields where women physicians already practiced and avoided male-dominated fields in order to feel socially comfortable (Quadagno 1976). This process went beyond the wish to avoid blatant discrimination and harassment. It involved the desire to be welcomed into a community and the sense that women are not welcomed into male-dominated environments.

On the one hand, the desire for acceptance inevitably led the women of the 1970s toward pediatrics because, prior to this point, American women physicians had historically clustered in this specialty. In the first half of the twentieth century, women physicians combated discrimination by embracing traditional gender differences. They argued that they were uniquely suited for pediatrics because of the female capacity to nurture, and they often focused their efforts on caring for the poor and disenfranchised and on providing public health outreach and education, as well as support services such as milk dispensaries (Riska 2001, 41; see also More 1999). Along with well-to-do women, female physicians campaigned for public support of such efforts and helped to bring about passage of the Sheppard Towner Act in the 1920s, which provided matching funds to states that created maternal and child health bureaus and provided outreach services. These efforts did not initially threaten male-dominated organized medicine and were thus allowed to flourish. During those years, the period More refers to as that of "maternalist medicine," women physicians cemented an identity as pediatricians. Women remained clustered in pediatrics throughout the mid-twentieth century, and so female medical students were most apt to find suitable role models in this field.

On the other hand, women who joined residency programs consisting of a majority of men found it harder to fit into the group, formally and informally. Women in such situations are often excluded from male-dominated socializing, since men are more likely to socialize with male colleagues after work, when these informal information-swapping sessions occur. When women are excluded from this vital interpersonal interaction, they are left without advice and social support that can make their transition into the work setting easier (O'Connell 2001, 44). The experiences of one woman participant in the MomMD Web site reflect this phenomenon:

> There was certainly a boys' club when I was in my fellowship in pain management—golf outings, nights out, stock trading tip sessions to which I was not invited. My case numbers were 50 percent of my male peers. The program director would not help. It was very frustrating. I completed the fellowship and stayed on as staff, but saw that I had no future. (Incidentally, I saw another female fellow after me having an even worse time than I had—she chose to go head-to-head with other fellows.... The following

year, no female fellows were admitted to the program.) I did leave and now
have a plum job which is incredibly rewarding. (posted February 10, 2003,
by Janet, an unregistered member)

A related experience is relayed by a student speaking about her efforts to
conduct and present medical research:

> I went to a neurosurgery conference—There was 1 woman neurosurgeon in
> the room, and me (F med student). The rest of the room was full of men. I
> was with a male med student. Who they chatted up. Me, not so much. It re-
> ally sucked. (posted to the Student Doctor Network Web site, June 22, 2006,
> by megalin)

In the 1970s and 1980s each specialty was strongly associated with a specific culture, and to a large extent those cultures persist today. In particular,
surgery has been the focus of a number of studies, all of which highlight its
traditionally masculine culture (Fox 1992; Pringle 1998; Katz 1999; Cassell
2000; Riska 2001, 92). The experience of one woman emergency medicine
physician who graduated in 1980 summarizes this situation. She told us:

> Surgery has always had a culture that was different than the rest of medicine
> that is…for lack of a better way to put it, macho-ism. It was something that
> I did [as a medical student] but had absolutely no interest in doing as a ca-
> reer. It is all about NEVER exposing the human caring side of you and doing
> procedures and getting the job done no matter what it takes. There was just
> no soft side to surgery back then and I still don't see much of it.…[Pediatri-
> cians are] just kinder and gentler. They are still ambitious but everything is
> cloaked in nicey nicey.…It translates into a more pleasant atmosphere.

In a similar vein, a woman who graduated from medical school in 1989
recalled how she chose her specialty: "It was really hard for me to choose. I
liked everything that I did except surgery, mostly because I found it so sexist that I found it difficult to bear. So I was torn between primary care and
rehab medicine."

Some quantitative research from the 1980s supports the link between social comfort and gender segregation by specialty. Weisman (1984) found
that female medical students who attended schools with more women
were more likely to select female-dominated fields, the idea being that such
women had a better understanding of the relief that social homogeneity
can provide because they trained in environments that were more gender
balanced. The social pressures on women to choose specific fields thus tran-
scend the behaviors of specific individuals.

The desire for social comfort should be especially strong among both female and male medical students selecting a specialty because of the routine
harassment that has long been a central component of medical training.

For example, a 1988 study found that 96.5 percent of all senior medical students reported experiencing some form of harassment, with public humiliation being the most common manifestation of inappropriate treatment (Baldwin et al. 1991). Although there appears to have been a decline in the overall frequency of medical student harassment, it remains a very common phenomenon. A multi-site study in 2003 found that 42 percent of students still experienced some form of harassment or belittlement during medical school (Frank et al. 2006).[1] Regardless of gender, people in such stressful situations would naturally seek emotional, social, and practical support from peers.

Anecdotal reports suggest that there really is strength in numbers. One graduate of an obstetrics residency program recounted that the women residents kept a steady supply of birth control pills, maxi pads, and Prozac pills in the call rooms. The environment was inevitably more "female" as a result of the critical mass of women residents. The remaining male residents simply had to cope with the changes. Harassment nevertheless endured even in this female environment. The same physician reported that the male chief resident, one of a handful in the program, would announce loudly that he was planning to make the call schedule the following evening and then ask if anyone would like to join him in the call room, thus insinuating that those who provided sex would be given fewer call-related responsibilities.

In addition, it is thought that women applicants to male-dominated residency programs have been persistently passed over because of the preference of male residency program directors for students like themselves, and because of a lack of reliable objective measures of residency applicants' potential (O'Connell 2001). One residency program director described the application process as follows:

> People are accepted into residency programs because they fit into the program for one reason or another, not because they're really better than someone who was not taken. He may even not be as good a candidate, but was taken because that is the type of person the program wanted, be it personality, or be it background, whatever is more important, whatever plays a greater role (O'Connell 2001)

If such discrimination still exists today, then it is likely to have been even more pronounced during the initial phases of women's entry into the profession. This subtle discrimination may account for the fact that women have historically had lower odds of acceptance into surgical residency programs (Iverson 1996).

Of course, the prejudice that women encounter when they seek admission to male-dominated residencies and fellowships may involve more than a simple desire on the part of directors to promote social homogeneity. It may involve an active dislike of women students. One woman surgeon who trained during the 1980s recalled how several of her attending supervisors would hold morning rounds in the men's bathroom and force her to enter. She was the only woman resident at the time. It is reasonable to believe that these men were not especially cordial to women seeking entry into their program. In a similar light, in the 2003 edition of *Forgive and Remember*, his study of a surgical training program, Charles Bosk admits that one of the residents who was not asked to continue training was the only woman in the program. He then suggests that the debate over this resident's progress and the decision to dismiss her was prejudicial:

> I look at the text [of the earlier edition of his book] and wonder how I could have left gender out. A good many of the points feminists make about male domination are present in the brief vignette [describing the discussion about whether to promote or dismiss her]: Dr. Jones is placed in the sick role and seen as a candidate for psychiatric care. ("She's totally out to lunch," "around the bend.") One physician even suggests, somewhat illogically since there had been no progression of symptoms, that "maybe she has a tumor." (Bosk 2003, 221)

Here again, it is hard to believe that the male attendings who so willingly labeled their troubled female resident as crazy were actively supportive of women seeking admission to their program.[2]

A final, and potentially most powerful, explanation for the initial gender differences in specialization stems from the manner in which medicine as a whole expanded. We noted in earlier chapters than one of the major reasons why women succeeded in entering medicine in the 1970s had to do with the dramatic increase in the capacity of U.S. medical schools. While all medical schools in the country theoretically offer a uniform education that prepares students for the full gamut of graduate-level medical training, medical education at the graduate level did not expand uniformly. In fact, data from the Association of American Medical Colleges on residency training indicates that residency openings in the fields that most attracted women increased at significantly higher rates than in the fields that persistently exclude women.

Figure 5.1 documents enrollment in pediatric and surgical residencies by gender and year from the late 1970s to 2004. It shows that the huge influx of women in pediatrics was accommodated almost entirely by a dramatic expansion in the availability of pediatric residency positions. In fact, between 1978 and 1998 the number of male pediatric residents declined only 10.5 percent, or by 328 individuals. At the same time, the number of female pediatric residents grew by 2,725, or 124 percent. In contrast, women entering surgery did so almost exclusively by "taking" a spot from a potential male surgical trainee. Between 1978 and 1998, the number of male surgical residents declined by 934 while the number of female surgical residents

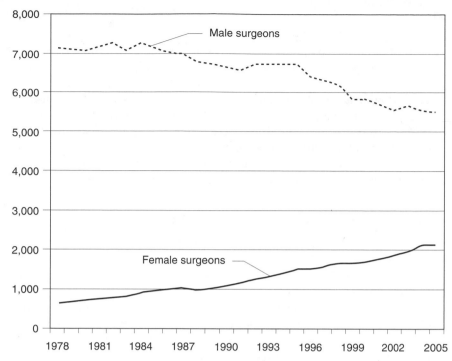

Figure 5.1a. Surgery Residents, by Gender, 1978–2005. *Source:* AMA Socioeconomic Monitoring System.

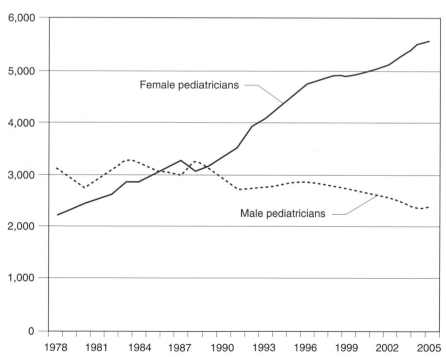

Figure 5.1b. Pediatric Residents, by Gender, 1978–2005. *Source:* AMA Socioeconomic Monitoring System.

grew by 1,001. The expansion of pediatrics over that period may have contributed to its more accepting and welcoming environment.

Thus women's desire for more controllable work schedules does not appear to provide a complete explanation for the initial gender differences in specialization. Instead we attribute these early differences to gender stereotypes, discrimination, and differences in the rate at which specific fields expanded. In other words, women gravitated toward fields such as pediatrics because they were most frequently encouraged and reinforced in these areas and because these areas could most easily accommodate them.

Contemporary Gender Segregation by Specialty

Does the research from the 1970s, 1980s, and 1990s continue to be relevant today? We have seen the continuity in the gender typing of specialties, with women clustering disproportionately in primary care, psychiatry, and a few other fields. Why do these patterns exist?

There are continuities in the culture and reputation of specialties that contribute to their enduring gender disparities. Specialties tend to be self-reproducing social organizations, and thus continuity over time is to be expected. One of the major reasons for the persistence of segregation involves momentum. Women initially entered specific fields primarily because of disproportionate social pressures. As a result, there are more female role models in those fields, who in turn helped to recruit more women.

A second reason for the persistence of segregation involves the ongoing gendered culture within medicine. Earlier we reviewed research from the 1970s which found a relationship between women's specialty choices and beliefs about the personalities best suited for specific fields. More recent research suggests that many of the gendered beliefs about medical work persist. For example, in a study of medical residents drawing on qualitative interviews, Hinze (1999) found that the high-prestige specialties are associated with active, interventionist hands and "balls," body parts that, arguably, are not gender neutral. Women continue to be discouraged from entering fields that are so strongly associated with masculine physical attributes and style of practice.

A third reason involves the persistent lack of objectivity in admissions to residency programs. Earlier we reviewed research which indicates that residency programs actively seek out students who will "fit in" with a prevailing culture. Since certain fields remain disproportionately male, women continue to confront subtle barriers to acceptance if they must "fit in" with a predominantly male culture. Also, although many observers believe that prejudices about women's stamina or capacity to succeed in male-dominated medical fields has declined, some programs still avoid female candidates for fear that they will become pregnant and seek maternity-related leave and benefits. The experience of Priya Krishna during her interviews for an otolaryngology residency demonstrates these types of concerns:

> "How many siblings do you have?" The interviewer asked, innocently enough.
> "None," I replied, not knowing where this line of questioning would lead.
> "Was that lonely growing up as an only child?"
> "Yes, I would have loved to have siblings, at least two or three."
> "So you probably want to have at least a few children to prevent them from having your own fate?"
> I answered enthusiastically with a big smile on my face, "Oh yes definitely."
> "Hmm...ok." The interviewer scribbled something in his file.
> My heart sank. I had succumbed to his well disguised illegal question.
> The rest of the interview was a blur for me and likely meaningless for him.
> (Chin 2002, 231)

Although discrimination against aspiring women residents is hard to quantify, it is clear that most residency programs are not prepared to support a pregnant resident, or any other resident with pressing family issues, and that there is every reason to believe that pressure exists on program directors to minimize such scenarios.[3] In fact, a 1994 survey of plastic surgery residents found that 36 percent of program directors actively discouraged pregnancy during residency (Van Diss 2004). This issue is examined in more detail in chapter 8.

A fourth reason for the persistence of segregation by specialty involves the inflexible structure of some of the more male-dominated specialty training programs. As we have seen, women are significantly more likely to withdraw from selective and demanding residency programs such as surgery or obstetrics and gynecology. Those women who withdraw do so most often because they feel that the demands of their training do not enable them to attend to their spouse's or children's needs (Bergen et al. 1998; Jancin 2002; O'Connell 2001). Research suggests that those women who do not withdraw to care for children usually leave their training in order to relocate for a spouse's job. Men who withdraw, in contrast, do so primarily in order to change specialties. Thus advocates of the "choice" perspective would cite this research as support for their theory. It appears that women are "electing" to avoid certain demanding specialties because they do not allow for controllable work schedules.

Discussions from the MomMD and Student Doctor Network Web sites often involve individual reflections about avoiding surgery in favor of more family-friendly medical specialties:

> I am so sorry that your experience has been so awful. I am now a practicing pediatrician...but as a former competitive athlete, I too had an interest

in ortho. I have always been used to competing against guys. But as my thoughts went to having children and family, I decided the surgical life was not for me. I got tired of busting the guys' XOXO. Besides, my mentality of compassion did not match the "cut and move on" mentality. (posted February 3, 2003, by rugrat)

Similarly, one woman answered others' questions about the potential to study orthopedics while having a family:

Orthopaedic residency is demanding and it's usually during the time in women's lives when they want to have children (mid 20's to early 30's)...if you can delay having kids until after your residency it would make your life much easier....Now there are other specialties with demanding residencies like general surgery, neurosurgery that pose the same problems for women who want to have families. Orthopaedic residencies FROWN UPON maternity leave and pregnant residents. If you decide to get pregnant during your residency, expect a backlash and quite a bit of hostility from your fellow residents and attendings. Residency is tough enough as it is....I for one do not want to pick up someone else's slack because they're pregnant or on maternity leave. Orthopaedics is not like other specialties where pregnant residents are acceptable. So keep this in mind. (posted December 2005 by asdf123)

So at least some women consider and reject male-dominated fields because they do not allow them to balance work and family. Indeed, the increased time demands of male-dominated specialties such as surgery, noted earlier, may be giving this old argument renewed credence.

We used data from the AMA patient care survey and the AMA Masterfile to assess the relationship between the percentage of women in a specialty and the average hours worked by individuals in that field. The correlation (Pearson r) between the percentage of women in a field and the average hours in professional activity for that field was −0.31 in 1989 and −0.43 in 1999.Therefore the evidence indicates that women cluster in fields with shorter average workweeks, and this relationship appears to be growing stronger over time.

Another way of approaching the issue of working time is that some specialties allow for greater flexibility in hours than do others. According to the 2004 CTS physician survey, female surgeons worked 96 percent as many hours as male surgeons. In contrast, female pediatricians work only 86 percent as many hours as male pediatricians. Thus there is more room for working a forty-hour-per-week schedule in pediatrics than there is in surgery. Nonetheless, part-time opportunities remain limited, a topic examined in more detail in chapter 8.

There may be a self-reinforcing aspect to this relationship. That is, women are selecting fields with lower average work hours, and then, as their presence in the field grows, average work hours decline further because, regardless of their specialty, women seek out more controllable work arrangements. But the modest correlation estimate suggests that the story is not entirely about women flocking to fields with more controllable lifestyles. The percentage of women in a field explained only .43 squared, or 18 percent, of the variance in work effort by specialty.

In other words, the disproportionate attraction of controllable work hours does not explain the entire gender gap in specialization. Similarly, data from the AMA socioeconomic monitoring system suggest that in 1999, the average neurologist spent 53.5 hours in professional work and the average pediatrician spent 54 hours. Nonetheless, women made up 49.6 percent of pediatricians but only 22.0 percent of neurologists.

In fact, research suggests that medical students are aware of how much physicians in various specialties work, and they generally do not view primary care specialties as affording a controllable lifestyle. These specialties are classified as offering either an uncontrollable or an intermediate lifestyle (Newton et al. 2005; Schwartz et al. 1989). Moreover, increases in the popularity of so-called controllable-lifestyle specialties such as dermatology, emergency medicine, and psychiatry have been driven by nearly equivalent changes in male and female preferences (Dorsey et al. 2005). To put these results another way, interest in primary care and psychiatry has been declining in recent years, but since it is declining at an equivalent rate among both men and women medical students, women continue to be overrepresented in both fields.

Another set of considerations has to do with constraints in the training process, as opposed to the actual experience of working in different specialty settings. The structure of medical training in the United States may be contributing to this gender gap in attrition. As a result, women medical students electing a specialty do not have as many choices as the choice advocates suggest.

The first problem involves the difficulty that resident physicians face if they wish to move geographically. Since the number of residency spots in a program is largely fixed, residents who seek to transfer into another program must find programs that have lost student physicians and are seeking to fill them. Although attrition occurs, it does not occur on a regular basis, nor does it occur evenly throughout the country, so residents usually do not have the option of transferring into another program. The fixed nature of residency training differs dramatically from the highly flexible nature of advanced graduate-level training. Students often complete dissertations away from the institution that ultimately grants them a degree.

The inflexible nature of residency training is not essential to the education of graduate-level student physicians. It is merely a byproduct of a system that evolved without significant planning efforts and without attention to the personal needs of student physicians. In fact, residents are often referred to as "house officers" because historically, they were expected to live in the hospital. Under such conditions, marriage was actively discouraged for the predominantly male population. In short, family concerns were not prioritized for either male or female residents. Nevertheless, since female physicians are significantly more likely than male doctors to have a spouse with graduate-level education and a prestigious occupation, they are more likely to have to accommodate the career of their spouse. (For details on gender differences in physicians' personal lives, see chapter 6.) So the geographically inflexible nature of U.S. residency programs puts women at a disadvantage.

The second and more important issue involves the intense work requirements for residents and physicians in some specialties. Research has also shown that surgery has become more attractive as a career for medical students of both genders, but especially for women, since the adoption of the eighty-hour-per-week work restrictions (Arnold et al. 2005). This finding suggests that it is the demands of the training process rather than that of the practice career which deters some women from pursuing a career in surgery.

Many will counter that the large work effort of surgeons and others is an inherent aspect of the profession. In particular, physicians in surgical professions cite the need for continuity of care as a major reason for requiring such long hours of residents. The idea is that patients benefit when there is less turnover among the staff, and resident physicians benefit from more experience and exposure to the entire course of an illness as well as an accompanying sense of professionalism that comes from "owning" patients (Van Eaton et al. 2005).

There is wide variation, however, in what is believed to constitute the ideal amount of effort needed to train surgeons. The European Union has adopted work restriction laws which are sparking significant resistance among academic surgeons (Scott-Coombes 2002). But even before these laws were adopted, European surgical residents were working significantly fewer hours than U.S. surgical residents. Under the European directive, trainees were not supposed to work more than fifty-eight hours per week in 2004, more than fifty-six hours a week by 2007, and more than forty-eight hours per week by 2009, in comparison with the eighty-hour maximum in the United States (Klingensmith 2003).

Determinants of Specialty Choice

We used data from the AAMC graduating and matriculating student questionnaires to analyze the determinants of interest in surgery and primary care pediatrics among medical school seniors who entered in 1998 and graduated in 2002. The results of these analyses are presented in Appendix Table 2.[4]

As recently as 2002, senior women medical students were only 31 percent as likely as their male colleagues to select a surgical specialty. Gender differences in the reasons offered for entering medicine that were reported when students were freshmen explain only 21 percent of the gender gap in interest in surgery. This analysis indicates that gender differences in interests and values that students bring to medical school matter, but less so than is assumed in many discussions in this area. For example, one might assume that gender differences in initial interest in pursuing surgery account for most of the gender gap in the choices of graduating seniors. But the responses to the question about intended field of specialization do not explain the gender gap in this area. The manual dexterity question is the value factor that most strongly predicts specializing in surgery. Questions regarding helping others and interest in being financially successful are also helpful in explaining the gender gap in seniors' choices.

In these analyses the gender gap in the choice of surgery was not due to gender differences in students' responses to a question about whether medicine restricts time for family. In other words, the disproportionate tendency for women to believe that medicine restricts time for family does not explain their tendency to avoid surgery. Instead, differences in why men and women come to medicine were more salient. In particular, the disproportionate tendency for men to say that the opportunity to use their manual dexterity has attracted them to medicine explains a sizable slice of the male interest in surgery.

Advocates of the choice perspective would interpret these results as evidence that gender gaps in specialization stem largely from differences in the interests of male and female medical students. Although they explain more than other factors, ultimately the values and goals that freshmen medical students bring with them account for only 21 percent of the gender gap in the choice of surgery. There is room for many social factors not measured here, or not fully captured by these measures, to influence the specialty selection process.

The next stage of the analysis considers experiences during medical school. Collectively, controlling for all elective experiences, such as differences in participating in a community health clinic or involvement in international health experiences, explained 6 percent of the gender gap in interest in surgery.

Surprisingly, gender differences in satisfaction with clinical rotations and experiences with mistreatment do not explain any of the tendency to enter surgery. Specific clerkships contribute to deterring women from pursuing surgery, but in a somewhat unexpected way: it is the draw of other specialties, rather than dissatisfaction with surgery clerkships per se, that tends to reduce women's persistence in surgery. There is, as one would expect, a strong positive relationship between satisfaction with the surgical clerkship and the odds of selecting surgery. But there is no gender difference in students' satisfaction with surgery clerkships. Women, however, are on average more satisfied than men with clerkships in pediatrics, psychiatry, and internal medicine. The more satisfied women are with these fields, the less likely they are to pursue surgery. Other research reports a similar pattern (Arora et al. 2006). Yet overall, the available factors explain only one quarter (26 percent) of this gender gap.

We repeated this analysis for pediatrics (see Appendix Table 2). The results indicate that in 2001, senior women medical students were 4.25 times more likely to elect to pursue primary care pediatrics. After controlling for all of the factors available, including initial specialty preference, career interests as measured on entry into medical school, medical school experiences, satisfaction with rotations, and students' perceptions of their ability to balance medicine and family, we found that women remained 3.26 times as likely as men to select a residency in pediatrics. Thus, as with surgery, the bulk of the gender gap, 81 percent, is attributable to factors that are not included in this analysis or are not sufficiently well measured. Like surgery, elective academic experiences and satisfaction with clinical rotations explain a small but significant portion of the gender gap. In particular, 8 percent of the gap stems from gender differences during medical school.

Furthermore, as with surgery, much of the explained gender gap is attributable to differences in the interests students express as freshmen. In particular, there is a negative relationship between interest in exercising manual dexterity as a freshman and intent to pursue general pediatrics as a senior, and there is a positive relationship between interest in contact with patients as a freshman and intent to pursue general pediatrics as a senior. Overall, gender differences in students' interests as freshmen explain 11 percent of the gender gap in interest in pediatrics.

As in the case of surgery, however, these data do not provide conclusive support for the choice perspective. Male and female medical students enter training with distinct preferences but without a clear sense of which specialty will enable them to realize their preferences. Along the way they gain an understanding that some fields offer more patient contact and less of an interface with technology. What they do not learn, however, is as important as what they do learn. The presentation of the various medical specialties to medical students is imbued with social norms surrounding those fields.

Thus, although it appears as if there is at least a kernel of truth to the idea that women cluster in different specialties because they prefer different specialties, gender segregation by specialty is not entirely a result of such gendered choices. In fact, as was noted earlier, there is ample evidence that women initially clustered in specific specialties because of social pressures. That is, they were discouraged from entering some fields because of social stereotypes and because there were relatively few training spots available in these fields. They were encouraged to enter other fields because of different stereotypes and because these specialties could often accommodate women without rejecting interested men. The unexplained variance in these models suggests that there is room for further refinement in our understanding of these issues.

Women Physicians and Medical Research

As noted in chapter 4, women physicians were overrepresented in medical research prior to 1990. The clustering of women in research may be surprising to some because social theorists have suggested that professionals engaged in academic work are among the most elite (Abbott 1988). So it is surprising that a socially stigmatized group would be overrepresented in a theoretically prestigious segment of a profession.

The tendency for women to be overrepresented in research stems from both push and pull environmental factors. Barriers to opportunities for women in other areas of medicine contributed to women's representation in research positions. Judith Lorber's research during the late 1970s and 1980s indicates that women physicians seeking to build their own practices encountered significant obstacles because they were excluded from informal referral networks and were unable to secure relevant financing. These obstacles may have made research the path of least resistance for some female physicians.

Another contributing factor was the historic overrepresentation of foreign medical graduates among women physicians. Language barriers and racial or ethnic bias of patients may have discouraged foreign female medical graduates from actively pursuing patient care and accordingly led them into research. Data indicating that foreign female physicians are more likely to specialize in internal medicine, the field with the strongest research opportunity, is consistent with this argument.

A third reason for the relative clustering of women physicians in medical research during this era was the dramatic disparity between the incomes of physicians in academia and those in private practice (Tierney and Kimball 2006; Taljanovic et al. 2003; Miller 1998). One study found that most academic radiologists experience more than a 100 percent increase in pay when they leave the academic setting for private practice (Taljanovic et al. 2003). This is not to say that the clustering of women in medical research caused declines in the salaries of academic physicians. The salary gap between academic medicine and private practice existed prior to the large-scale entry of women into medicine. Instead, since women are slightly less motivated by money, they were probably less discouraged from research careers as a result of this salary gap.

The decisive consideration, however, was probably the growth of opportunities in this area of the medical profession. Recall that prior to 1990, opportunities for medical researchers were expanding. (Details of this issue were discussed in chapter 4.) Since medical researchers were actively recruiting physicians, they were probably willing to overlook women's status as minorities or outsiders, and so women were relatively well received in the research community.

The 1990s and Beyond

Many policymakers, physicians, and researchers have suggested that women's underrepresentation among physician researchers in the years since 1990 stems primarily from differences in the priorities of male and female physicians (Andrews 2002). The idea is that women do not pursue research because they do not wish to maintain the schedule of a typical physician researcher. In contrast to this view, we suggest that trends in research stem as strongly from discrimination and generational and structural changes in medical research as from individual choice. What is required is an explanation that would account for why women's overrepresentation in research prior to 1990 turned into a female deficit after 1990.

The overall decline in the numbers of physician researchers contributes to this pattern. As we saw in chapter 4, physician scientists have become a progressively smaller minority of those seeking and obtaining NIH project support. The role of physicians in federally funded medical research has been declining. Historically, socially stigmatized groups have not fared as well during periods of declining opportunities.

The Rise of the Clinical Educator Track

The considerations just discussed all focus on the underrepresentation of women in research. The data, however, suggest that women report a high level of interest in academic careers. Can women medical students' greater interest in academia be consistent with their lower representation in research? The emergence of the clinical educator track helps to explain this paradox.

The dynamic behind gender inequity in academic medicine becomes even more complex than might be assumed at first glance because of the emerging internal hierarchy of academic medicine. Over the past several decades academic medical faculties have become increasingly divided. Changes in the financing of medical care, which began in the early 1970s, forced academic medical centers to rely on clinical revenues for increasingly large portions of their total operating budgets (Barchi and Lowery 2000).

Academic medical centers and associated medical schools responded to increasing needs for clinical income by creating the clinician or clinician educator tracks and then hiring increasingly large cadres of standing medical faculty to fill these positions. In recent years most medical schools have had at least two tracks for faculty: a clinician or clinician educator track and a physician scientist track (Barchi and Lowery 2000). Although distinct university policies govern the precise allocation of time for clinician educators, these faculty members universally devote significantly more time than their physician scientist colleagues to the relatively low-prestige activities of seeing patients and mentoring students (Abbott 1988; Barchi and Lowery 2000).

The rise of the clinician educator track explains how women are overrepresented in academia (or at least among those planning to enter academia) while being underrepresented in research. While women are underrepresented in the research track for reasons of both personal preference and social exclusion, these factors are likely to play out very differently in the clinician educator context.

Although no nationally representative studies have been conducted to assess the relationship between gender and faculty track, and no concrete evidence suggests that women are being *recruited* disproportionately for clinical track positions, evidence from single-school assessments suggests that women are overrepresented on the clinical track (Nickerson et al. 1990). Furthermore, disproportionate representation in the clinical track seems a plausible explanation for the clustering of female academic physicians at the bottom of the career ladder.

Students with altruistic motives should be drawn to clinician educator positions because of the normal expectations associated with such jobs. Physicians in clinician educator jobs are expected to care for the patients who frequent teaching hospital clinics. Since these patients are usually underserved and low status, students who are drawn to medicine primarily because they believe they can help others ought to find academic positions especially attractive.

Whether the clinician educator track is helpful in the area of work and family is another matter. Unlike their colleagues in private practice, physicians on the clinician educator track have relatively few weekend and after-hours clinical responsibilities, primarily because medical students and residents attend to these demands. In theory, universities are well situated to offer clinician educators reduced-hour schedules. Because these institutions enjoy large economies of scale, they can also distribute the additional malpractice costs of their part-time workers over a larger number of patient visits. And anecdotal evidence suggests that this is actually happening. In

2007 about 210 of the 400 clinician educators at Stanford Medical School worked reduced hours (Kunz 2007). On the other hand, physicians in research-intensive positions normally have to work at least as hard as their colleagues in private practice and must make themselves available for the inevitable late nights associated with grant writing and delayed laboratory experiments. One survey of surgery faculty at a large Midwestern academic center found that general surgery faculty worked an average of 74 hours per week, trauma surgery faculty worked an average of 88 hours per week, and subspecialty surgery faculty worked an average of 67 hours per week. These estimates are considerably higher than the estimates for all surgeons (Klingensmith 2003). Not surprisingly, physicians on the research side of academic medicine have very low rates of part-time work. Fewer than 20 of the 784 tenure track, non–tenure track, or Medical Center Line faculty at Stanford have less than full-time schedules (Kunz 2007).

Explaining the Gender Gap in Research

We sought to explore the processes related to the selection of careers in research and academia using data on medical school students. We followed the students who entered medical school in 1998 and graduated four years later to see what factors might help to explain these career decisions.

Figures 5.2 and 5.3 document trends in graduating medical students' intent to pursue full-time academic careers and intent to pursue research. Results are separated by gender.[5] Figure 5.2 indicates that upon graduation,

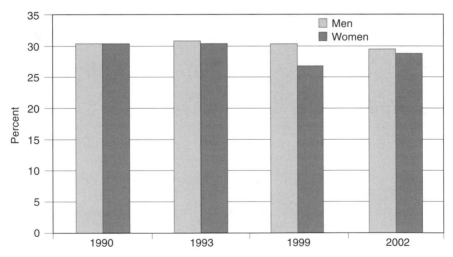

Figure 5.2. Medical Graduates' Intent to Pursue Full-Time Academics, 1990–2002. *Source:* AAMC Graduating Student Questionnaire.

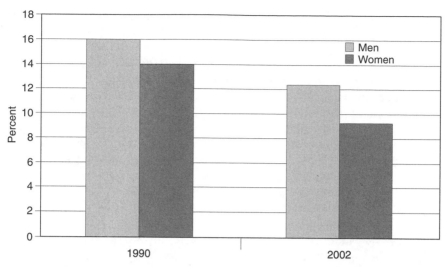

Figure 5.3. Medical Graduates' Intent to Pursue Full-Time Research, 1990–2002.
Source: AAMC Graduate Student Questionnaire.

roughly the same fraction of male and female medical school graduates (about 30 percent) intend to pursue careers in full-time academic research and teaching. Figure 5.3 indicates that substantially fewer students express an interest in a research-oriented career, and fewer female students intend to pursue extensive involvement in research (14 percent for men versus 9 percent for women in 2002). Furthermore, the gender difference in research did not change substantially over the twelve-year period from 1990 to 2002. Finally, there appears to have been a slight decline in the percentage of students intending to pursue exclusive or extensive involvement in research.

Appendix Table 3 summarizes the results of two sets of nested multivariate models.[6] The first set assesses the determinants of the intent to pursue a full-time academic position. The second set examines the same issues regarding the intent to be exclusively or significantly involved in research. These models suggest that students' motivations to study medicine and students' experiences in medical school play major roles in explaining gender differences in the intent to be extensively or significantly involved in medical research. They are also critical to our understanding of gender differences in academic medicine.

The story begins with attitudes and values of entering medical students. More specifically, altruism is negatively associated with the decision to pursue a career in research. In other words, those physicians who indicate that helping others is an important factor in their choice of a career are less likely to pursue careers in research. Since women tend to express higher levels of interest in altruism than do men, this differential can account for some

of the gender gap in interest in research. When we control for gender differences on the MD altruism scale, we explain 39 percent (14 points of the
36-point gap) of the gender difference in intent to be extensively involved in
research.[7] Thus, while these results support the "different voice" thesis, this
factor does not account for the majority of the gender gap.

These results also suggest that medical school experiences are salient in
students' intent to pursue medical research. More specifically, students who
submitted a paper for publication as an author, wrote a thesis, worked on
research with a faculty member, or completed an independent study during medical school were all more likely to express an interest in research
careers following graduation. Male medical students were more likely to
report each of these experiences. Specifically, men were 5 percentage points
more likely to take an independent study course during medical school
(38 percent versus 33 percent), 8 percentage points more likely to work on a
research project with a faculty member (58 percent versus 50 percent), and
9 percentage points more likely to author an article during medical school
(37 percent versus 28 percent). Thus the gender disparities in these medical
school experiences also contributed to differences in interest in research.
Our analysis indicates that these factors explain 31 percent of the gender
difference in intent to pursue research-oriented careers. These results suggest that experiences during medical school are roughly as important as the
values and goals that students hold upon entry into medical school.

It should be noted that the effect of these medical school experiences take
into account prior measures of preferences and career interests. In other
words, it is not simply that men were more interested in pursuing research
and therefore sought out more research opportunities during medical
school. Even after taking freshman-year interest in pursuing research into
account, we found that men are nonetheless more likely to obtain formal
research opportunities during medical school than are women. We suspect
that gender differences in informal communication with faculty contribute
to these disparities.

This analysis also suggests that gender differences in students' chosen
specialty explain the remaining difference in the odds that male and female
medical students will be interested in research-oriented careers. In other
words, the specialties that women are interested in tend to offer fewer research opportunities than do more male-dominated fields. Controlling for
the disproportionate tendency for women students to select specific medical specialties upon graduation accounts for an additional 19 percent of the
gender gap. Once specialty is taken into account, the gender differential in
interest in research is no longer statistically significant.

The same factors are related to interest in academic careers. Since women
and men start out at roughly the same point, however, controlling for these
factors *increases* women's position relative to men. That is, once initial in-

terest, medical school experiences, and specialty are statistically controlled for, women are considerably (28 percent) more likely to express interest in pursuing an academic career than are their male counterparts.

The analysis we have presented in this section suggests that, once relevant covariates have been accounted for, graduating female medical students are significantly more likely than their male peers to express an interest in full-time academic careers but significantly less likely to intend to be exclusively or extensively involved in research. As suggested earlier, although the representation of women among medical students has increased dramatically, women are still strikingly absent from the higher echelons of the profession. This gender inequity is especially prominent in academic medicine, where significant gender differences exist in the odds of promotion and in mean lapse of time to promotion.

This research suggests that one possible reason for gender differences among medical school faculty may stem from gender differences in the interests of those who pursue academic medical careers. More specifically, if women entering academic medicine are less likely then their male colleagues to express interest in research-oriented careers, it is possible that they are less likely to produce the type of research that has historically been tightly linked to academic promotions.

This analysis also suggests that experiences during medical school are significant correlates of students' ultimate career goals. In particular, we find that participating in research during medical school significantly enhances the odds that students will express an interest in research and academic medicine. This relationship persists even when students' perceived motivations for entering the medical profession are taken into account. We also find that these experiences explain a significant proportion of the gender difference in intent to pursue research and reveal a gender difference in interest in academic medicine.

This chapter has highlighted the role of social pressure, momentum, and structural change during medical training as determinants of gender differences in status. The individual choice or "different voice" argument is not sufficient to explain in full the status gap between men and women in the medical profession. In fact, gendered choices play a more limited role in creating such segregation and ultimately need to be understood in a broader context. Men and women make different choices as medical students, but they also have different options. Further, over time, structural changes in medicine have had different implications for men and women physicians and medical students because they initially occupied distinct positions in the medical profession. Since men and women aspiring physicians exist in unique social worlds, it is not surprising that they make different choices. Although medical specialties remain highly gendered, we are cautiously optimistic about long term social change. One recent male graduate of a neurosurgery program described the shock on the face of one of his more traditional attendings, a man who had spent several years in the military and had served in Vietnam, when he entered the neurosurgery resident work room and found the program's two female residents looking at pictures of wedding gowns on the internet. He immediately left the room in disgust mumbling under his breath, "What will they think of next?" Historically, neurosurgery call rooms were bastions of male culture that included, among other thing, plentiful supplies of pornography. Clearly, women remain in the minority in neurosurgery programs and anti-female sentiment is still prevalent in surgery. Nevertheless, as their presence increases, women are inevitably changing their environments in ways that will ease the experiences of women who follow them.

6

Work, Family, Marriage, and Generational Change

Over the previous chapters we have covered a great many aspects of women's dramatic entry into medicine and the enduring differences in the practice patterns between male and female physicians. Women doctors continue to be underrepresented in certain specialties and in the upper echelons of the profession, and they earn significantly less than their male counterparts.

Now we turn our attention to how gender affects physicians' lives outside of work. We explore how differences in the family life of male and female physicians have evolved as women's presence in the profession has grown. What kinds of personal lives do male and female physicians lead? How many of them form families? Are they more or less likely to marry and have children than comparably educated men and women? When they do marry, how do they negotiate work and family life with their spouses?

A more complete understanding of physicians' family lives might also help us assess the potential for real integration of women within medicine and the possibility for gender equality in high-status couples more generally. In other words, in this chapter we begin to reverse the work-family equation. Thus far we have examined the work-family nexus from the point of view of professional success. We focused on the extent to which marriage and especially motherhood are responsible for the gendered pattern of specialization in medicine and the gender gap in the attainment of earnings and other markers of career accomplishment among physicians. In this chapter we shift our focus from the office and the hospital to the family.

We begin by exploring whether new generations of female physicians approach work differently. Are members of the most recent generation of physicians more determined to find a new balance between work and family? Are they dropping out of the labor force when their children are young? In the words of Lisa Belkin (2003), are women physicians "opting out" of professional careers in order to be fully engaged mothers? Are they demanding more flexible and part-time arrangements than did previous generations of women physicians, as some have suggested (Bickel and Brown 2005)? Are they forgoing the long workdays that have been emblematic of practicing physicians since the days of house calls? We then reverse the work-family relationship by asking whether professional success requires the sacrifice of a satisfying family life. Are women physicians able to get married, stay married, and have children?

Sociologists have been fascinated with generational shifts at least since Karl Mannheim's (1952) classic essay on the topic. The underlying idea is an appealing one: we are formed by early-life experiences, and thus changes in social life are not linear responses to circumstances but can take the form of more discrete changes as different generations with different experiences take center stage.

Glen Elder (1974) has written persuasively about the distinctive experiences of the generation that grew up during the Great Depression. Economist Claudia Goldin (1997; 2004) has developed an argument along these lines in her analysis of the experiences of college-educated women in the United States. She maintains that the first generation chose between work and family, while those who followed tended to pursue family then work as discrete stages in their life course. The most recent generation, those graduating from college since 1980, is the first to try to combine work and family simultaneously.

The generation shift thesis has been applied to the case of medicine most visibly by Janet Bickel (Bickel and Brown 2005). Her thesis is that the recent generation of women entering medicine has a different set of values and priorities from those of their predecessors. According to Bickel, members of the Baby Boom generation, or those currently at the highest tiers of the medical hierarchy, work hard out of loyalty, respect authority, believe that self-sacrifice is a virtue, and expect a long-term job. Members of Generation X and those currently seeking to enter academic medicine and percolate through its ranks question authority, expect to change jobs periodically, work hard only if balance is allowed, and believe that self-sacrifice may have to be endured occasionally. She suggests that fewer Generation Xers are electing careers in academic medicine because they do not want to make the associated sacrifices and because the rewards offered by medical academia are fewer today than in the past. She then suggests that academic health centers need to make a stronger effort to recruit and nurture the next generation of faculty by creating programs that meet their unique expectations for work-family balance and mentoring.

We find little support for the "opt out" thesis. Women physicians are fully committed to their careers. We also find little evidence that women physicians are cutting back on the hours they devote to the profession. Indeed, in some respects the level of professional commitment has continued to increase over time.

As to whether women's careers come at a great personal price, the answer we offer is more mixed. On the one hand, women physicians are marrying and having children at a rate similar to other women: since the 1980s women physicians have narrowed or reversed the gaps in family life between themselves and their female counterparts outside medicine. On the other hand, it remains true that male physicians are more likely to be able to combine work and family than are their female colleagues.

Employment Rates

It is no secret that women's labor force participation has grown dramatically over the past half century. In 1950, 24 percent of married women worked for pay. By 1994 the number had more than doubled, so that 60 percent of married women reported some degree of employment.[1] This same level was evident in 2004 as well (U.S. Department of Labor 2004). Several indicators of women's labor force participation peaked in 1997 during the very tight labor market conditions under the Clinton administration. Beginning in 2000, the labor force participation rate of mothers of young children began to level off. In 2005, 68 percent of married mothers with children under eighteen were in the labor force, including 65 percent of married women with children aged three to five and 57 percent with children under age three (Cohany and Sok 2007).

Recently, however, there has been a growing sense that mothers are deciding to forgo employment in order to devote their full attention to nurturing children. In particular, Belkin (2003) asserted that highly educated women are increasingly likely to stay home full-time with children. Data from the U.S. Census Bureau appear to confirm some of what Belkin found from in-depth interviews. The labor force participation rates of mothers with infant children fell from a record-high 58.7 percent in 1998 to 54.6 percent in 2004, the first decline since the Census Bureau developed the indicator in 1976 (Dye 2005).

Although these declines in labor force participation among mothers of the youngest children are real, they are substantively small. And it is too early to tell if they reflect a long-term change or a temporary blip. Nevertheless, this trend in women's labor force participation, especially among the most highly educated, has sparked questions about the potential of professional women such as physicians to fulfill society's needs, and about the meaning of professional work for women, many of whom are married to successful men. (See Pamela Stone's 2007 book *Opting Out?* for an illuminating study of professional women who have left the labor force, often temporarily.)

In this section we examine the validity of Belkin's claim with regard to female physicians. By tracking trends in employment among married doctors, we not only begin to assess whether female physicians take advantage of their training but also uncover trends in the status of male physicians' marriages. A more complete understanding of work and family issues among male physicians will help us to understand what female physicians are up against as they struggle to balance their professional and family lives and achieve true equality at work.

We drew on data from the U.S. Census to document the labor force participation rates of married physicians. Our results demonstrate that married physicians, both male and female, have extremely high labor force participation, regardless of either their spouse's qualifications or the presence of children, and that married female physicians are only slightly less likely than married male physicians to work for pay. Thus, like their male counterparts, female physicians utilize their training regardless of whether their spouse has high earning potential or whether they have children.

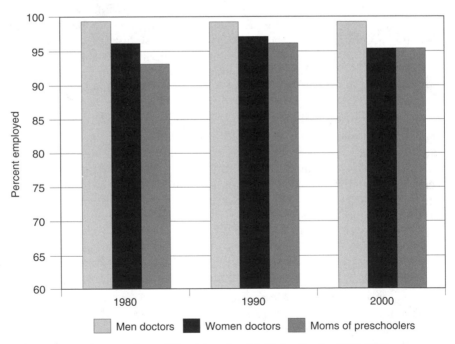

Figure 6.1. Employment Rate of Physicians Age 30–50, by Gender, 1980–2000.
Source: U.S. Decennial Censuses.

Figure 6.1 illustrates this pattern by focusing on employment rates for married physicians between thirty and fifty years of age.[2] Since these are the peak childbearing and child-rearing years, this age group would be the most likely to show exits from the labor force. In 2000, 99 percent of married male physicians in this age group were employed, along with 96 percent of their female counterparts. There was only a limited difference between the physicians who were mothers of preschool children and all women: 94 percent of physicians who were mothers of young children were employed, while 96 percent of all female physicians were employed. Indeed the employment rate of mothers of pre-school-age children was up slightly between 1980 (93 percent) and 2000 (94 percent).

Thus the vast majority of women trained in medicine are in active practice, even those with young children at home. These trends compare to 79.2 percent for women and 91.0 percent for men of the same age in the general population. The employment rates for physicians of all ages and household compositions are extremely high. We found nothing in the census data that points to a major retreat from the labor force on the part of women physicians. Data from the AMA Masterfile on physician inactivity also support the contention that women physicians maintain a strong connection to medical work.[3]

Parenting and Work Hours

The pattern with respect to working time is even stronger than that for labor force participation. Women physicians are putting in longer workweeks than ever before, not increasingly cutting back on their work. These results provide no support for the notion that women physicians are opting out of their professional commitments.

Overall, female physicians aged thirty to fifty work fewer hours than their male counterparts. In 2000, women worked an average of forty-seven hours per week, compared with fifty-five hours per week for men in the same age group. This gap in the work week of eight hours, however, is concentrated among women physicians who are married and have children at home. Single childless women in this age group put in nearly as much time on the job as their male counterparts. In 2000 they worked fifty-one hours per week compared with fifty-three hours per week for the men. Married but childless women worked fifty-one hours per week—just two hours less than similarly situated men. Married women physicians with children under eighteen at home worked an average of forty-five hours per week. While parenthood cuts into the workweek for these women, fathers actually put in longer hours on the job than do other men (fifty-six hours per week compared with the average of fifty-five hours). Thus the arrival of children tends to heighten gender differentiation among physicians, reducing women's workweek by a few hours while adding slightly to men's workweek. It is notable that female physicians who find themselves single mothers work as many hours per week as the average woman physician (forty-seven hours).

Figure 6.2 displays these trends for married male doctors, female doctors, and doctors who are mothers of pre-school-age children. These patterns changed very little during the last two decades of the twentieth century, the very period during which professional women's retreat from work is supposed to have taken place. The workweek for women physicians actually edged upward during this period of time, from forty-three to forty-six hours; the workweek for men also edged up three hours during the same period. This increase was evident among married women with young children, whose workweek increased from forty-one to forty-five hours per week during this period. Thus the extent of professional commitment on the part of the most recent generation of women physicians has not declined, in terms of either their rate of employment or the hours they put in on the job.

Over the last several decades the work effort of female physicians has come to resemble more closely the work effort of men who share their household composition. The trend is driven primarily by increases in the work effort of women physicians regardless of their personal lives rather than by declines in the work effort of male physicians.

Finally, although the work effort of employed female physicians came to resemble more closely the effort of their male colleagues during the 1990s,

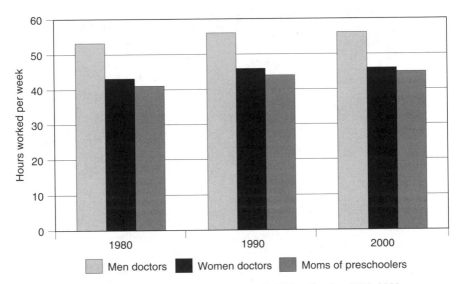

Figure 6.2. Average Workweek of Physicians Age 30–50, by Gender, 1980–2000. *Source:* U.S. Decennial Censuses.

this trend raises questions as to whether medicine is becoming a more family-friendly profession. Physicians work significantly longer hours than the general population. In 2000, for example, employed male physicians reported an average workweek of fifty-five hours. The comparable figure for all employed men of the same age was only forty-five. Similarly, in 2000, employed female physicians between thirty and fifty reported an average of forty-seven hours of work per week. This compares with thirty-eight hours for employed women of the same age in the general population. Increases in work effort may signal increasing pressures on female physicians with regard to their lives outside of work. Trends in work effort are especially interesting in light of trends in marriage and family discussed earlier. We examine the issue of family-friendly employment opportunities at greater length in chapter 8.

The Impact of Work on Family Life

In this section we track changes in family formation, work effort, and earnings among physicians since the 1980s. Before the large-scale entry of women physicians, the medical profession had been built on the model of the male breadwinner family. The physician husband could devote himself exclusively to his career knowing that his stay-at-home wife would attend to their children, their home, and their social life. This arrangement enabled physicians to spend long hours at the office and in the hospital, and to be on call at nights and on weekends.[4]

How do women physicians fit into this picture? Are they as likely to marry as their male counterparts, or do many end up trading off a family life for professional success? Previous research suggests dramatic differences in marriage, divorce, and fertility for male and female physicians such that women doctors are less likely to be married, more likely to be divorced, and less likely to have children (Uhlenberg and Cooney 1990; Hinze 2004). These results are not surprising given the long period of medical training, which coincides with the period of family formation and childbearing, as well as the strong career penalty that appears to be connected to family formation for women physicians. We seek to build on these analyses to see how these patterns are evolving with the entry of steadily larger cohorts of women physicians.

We also build on previous research (Hinze 2004) by presenting these trends in the context of three different benchmarks: we compare women physicians' experiences today to those of their counterparts a generation earlier, to those of their male counterparts today, and to those of other women in the general population. Each of these three different vantage points provides valuable insights and helps us offer a more complete picture of what has changed, and what has not, for female physicians.

Women physicians increasingly resemble other women with respect to marriage, divorce, and childbearing. Indeed, whereas women physicians in 1980 trailed other women in marriage and childbearing and led in divorce, all of these comparisons are now more favorable to women physicians.

Figure 6.3 documents marriage rates for physicians aged forty to forty-nine, drawing on the 1980, 1990, and 2000 censuses.[5] Overall trends throughout American society have left fewer Americans married than was the case in the 1970s. Physicians, however, have been less vulnerable to these trends than have those in other fields. Women physicians in 2000 were slightly less likely to be married than were women physicians twenty years earlier. For example, among women aged forty to forty-nine, 71 percent of female physicians were married in 2000, compared with 74 percent in 1980. Male physicians also experienced a slight decline in marriage rates, from 90 percent in 1980 to 87 percent in 2000. If the percentage of married women physicians is taken as one indication of how family-friendly the profession is, then medicine would seem to be even less family-friendly today than it was a generation ago.

Another useful point of comparison, however, involves comparing women physicians with other women. Here we get an additional perspective from which to understand the experiences of women physicians. The data indicate

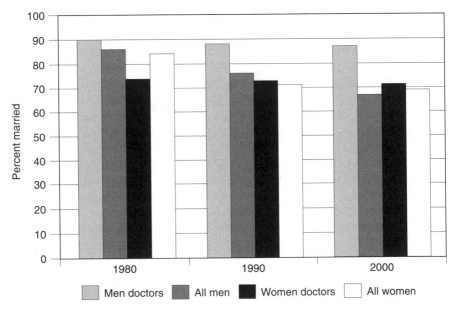

Figure 6.3. Percent Married, Physicians and General Population, Age 40–49, 1980–2000.
Source: U.S. Decennial Censuses.

that the decline in marriage among women in the general population has been much sharper than was the case for women physicians. Among the same age group of women forty to forty-nine, 69 percent were married in 2000, down from 86 percent in 1980. As a result, whereas female physicians trailed other women in marriage rates in 1980, they have eliminated this differential and are now at least slightly more likely than other women to be married (71 percent versus 69 percent). This conclusion is consistent when various age groups over thirty are examined.

A final approach involves comparing women physicians with their male counterparts. This is another useful yardstick for assessing recent trends. The data in Figure 6.3 indicate that the decline in marriage is evident among both male and female physicians. Among male physicians aged thirty-five to thirty-nine, 78 percent were married in 2000, down from 87 percent in 1980. In other words, if we ask what the differences in the experiences of male and female physicians are today, the answer is that the gender gap in marriage rates has narrowed.

On the one hand, professional success for women physicians is associated with a lower likelihood of being married than for men. While not all women seek marriage, the lower marriage rate of women physicians suggests that marriage continues to mean different things for male and female physicians, and that it remains harder for women to combine these roles than it is for men. On the other hand, careers in medicine now no longer pose a greater obstacle to marriage than do other jobs. The decline in marriage rates that has occurred among women physicians has been less extreme than in the general population. Thus, while combining marriage and career is no more likely for women physicians today than it was in 1980, the gap between women physicians and other women in marriage rates has been eliminated to the point where women physicians have a small advantage.

These results give us a mixed answer to the question of generational comparisons. The declining marriage rate among female physicians does not herald a return to traditional family arrangements, since the current generation of women physicians is not more likely to marry and have children than their counterparts a generation earlier. Yet the marriage experiences of female physicians are now more in line with those of other women. The case that Generation X female physicians are seeking a new balance between work and family could be made in relative terms, that is, relative to the experiences of other women.

Divorce appears to be less frequent among women physicians now than among other women. Cross-sectional data on divorce need to be treated cautiously because incidence and persistence are impossible to separate. In other words, if women physicians are more likely to be divorced than other women in the same age group, it may be due to a higher divorce rate, or it may be due to women physicians remarrying at a lower rate than their female counterparts, and therefore remaining divorced for a longer period of time.

As a result of changes in the broader society, female physicians are now markedly less likely to be divorced than are women in the general population. In 1980 women physicians aged forty to forty-nine were 2 percentage points more likely than other women their age to be divorced (results not shown in a separate figure). By 2000, women physicians aged forty to forty-nine were actually 7 percentage points *less* likely than other women their age to be divorced. Divorce has declined among female physicians under forty but has remained at a constant rate among those over forty. The pattern for divorce resembles that for marriage in that there has been an improvement in both respects in the position of women physicians relative to other women.

At the same time, the divorce rate has declined for male physicians. As a result, the gender gap in divorce among physicians actually increased slightly between 1980 and 2000. In 2000, 13 percent of women physicians aged forty to forty-nine were divorced, compared with 6 percent for men. This 7 percentage point gap was up from a 5 percentage point gap in 1980.

Sorting out among possible alternative explanations for the decline in divorce among physicians is not possible, given the limitations of these data. One explanation is that male physicians are marrying later and thus reducing their chances of divorce by choosing more carefully or waiting until they can spend more time on their marriage. An alternative possibility is that because male physicians marry later, their years of risk of divorce have decreased.

The trends in both marriage and divorce highlight the importance of putting the experiences of women physicians in the broader context of trends occurring in American society. In both cases, focusing on trends in the experiences of women physicians by themselves would not suggest that major changes have occurred during this period. The census data discussed earlier indicate that, relative to their male colleagues, women who enter medicine continue to marry at significantly lower rates and divorce at higher rates. Comparing women in medicine to women in other pursuits, however, suggests an improvement in the relative position of medicine in terms of the compatibility of work and family.

We find the same pattern of improvement among women physicians relative to other women in American society when we turn to the issue of parenthood (results not shown in a separate figure). Fertility rates (as reflected in the presence of children at home) for female physicians increased slightly between 1990 and 2000. Overall, 81 percent of married female physicians between thirty and fifty had children at home in 2000, compared with 79 percent in 1990. Comparing women physicians to other women in terms of childbearing is less informative because other women are more likely to have their children at younger ages than women physicians. Nonetheless, we actually see the gap between the fertility of female physicians and women in the general population narrowing between 1990 and 2000. In fact, in 2000, married women physicians aged thirty to fifty were 2 percentage points more likely to report having a child at home than women in the general population. The differential between women physicians and other women is now confined to single mothers. Single women outside the medical profession are far more likely to have a child than are single women physicians (45 percent of single women aged thirty to fifty in the general population had a child at home in 2000, compared to 27 percent of single women physicians).

Male physicians were more likely to have children at home than were female physicians throughout this period. Again, combining this demanding career with having a family remains easier for men than for women physicians. But since fertility decreased slightly for the families of male physicians between 1990 and 2000, the gender gap in parenting narrowed for physicians during this period. While this trend certainly signals increasing gender equality in fertility among younger physicians, it does not necessarily imply increasing equality in total fertility. The recent tendency for male physicians to delay marriage may also have caused male physicians to delay becoming fathers, and it is possible that the ultimate family size of male physicians will deviate little from that of the past.

The number of children of physician parents has declined slightly. In 1980 male physician parents between thirty and fifty reported an average of 2.33 children. Women physician parents in the same age range reported 2.03 children on average. By 2000 these numbers had declined to 2.25 and 1.96, respectively. While these declines may be related to the inflexibility of the medical workplace, the fertility of female physicians is not uniquely low. The total fertility rate (TFR), or average number of children per woman given current birthrates, was 2.1 children per woman in 2005. The TFR was 1.8 for non-Hispanic whites and 1.9 for Asians and Pacific Islanders.[6] According to the 2000 census, 90 percent of female physicians were either white or Asian in ethnicity, so these total fertility rates offer the best benchmark for women in medicine.

The trends in marriage, divorce, and fertility present a mixed picture with respect to gender inequality among physicians. Male and female physicians have become closer to each other in terms of marriage and parenting, but the gap in terms of divorce has grown marginally. In contrast, comparisons between female physicians and the general population of women yield a clear conclusion; over time, women physicians are becoming relatively more likely to combine work and family. Female physicians are less likely to be married today than they were thirty years ago, but this decline is significantly less than the corresponding decline in the general population.

Similarly, female physicians' odds of divorce have actually declined relative to the corresponding odds for women in the general population. Finally, our data suggest that the odds of becoming a parent are increasing for female physicians, and that they are coming to resemble more closely women in the general population.

Physicians' Marriages

The relative position of women within marriage is improving. This is evident in the marriages of female physicians as well as male physicians. Table 6.1 displays data on the education, occupation, employment rate, and hours worked of physicians' spouses.

Turning first to the husbands of women physicians, over time there has been a decline in the proportion of husbands with a postgraduate degree. The level declined by roughly 10 percentage points, from 80 percent in 1980 to 70 percent in 2000. This decline reflects the growing education levels of American women: as women begin to surpass men in the level of schooling completed, it becomes increasingly difficult for women to find men with the same or higher level of education. Nonetheless, female physicians remain more likely to have highly educated spouses than do their male counterparts. The same pattern is evident with respect to the occupations

Table 6.1. Attributes of Physicians' Spouses, 1980–2000

Year	Wives of Male Physicians	Husbands of Female Physicians
Percent of Spouses with Post graduate Education		
2000	0.40	0.70
1990	0.32	0.72
1980	0.22	0.80
Percent of Spouses in Professional or Managerial Occupations		
2000	0.56	0.81
1990	0.55	0.83
1980	0.41	0.89
Spouses' Employment Rate		
2000	0.59	0.93
1990	0.61	0.95
1980	0.44	0.96
Spouses' Hours per Week of Paid Employment		
2000	35	47
1990	33	47
1980	30	47

Note: All married physicians under age 65.
Source: U.S. Decennial Censuses.

of physicians' spouses. Historically the overwhelming majority of the husbands of female physicians were professionals or managers. For example, in 1980 nearly nine in ten husbands of women physicians fit this profile. There was erosion in this pattern over the next twenty years, however, with the proportion of women physicians married to husbands with professional or managerial careers declining to just over 80 percent.

With respect to the employment rate and the length of the workweek, there has been relatively little change in either husbands' employment rates or hours worked. Nearly all of the husbands of female physicians are employed and work more than a standard full-time schedule. In 2000, 93 percent of the husbands of female physicians were employed. This was down a few percentage points from 1980, but that drop primarily reflects the fact that some women physicians in their fifties and sixties are married to men who have reached retirement age. Among women physicians in their thirties and forties, very few are married to stay-at-home husbands. The typical husband of a female physician puts in forty-seven hours per week on the job.

Thus most women physicians find themselves in dual-career families, and few have the stay-at-home spouse that male physicians have historically relied on. At the same time, women physicians are increasingly the better-educated partner and increasingly are the partner with the higher-status profession.

A countervailing trend is evident for male physicians. There has been movement toward greater equality in the marriages of male physicians as their wives have become increasingly educated and are more likely to be employed full-time in professional or managerial careers. In 1980 about one in five male physicians had a wife with a postgraduate degree; by 2000 this fraction had doubled to two in five. This trend in part reflects the growing educational attainment of women in the United States as well as a trend toward for educational homogamy, that is, the pattern of spouses to have similar levels of education.

The wives of male physicians were more likely to be engaged in a professional or managerial occupation in 2000 than was the case twenty years earlier. By 2000 a majority of male physicians were married to women whose occupations were in the professional or managerial ranks.

The data in Table 6.1 show that by 2000 the traditional model of the male breadwinner with a stay-at-home wife no longer characterized the majority of the families of male physicians. A clear majority—roughly three in five—of the wives of male physicians were employed in the paid labor market. The change occurred mostly during the 1980s. And these wives were more likely to put in a longer workweek than was the case in the past (thirty-five hours per week in 2000 compared with thirty in 1980).

We draw two main conclusions from these data. First, married male and female physicians experience married life very differently. Female physicians rarely have a stay-at-home husband or one who works part-time. They nearly always are married to men who themselves put in very long workweeks. The challenges of dual-career families can be daunting when both spouses work fifty or more hours per week. This is an American pattern: very few couples in western European countries are in relationships in which the joint hours of paid employment exceed one hundred hours per week (Jacobs and Gerson 2004). The career decisions of female physicians who are married need to be understood against the backdrop of these relationships.

Another important conclusion, however, is that the marriages of male physicians are moving away from the traditional male breadwinner model toward dual-earner arrangements. There has been an increase in the economic position of the wives of male physicians, as indexed by trends in education, occupation, and employment.

It appears as if the increasing tendency of having an employed wife is affecting male physicians' work lives, but in fact spousal employment exerts a significantly greater effect on female physicians. In additional analyses not shown, we used census data to conduct regression analyses to assess how spousal employment influences male and female physicians' work effort. Overall we found that married male physicians with an employed spouse worked an average of 1.5 hours less in 1990 and 2.25 hours less in 2000 than their colleagues with an unemployed wife. By contrast, married female physicians with an employed spouse worked an average of 8.3 hours less in 1990 and 8.0 hours less in 2000 than those with a stay-at-home partner. We reiterate, however, that having a stay-at-home husband remains a rarity for female physicians.

We hasten to add that the dual-income marriages of male physicians remain far less equal in an economic sense than the dual-income marriages of female physicians. As we will see in the next section, the wives of male physicians rarely make the same financial contributions to the family's well-being as do their husbands.

Financial Contribution of Spouses

In the male breadwinner family, the husband earns the salary and the wife manages the household. As we have seen, this pattern holds for a diminishing but still significant share of male physicians' families. Meanwhile, married female physicians have rarely had the support of a stay-at-home husband.

In this section we focus on the relative financial contribution of husbands and wives. If men are no longer the sole breadwinners, do they nonetheless contribute the lion's share of the family's financial resources? Do female physicians earn as much as or more than their husbands?

Financial contributions can be influential in setting the terms of the relationship between spouses. Family researchers have long maintained that power within families in part reflects the relative financial contribution of spouses. An examination of the financial division of labor within physicians' households will thus shed light on the extent of change in these families.

Over the twenty years from 1980 to 2000, female physicians moved from being the secondary to the primary earners in their families. In other words, in 1980 women physicians were earning less than their husbands, on average, while by 2000 they were typically earning more than their husbands. Specifically, in 1980 the average female physician earned 20 percent less than her husband. By 2000 she was earning 10 percent more than her husband. This reflects the change in the types of men whom female physicians are marrying. As we will see in the next section, this conclusion differs sharply depending on whether the husband is himself a physician.

Even though male physicians are no longer the sole earners in their families, they remain the principal source of the family's income. In 2000 male physicians in dual-earner households earned 4.5 times as much as their wives. While these marriages remain far from financial equality, they are nonetheless much more equal than had been the case twenty years earlier, when physician husbands earned eight times as much as their wives. It is also worth noting that because the average physician's educational debt has increased dramatically, the earnings gaps for male and female physicians are somewhat misleading. After loan payments, which often rival a family's mortgage payment, are subtracted from both the male and female physician's income, disposable earnings ratios inevitably change. Given their lower incomes, the burden of loan payments is probably heavier for women physicians.

Physician-Physician Marriages

Marriages in which both the husband and wife are physicians would seem to represent an interesting special case, since such marriages would seem to hold out the prospect for true equality. If both partners are in the same occupation, have gone through the same training, and have had the same experiences, then perhaps there would be the basis for a true partnership with similar levels of financial contribution from both parties. Moreover, such an arrangement might also imply more equal contributions in terms of the unpaid labor of housework and child care.

Are physician-physician couples more common today as the number of women physicians has increased? Are these couples more financially equal than those families in which the spouse is not a physician?

Historically it was quite common for female physicians to marry within the profession. In a sense, medical schools provided a husband-rich field of opportunity. While we would not suggest that women entered medical school in search of a husband, many nonetheless often found their partner in this way. In 1980 fully half of all married female physicians under age fifty were married to a male physician.

This pattern makes sense in the context of a male-dominated profession in which these female physicians represented members of a small minority. A female medical student or resident was in her late twenties or early thirties. Her medical training consumed most of her time, limiting her opportunity to meet men in other fields. And there were eight or nine men for every woman. In this situation it should not be surprising that many of the women physicians would find a partner in the profession. Sometimes marriage would involve a male physician who was in a more senior position in the hospital rather than a classmate.

As the gender composition of medical classes has moved toward parity, the likelihood of female physicians' finding a husband in medicine has declined. In 2000, among physicians under age thirty-five, just over one third (34 percent) of female physicians were married to a male physician (see Figure 6.4).

The same demographic changes had the opposite effect on the marriage prospects of male physicians. With more female classmates, the chances of marrying a female physician increased. In 1980 the scarcity of female classmates meant that only 7 percent of male physicians under age thirty-five

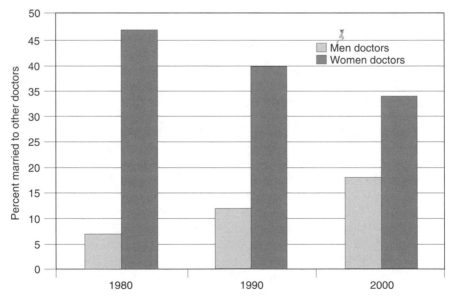

Figure 6.4. Physician-Physician Marriages under Age 35, 1980–2000. *Source:* U.S. Decennial Censuses.

married a female physician. By 2000 this fraction increased to 18 percent. In 2000, for the first time, male physicians were more likely to marry a female physician than they were to marry a nurse (10 percent, down from 18 percent in 1980). This certainly represents a notable shift in the type of relationship experienced by male physicians.

Dual-physician marriages are busy ones. On average, in 2000, the two-career, two-physician family worked one hundred hours per week, while the average for two-career families with a male physician and non-physician spouse was only ninety hours and the average for two-career families with a female physician and non-physician spouse was ninety-five hours.

Do both partners make equal financial contributions in doctor-doctor marriages? In dual-physician families the wives earn far less than the husbands. In 2000 female physicians earned just 60 percent as much as their male physician husband. Among parents, women earned 55 percent of what their husband earned. The gender gap was much smaller among couples with no children at home.

One informative way of summarizing the financial position of women in marriages is to examine the percentage who earn more than their husband. Overall, 46.5 percent of all married female physicians between thirty and fifty earn more than their husband. This figure far exceeds that for working women as a whole, for whom fewer than one quarter out-earn their husband. Among physicians, 28 percent of married female physicians with a physician spouse earn more, and 59 percent of female physicians with a non-physician spouse earn more. In summary, marriages between physicians have not resulted in equal financial contributions by husbands and wives, while marriages of female physicians to non-physicians are beginning to tip in the direction of greater earnings contributions by the physician wife.

Although male physicians in dual-physician marriages earn more on average, previous research on dual-physician marriages indicates that having a physician spouse involves reductions in work effort for physicians of both genders. One U.S.-based study of 1,782 married pediatricians found that having a physician spouse was associated with a significant reduction in work effort for male and female physicians (Brotherton and LeBailly 1992). A similar study of Canadian family physicians found similar results. On average, female family physicians in physician-physician marriages worked about five fewer hours weekly than other female physicians, and male family physicians worked about three fewer hours weekly than other male physicians (Woodward 2005). Thus the considerable earning potential of dual-physician marriages may provide an opportunity to reduce the work commitments of both partners, and thus may offer the opportunity for a lifestyle more evenly balanced between work and career. However, since these studies focus on physicians in the less well remunerated specialties, their tendency to reduce work effort may also capture the fact that these physicians are likely to be the partner with the lower earnings prospects. One study of physician marriages that was not limited to specific specialties found that although female physicians with a physician spouse worked less than their female colleagues with a spouse outside of medicine, male physicians' work habits were not influenced by their spouses' occupation (Sosbecks et al. 1999).

We find that physicians work less if their spouse is a physician, but this effect is quite small. For example, in 2000, male physicians worked 0.5 fewer hours per week if their wife was a physician, all other things being equal, while female physicians worked 1.2 fewer hours per week if their husband was a physician.

In this chapter we find that although women physicians continue to pursue very distinct lives at home and at work, there is a general drift toward equality. These trends should eventually enhance equality in the profession by evening the playing field at home. There is a long way to go before physicians reach this point, but, barring unanticipated developments, these trends should create further pressure for the adoption of family-friendly supports, since male and female physicians will have more similar needs for flexibility at work.

In particular, the evidence does not indicate that female physicians are opting out of work in a significant way. While the rate of women who were not working for pay ticked up slightly during the 1990s, the overwhelming majority of women physicians, even those with young children, are professionally active. Overall, the "opt out" revolution has not significantly affected the medical profession.

Furthermore, although women physicians continue to work less than their male colleagues, the extent of this gap is declining over time. The drift toward equality is occurring even among parents and is driven primarily by increases in work effort. Our data do not support the generational shift arguments discussed earlier.

We also suggest that although medical work continues to represent a more significant barrier to personal life for female physicians than male physicians, trends are mostly drifting toward equality. In particular, although women physicians are still less likely to marry and become parents than their male colleagues, the gender gap is closing on both measures. In addition, over time, the gap between women physicians and their female peers with respect to marriage has closed completely. Women physicians are now more likely to be married than their peers in the general population.

Still, marriage rates of female physicians need to be understood in the context of overall declines in marriage. The improvement in women's relative status with respect to marriage has occurred amidst a decline in overall marriage rates; it does not necessarily denote an increase in the tendency for women physicians to meld marriage with professional life. (The trends in fertility, by contrast, are slightly positive for female physicians.) So it appears that women physicians continue to struggle to blend personal and professional lives but that their struggle is increasingly shared by other women, especially professional women, to a much greater extent than it was a generation ago.

In addition to the general trend toward equality in work effort, we also note a drift toward greater equality in the types of marriages maintained by male and female physicians. In particular, over time, the tendency for female physicians to wed physicians and other professionals has been declining, while male physicians are increasingly likely to marry highly educated, employed women. Nevertheless, since a dramatic gap remains between the work lives and earnings of male and female physicians' spouses, it is reasonable to believe that male physicians continue to enjoy significantly more support at home than their female colleagues.

Looking to the future, we believe that one possible engine of change may derive from the fact that male physicians are no longer in exclusively male breadwinner marriages. As the men find themselves married to female physicians and other women with their own demanding careers, perhaps the traditional expectations regarding a physician's work schedule and career may begin to change. Without a full-time stay-at-home wife for support, it is difficult if not impossible for a male physician to sustain a career working sixty, seventy, or eighty hours per week. Understandings of the "ideal" physician, in terms of hours worked per week and career continuity, may thus evolve. In other words, we expect that changes in men's experiences might begin to be a significant force in altering the work-family equation for all physicians. We revisit the issue of medicine as a family-friendly career in chapter 8.

7

Women Physicians
Caring for Patients

In this chapter we examine how gender is related to the nature and quality of care provided to patients. As the presence of women in American medicine has grown, researchers have repeatedly speculated about their impact on the practice of medicine. As an article in the *New York Times Sunday Magazine* once posed the question, "Are Women Better Doctors?" (Klass 1988). Discussions in the medical press and among academic researchers have been drawn to the same question (Bluestone 1978; Hayes 1981; Abel 1992; Lorber 1984 and 2000; Levinson and Lurie 2004). One prominent theme in these discussions is that women physicians are more empathetic with patients (Bluestone 1978; Levinson and Lurie 2004). It is often suggested that as their overall representation increases and, more specifically, as their presence in leadership grows, women physicians will transform American health care, making it a more caring, patient-centered institution (see especially Levinson and Lurie 2004).

In contrast to this emphasis on gender differences, we stress the similarities between men and women in how they diagnose and treat individual patients. Even stylistic differences between males and females in treatment patterns, such as communication and empathy, are smaller than many might suspect. We emphasize the context in which interactions are taking place and note the importance of training in influencing the practice behaviors of both men and women. Rather than predicting a future of patient-centered care, we point out some troubling trends regarding the exodus of physicians, both male and female, from primary care settings. Ultimately, gender differences in practice appear strongly tied to differences in the social pressures and structural realities that male and female physicians confront in the everyday practice of medicine.

We begin by examining a basic question: When confronted with the same information, do male and female physicians take the same course of action? Drawing on data from the Community Tracking Study, the analysis examines how physicians respond to six treatment vignettes. We focus our attention on whether differences between male and female physicians emerge in cases involving personal privacy. Turning to the nature of the doctor-patient relationship, we synthesize the findings of numerous studies on gender and communication, empathy, and the duration of office visits. We present our own analysis regarding concerns over the amount of time physicians spend with patients.

Physician Gender and the Treatment of Patients

Although many researchers have examined the connection between gender and physician-patient relationships, there has been much less attention to whether the growing number of women in the profession will influence the administration of specific treatments. The standard medical view is that the sex of a physician does not affect the provision of care to patients. Because physicians are carefully screened and rigorously trained, patients can count on physicians to diagnose, treat, and refer patients as medically indicated regardless of whether they wear shirts or blouses under their medical garb.

Nevertheless, advocates of the "different voice" perspective might suggest that women physicians are more attentive to prevention, more accepting of holistic or alternative medicine, more adept at diagnosing psychosocial problems, and less likely to employ technology-intensive procedures. All of this behavior would stem from women's presumably more nurturing orientation.

Advocates of the discrimination perspective might counter that differences in the treatment offered by male and female physicians stem from differences in the types of environments where male and female physicians work. In particular, the well-documented (Collins et al. 1997) tendency for women to work in managed care environments may contribute to an emphasis on prevention, since studies have linked managed care and preventive medicine (Haas et al. 2002). Consequently, gender differences in practice patterns related to prevention may result from differences between the environments where male and female physicians practice rather than gender per se.

Cohort differences may also contribute to gender differences in practice. Since women's entry into medicine is for the most part a relatively recent phenomenon, women physicians are on average younger than their male counterparts. Thus behaviors that appear to be linked to gender may simply reflect generational shifts in the way medicine is practiced. Generational and regional differences in practice have been well documented (Pai et al. 2000; Detsky 1995; Jacobsen et al.; Barnsley et al. 1999). Researchers have indeed found that women physicians may offer more preventive care because they are younger than their male colleagues, and younger physicians are more oriented toward prevention (Franks and Clancy 1993).

In fact, research on how gender affects actual treatment patterns is much less complete than research on physician gender and communication style. Some studies of gender-neutral conditions suggest that physicians' gender has only a limited influence on the treatment of patients with conditions such as heart disease and diabetes (Case et al. 1999; Rathore et al. 2001; Kim et al. 2005). It even appears that gender does not affect the ability of physicians to diagnose and treat the psychosocial problems of children (Scholle et al. 2001; Bowman and Gehlbach 1980). We refer to all of these conditions as gender neutral because both men and women suffer from them. Although physician gender does not relate to the treatment of heart disease or the tendency to advise patients to quit smoking, there is a significant association between patient gender and access to these treatments. Research suggests that male patients receive consistently more active care regardless of the gender of their physician (Rathore et al. 2001; Young and Ward 1998). The relationship between provider gender and treatment, however, is far from clear simply because too few studies have been done, and some of the available literature focuses on a select nonrepresentative group of medical conditions.

Do women physicians concentrate more time and attention on prevention-related consultation and services? Research on the association between physician gender and gender-neutral screening and preventive services such as cholesterol and blood pressure tests has yielded mixed results (Henderson and Weisman 2001; Flocke and Gilchrist 2005; Cassard et al. 1997; Franks and Bertakis 2003) and suggests at most only a limited advantage for the patients of female physicians in some specialties which centers on their odds of receiving adult immunizations. Similarly, research on counseling and advice for gender-neutral conditions such as weight management or diet counseling has also reached different conclusions (Henderson and Weisman 2001; Franks and Bertakis 2003). Research on counseling against drug use has also produced conflicting results. Some studies find that male physicians spend more time discussing substance abuse with patients (Bertakis et al. 2003), while other studies find the opposite pattern (Frank and Harvey 1996). The fact that gender does not influence preventive care in HMOs (Schmittdiel et al. 2000) raises the possibility that other evidence of gender effects are due to the HMO practice environment rather than gender per se (Flocke and Gilchrist 2005).

Personal Privacy and Gender Concordance

Another possibility is that gender differences are most likely to emerge in the treatment of diseases or conditions that are socially sensitive and explicitly sexual, especially those involving personal privacy. In other words, it has been suggested that male physicians provide higher-quality and more cost-effective care to male patients and that women provide higher-quality and more cost-effective care to female patients. We refer to this idea as a situation of physician-patient gender concordance.

There are at least three possible mechanisms through which gender concordance may influence medical care. These hypotheses are not mutually exclusive. The relationship between gender concordance and gender-specific treatment may depend on the particular scenarios being examined, and multiple factors may contribute to the relationship between gender concordance and gender-specific treatment.

Gender concordance may lead to greater training, familiarity, and confidence. On average, female primary physicians get more experience treating women patients in training, treat more women in practice, and thus are more confident performing female-specific preventive examinations and screenings (Powell et al. 2006; Emmons et al. 2004; Bensing et al. 1993; Orzano and Cody 1995; Britt et al. 1996; Lurie et al. 1998). Concomitantly, research indicates that male primary care physicians appear more confident and experienced providing male-specific preventive screenings (Lurie et al. 1998; Levy et al. 1992). Thus gender differences in confidence and experience may explain why research has consistently shown that primary care providers offer more gender-specific screenings to patients of their own sex (Lurie et al. 1997; Lurie et al. 1998; Flocke and Gilchrist 2005; Andersen and Urban 1997; Franks and Bertakis 2003; Levy et al. 1992). Differences in experience with female patients may also explain the limited evidence suggesting a greater tendency for female than male primary care physicians to treat female urinary incontinence (Sandvik and Hunskaar 1990). Since only one Swedish study correlates provider gender and the treatment of urinary incontinence, this assertion, however, remains tentative.

Gender differences in experience may also explain apparent differences in how male and female general surgeons treat older women with early stage breast cancer. Several studies have found that male surgeons are more likely to recommend a mastectomy, while female surgeons favor lumpectomy and adjuvant therapy for these patients (Mandelblatt et al. 2001; Silliman et al. 1999; Cyran et al. 2001). One possible reason for this relationship could involve gender differences in the tendency to specialize. Research has repeatedly shown that surgeons treating twenty or more breast cancer patients per year are more likely to employ breast-conserving surgery than those who do not specialize in breast cancer (Kotwall et al. 1996). Although systematic data on specialization rates by surgeon gender are not available, some evidence suggests that female general surgeons are more likely to specialize in breast care (Cassell 1998; Yutzie et al. 2005). So it is possible that gender differences in practice stem in part from differences in experience.

An alternative possibility is that gender concordance stems from gendered patient expectations. In other words, situations involving physicians and patients of the same gender may lead to greater patient comfort and trust. For example, Dulmen and Bensing (2000) found that the patients of female gynecologists volunteered more information for which male physicians had to probe. As a result, they observed that female obstetrician-gynecologists actually spent less time with patients, engaged in less facilitative communication, and made fewer expressions of concern than did the male doctors (see Roter et al. 1999 for additional evidence). This finding may stem from greater patient comfort levels in the gender-concordant situation. Research suggests that a sizeable percentage of men and women prefer to see same-sex providers for the treatment of sexually sensitive conditions (Heaton and Marquez 1990; Ivins and Kent 1993).

Finally, gender concordance effects could also result if providers are better able to empathize with patients who have conditions that they themselves can contract and experience. The idea here is that male providers offer higher-quality care to patients suffering from male conditions such as erectile dysfunction because they have a deeper, more emotional understanding of the negative implications of such a condition. And in a similar vein, women can empathize with female patients who have gender-specific problems such as premenstrual dysphoric disorder. In fact gender differences in empathy may contribute to the relation between providers and gender-specific preventive screenings. Some research suggests that female primary care physicians feel greater "personal responsibility" for ensuring that their female patients receive gender-specific screenings such as mammography and Pap tests (Lurie et al. 1998), and evidence also indicates that female obstetrician-gynecologists feel greater responsibility for treating premenstrual dysphoric disorder (Hill et al. 2001).

There is also evidence of male physicians' empathy with their male patients. Researchers find that male physicians trained before 1974 were more likely than either younger men or women physicians of any age to recommend prostate (PSA) screening to male patients of appropriate age (Edlefsen et al. 1999). Consistent with a personal empathy interpretation, older male physicians, those with the highest personal risk of prostate cancer, were most likely to recommend screening for the condition.

While evidence exists to support all three justifications for a gender concordance effect in the provision of gender-specific medical care, it should be noted that none of these theories fully supports the "different voice" perspective. The gender concordance hypothesis suggests that empathy is elicited in specific situations, and favors males in some cases, rather than implying a fixed relationship between gender and empathy.

Physicians' Gender and Treatment Vignettes

We drew on data from the 1996 Community Tracking Study physician survey, a nationally representative sample of adult primary care physicians. The survey included six vignettes of model patients with presentations designed to have multiple appropriate treatment plans. Four of the vignettes involve no major issues of personal privacy.

In the first scenario, a fifty-year-old white male complains of chest pains. After six minutes of exercise during a stress test, the patient shows signs of potential heart problems (specifically, 2 millimeters of ST depression in three of the leads). In these circumstances, should the physician recommend a cardiac referral? The second vignette involves a thirty-five-year-old man who develops back pain after shoveling snow. An office visit reveals a new left-foot drop. The question for the physician is whether further tests (an MRI) would be recommended in this circumstance.

The third model male patient is a sixty-year-old white man with no family history of prostate cancer, who reports no symptoms. Physicians are asked for what percentage of such patients they would recommend a PSA test. The fourth patient, aged fifty, has high cholesterol (cholesterol is 240; LDL is 150; HDL is 50; Total/HDL is 4.8) but no other cardiac risk factors. Should the physician recommend cholesterol-lowering drugs?

In the first explicitly sexual case, a forty-year-old monogamous woman reports vaginal itching and a thick white discharge. She reports no abdominal pain or fever. The question here is whether an office visit to evaluate the patient is in order. The other case involving sexuality is a sixty-year-old white man experiencing bothersome symptoms of benign prostatic hyperplasia (BPH). The question here is whether the patient needs a referral to a urologist.

We distinguish between this final case and case three, the other white sixty-year-old patient with urologic issues, because the patient in case three is not being considered for an explicitly sexual procedure. Whereas the PSA test is a blood test that can be ordered by a physician and administered by a nurse, diagnosis of BPH requires the physician to insert a gloved finger into the patient's rectum to feel the prostate. Table 7.1 describes the vignettes in further detail.

We began our analysis of physicians' proposed treatments for these model patients with a simple comparison of male and female doctors' responses to the vignette questions (see Figure 7.1). In two of the six cases we found no statistically significant differences in the responses of male and female physicians. In particular, there was no difference in how female and

Table 7.1. Summary of Treatment Vignettes

Patient	Chief complaint/condition	Medical history	Treatment: physicians are asked for what percentage of such patients
50-year-old white man	exertional chest pain	No medications. After 6 minutes of exercise, patient develops a key sign of heart disease, 2 millimeters of ST depression in leads II, III and F.	they would recommend a cardiology referral
35-year-old man	back pain	Man developed back pain after shoveling snow. On examination, there is a new left foot drop.	they would recommend an MRI
60-year-old white man	n/a	No family history of prostate cancer and a normal digital rectal exam.	they would recommend a PSA test
50-year-old man	high cholesterol	No other cardiac risk factors. Cholesterol is 240; LDL is 150; HDL is 50; Total/HDL cholesterol = 4.8.	they would recommend cholesterol-lowering agents
40-year-old woman	vaginal discharge	Monogamous married woman has no abdominal pain or fever. Patient has had thick white vaginal discharge for two days.	they would recommend an office visit to evaluate the discharge
60-year-old white man	bothersome BPH symptoms	Man has no evidence of renal compromise or cancer.	they would recommend a urology referral

Source: 1996 Community Tracking Study (CTS) data.

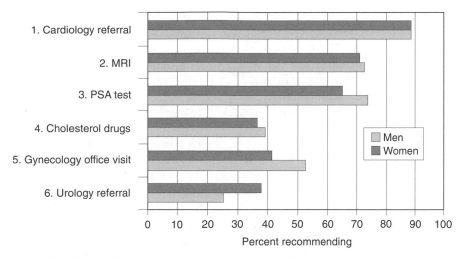

Figure 7.1. Physician Gender and Treatment Outcomes. *Source:* 2004 CTS data.

male physicians reacted to the vignettes involving the cardiology and MRI referrals. Male and female physicians recommended a cardiology referral (88.8 percent and 89.9 percent, respectively) for the fifty-year-old man with exertional chest pain. And male and female physicians recommended an MRI (71.7 percent and 70.3 percent, respectively) for patients with symptoms like those in the fifth vignette, the thirty-five-year-old man with back pain and left foot drop. Neither of these differences was statistically significant.

By contrast, for the two vignettes involving preventive tests, we found a tendency for male physicians to pursue a more active path of treatment. In both of these cases, however, the apparent gender disparities were due to differences in practice settings or physicians' attributes other than gender per se. Before any controls were included in the analysis, we found that male physicians were more likely to recommend the PSA test for prostate cancer, 73.1 percent versus 64.4 percent for female physicians. Similarly, male physicians were slightly more likely to recommend cholesterol-lowering agents for the fifty-year-old man with no other cardiac risk factors (39.4 percent versus 36.4 percent). Nevertheless, both of these apparent gender disparities were erased when other factors were taken into account.[1] We found that the entire gender difference in the tendency to offer a PSA test and to prescribe cholesterol-lowering drugs was attributable to differences in physicians' personal characteristics such as age.

We also found gender disparities in the treatments prescribed in the two vignettes pertaining to sexually sensitive issues. In both cases, treatments are apparently more active or aggressive when the patient is of the opposite sex rather than in gender-concordant situations. Male physicians were more likely to recommend an office visit for the forty-year-old woman with a vaginal discharge (52.7 percent versus 40.6 percent). Similarly, female physicians were more likely to recommend a urology consult for the sixty-year-old man with symptoms of BPH (37.5 percent versus 24.9 percent). Unlike the differences in administration of the PSA test and the anti-cholesterol drugs, differences in treatment for BPH and vaginal discharge are not fully explainable by available covariates.

Thus it is not a matter of male physicians consistently being more aggressive in their approach to treatment or more likely to refer patients for a visit or a referral. And it does not appear that the disproportionate tendency for women to work in certain types of environments accounts for this particular gender differential. Rather there seem to be differences that pertain to gender-specific conditions. Female physicians are more aggressive in pursuing a referral for the condition affecting men's private areas, while male physicians are more aggressive in soliciting an office visit for conditions affecting women's private areas. These results suggest that gender differences in experience rather than gender differences in empathy are influencing care. If gender-concordant empathy were the motivating factor, women physicians should treat women more actively and men physicians should treat men more actively, when in practice, we see the reverse scenario.

It may be that doctors are more likely to solicit additional information under conditions of uncertainty. Previous research indicates that physicians use more resources if they are uncertain (Davis et al. 2000). If physicians feel less certain about how best to treat these opposite-sex conditions, then this might explain their increased likelihood of pursuing additional information. These results cast doubt on the premise that men and women treat same-sex conditions differently because they are inherently more interested in patients who share their gender.

We used available covariates to attempt to explain gender differences in treatment. As the results in Appendix Table 4 indicate, we could explain only one third of the gender difference in treatment of the fifth hypothetical patient, the otherwise healthy, monogamous forty-year-old female complaining of a white vaginal discharge.[2] Virtually all of the explainable portion of the gender difference in treatment of vaginal discharge is attributable to the younger age and more limited experience of women physicians. Specifically, nearly 4 percent of the 10.4 percent gender difference in the tendency to request an office visit is attributable to the fact that female physicians are younger and/or less experienced. (We cannot separate age and experience in this analysis since the younger physicians are almost uniformly less experienced.) The gender disparity regarding the urology consultation was even more resilient in the face of control variables. In other words, most of the female advantage in urology referrals remained even after practice location and other physicians' attributes were taken into account.

Thus male physicians may be more inclined to recommend an office visit for women with vaginal itching because they are less confident diagnosing and treating female-specific conditions by phone. The two most common possible diagnoses for the model female patient with white vaginal discharge would be yeast infection and gonorrhea. Male physicians may also be less confident in women's abilities to treat themselves or less willing to trust women's accounts of their sexual history and therefore less willing to forgo a gonorrhea test. Furthermore, male physicians may be more distrustful of women's partners, and may suspect that the model patient has gonorrhea as a result of male infidelity. Similarly, female providers may be more likely to refer patients with the prostate condition (BPH) because they are less experienced and less confident in performing rectal examinations on men. They may also refer patients because they believe that their older male patients might prefer to be treated by a male provider. In both cases the persistence of gender as a factor in treatment can be directly related at least in part to other factors rather than to essential differences between male and female physicians in interest or treatment. The disproportionate training that male and female primary care physicians receive in treating patients of their own sex leads them to have more confidence with these populations.

Our findings were limited by our inability to assess several factors that include but are not limited to specific, detailed characteristics of physicians' training; the exact profiles of physicians' patient panels; and the extent to which physicians come to know their patients over time. The study is also limited by its focus on vignettes rather than actual practice patterns. Furthermore, we were limited in our capacity to investigate the role of provider gender on treatment of gender-neutral conditions because we did not examine reactions to model patients of both sexes with equivalent gender-neutral presentations.

Nevertheless, collectively our analyses suggest that existing gender differences in practice stem largely from differences in the experiences of male and female physicians during training and practice. These results raise questions for medical educators about whether and how to ameliorate gender differences in access to hands-on medical education. Our results are largely at odds with the gender-specific empathy thesis, since the patterns are directly opposite to the predictions of this hypothesis. Of course, it may be that gender-specific empathy does occur in some cases. The evidence presented here suggests, however, that other factors, such as familiarity and uncertainty, are likely to be as powerful, if not more powerful, in many circumstances. Further research is necessary to flesh out more fully the types of situations that might elicit empathy effects.

Empathy and Communication with Patients

There is an extensive research literature suggesting that women physicians employ a more humane approach to patients. Women physicians appear to have stronger empathic skills in dealing with patients. In particular, four aspects of the doctor-patient relationship have received close attention (Roter and Hall 1998 and 2004).

First, female physicians use more partnership statements in their routine communication, thereby encouraging the patient to take a more active role (Hall et al. 1994; Roter and Hall 1998, 2004). Soliciting opinions as well as checking for understanding and listening attentively exemplify partnership building (Roter and Hall 1998, 2004). Research indicates that such behaviors encourage patient assertiveness, which in turn causes physicians to offer more medical-related information (Street et al. 2005). Second, women physicians are more likely to consult a colleague or a reference book during a visit and are therefore less protective of their professional status (Shapiro and Schiermer 1990; Roter and Hall 1998). Third, female physicians tend to be less verbally dominant than male physicians. Female physicians talk more than male physicians, but their patients talk more as well, so the ratio of physician to patient statements is more equal in the visits of female physicians (Roter and Hall 1998; Roter et al. 1991). Fourth, female physicians do more probing of issues of a psychosocial nature and provide more psychosocial counseling (Roter and Hall 2004; Riska 2001, 88). Researchers also find that female physicians tended to communicate higher degrees of empathy in response to opportunities created by patients (Bylund and Makoul 2002; Street 2002).

Moreover, the empathy and collegiality offered by female physicians are not reserved for female patients. Women primary care physicians use a more participatory approach regardless of patients' gender (Cooper-Patrick et al. 1999), although some evidence suggests that the most collegial relationships are between female primary care physicians and female patients (Roter and Hall 2004). As we discussed earlier, however, interactions with gynecologists do not follow this trend.

Does empathy translate into greater patient satisfaction? Overall, research on physician gender and patient satisfaction yields conflicting results (Roter and Hall 2004). One study indicates that patients of female physicians are more satisfied (Bertakis et al. 2003), while another suggests that, among HMO patients who choose their physicians, female patients choosing female doctors are the least satisfied and male patients choosing female doctors are the most satisfied (Schmittdiel et al. 2000). And some evidence suggests a youth and gender interaction such that patients of young female physicians are the least satisfied (Hall et al. 1994). A study of patients in the emergency department indicates that female patients are more satisfied if they are cared for by female physicians but that male satisfaction is not affected by provider gender (Derose et al. 2001). Our summary, then, is that the female advantage in collegiality is more clearly supported by the research than is any female physician advantage in patient satisfaction.

A More Empathetic Profession?

Studies in various countries across the industrialized world suggest that women doctors exhibit more "humane" behavior with patients than do their male peers (Riska 2001). Thus one might expect that as the number of women in practice grows, the use of empathy in practice will grow as well. In this scenario the feminization of medicine would deemphasize the scientific authority historically associated with male physicians and highlight instead a collaborative approach to healing illness.

Those who suggest that the increasing presence of women in medicine will result in reforms in overall professional practice often base their claim on this substantial body of research. The most important idea here is that as the likelihood of having a female provider increases, the odds of receiving more humane care will also grow. An even more optimistic projection is that the growing presence of women in medicine will encourage men to adopt a more humane approach to patient relations both by changing patients' expectations (male physicians will have to keep up with their competition) and by providing more caring role models for both male and female medical students.

We are frankly skeptical about this rosy scenario. We believe that the implications of this research for the practice of medicine are much more limited than current debates suggest. We maintain that physician empathy and communication style are primarily determined by social forces such as educational experiences and daily interactions with patients and colleagues rather than by fixed, biologically determined characteristics. We also suggest that independent changes in the structure of medicine are constraining the ability of physicians to provide patient-focused care regardless of their personal desires and proclivities.

Although the research on physician gender and empathy is largely consistent, its implications for practice and the structure of the medical profession are less clear. To begin with, even researchers who have extensively investigated the communicative performance of men and women acknowledge that gender differences, while apparent, are small in magnitude, and that male and female clinicians are generally more similar than different in their communication with patients (Street 2002).

Moreover, although women physicians employ a more collegial approach than men and feel slightly more empathy toward patients, physicians of both genders are lacking in communication skills (Wissow et al. 2005; Levinson et al. 2000). In a study of the capacity of primary care physicians and surgeons, Levinson and colleagues (2000) found that all physicians, regardless of gender or specialty, scored low in their ability to recognize and respond to cues from patients.

Another large body of research literature indicates that both physician empathy and physician communication respond to educational and social interventions. For example, Alexander and colleagues (2006) found that a short, intensive communication course can improve residents' skills involving end-of-life patients. Similarly, Roth and colleagues (2002) found that a series of videotaped interactions between residents and standardized patients could be used to enhance residents' communication skills. Some research also indicates that the effects of well-designed communication skills programs are long lasting (Roter et al. 1995).[3] Collectively these studies suggest that the focus on essential gender differences in communication is clinically inappropriate and politically misleading. A greater emphasis on communication skills during medical training could improve relationships with their patients for all physicians and would further reduce the small differences observed between male and female doctors.

Another contributing factor that is not often addressed by researchers is the gendered expectations of patients. Previous studies suggest that patients generally believe that female physicians are less likely to use aggressive communication strategies (commands, directives, negative opinions, controlling behaviors) than are male physicians (Burgoon et al. 1991). This expectation may explain why both male and female patients tend to talk more, reveal more psychosocial information, ask more questions, and are more involved in the decision-making process when interacting with female health care providers (Hall et al. 1994; Roter et al. 1991; Street 2002; Roter and Hall 2004). Differences in patient expectations may explain why the patients of female physicians are not necessarily more satisfied with the more collegial and empathetic care that they receive.

And finally, the optimistic vision of feminine-inspired patient-centered medicine must be squared with a series of changes to American medicine, including increasing pressures on physicians to maximize efficiency and productivity and the flight from primary care that worries many leaders in the medical profession today. As we have suggested throughout the book, the implication of women's increasing presence in medicine needs to be understood in the context of other changes in the U.S. health care system.

As we discussed in chapter 2, physicians increasingly find themselves having to cope with declining reimbursements. There is increasing pressure to limit the time spent per patient so that they can see more patients every hour and maintain their incomes. At the same time, the heightened use of clinical protocols has increased expectations for each individual visit. Today, physicians are expected to address an ever increasing list of concerns every time they encounter their patients (Mechanic 2003). While little research exists on long term changes in communication during clinical encounters in the United States, one recent study examined this topic among Dutch family practitioners in 1986 and 2002. In their analysis, Bensing and colleagues (2006) confirmed that primary care encounters in the Netherlands have not become more collegial and communicative. In fact, consultations in 2002 were more task oriented and businesslike than sixteen years earlier (Bensing et al. 2006). As we note in chapter 3, in 2004 women made up a 38.4 percent of the medical profession in the Netherlands. In short, the feminization of medicine in the Netherlands was by itself insufficient to generate a more empathetic profession.

Recent research has documented a dramatic decline in the tendency for American-born graduates of U.S. allopathic medical schools to pursue careers in primary care medicine (Lambert and Holomboe 2005; Kirk 2006). The declines are evident among both male and female medical students. Increases in attrition out of primary care fields through both career changes and accelerated retirement have also been documented (Kirk 2006). As we discuss in more detail in the conclusion of the book, this trend has raised the question whether primary care will continue to be provided by physicians, or whether other medical professionals such as nurse practitioners and physicians' assistants will become the most common point of first contact for patients seeking treatment.

In the meantime, the flight from primary care is leading to significant increases in the absolute and relative presence of foreign medical graduates among U.S. primary care physicians, especially those in adult medicine. In 2007 only 57 percent of those who matched into internal medicine residency programs were seniors at U.S. medical schools (National Resident Matching Program 2007b). And research on international medical graduates indicates that the representation of native English speakers in this population is declining (Whelan et al. 2002). In particular, in 1999, 39 percent of all international medical graduates seeking certification to practice in the United States were native English speakers. By 2001 that number had declined to 22 percent (Whelan et al. 2002). The communication patterns of foreign medical graduates have not been well researched. Nevertheless, it is reasonable to suspect that country of origin and language of preference will influence both male and female physicians' approach to patients. In addition, there is an increasing disconnect between the country of origin and language of preference for physicians and for patients. On the one hand, physicians are increasingly likely to come from Asia. As recently as 2001, 26 percent of all international medical graduates seeking permission to practice in the United States were from India or Pakistan (Whelan et al. 2002). On the other hand, patients, especially pediatric patients, are increasingly likely to be of Hispanic origin. These two trends should exacerbate communication problems, especially in pediatrics, the field in which women are most likely to practice.

As the representation of foreign physicians grows in the country's primary care physician workforce, so too do the demands on these practitioners. Research indicates that physicians perceive increasing pressures to see more patients in less time and that expectations surrounding the content and tenor of patient visits have expanded (Mechanic 2003). Further evidence indicates that foreign physicians are most likely to practice in poor areas and to treat disenfranchised patients, whose needs for clear communication are most pronounced (McMahon 2004). Thus foreign physicians whose language of preference is not English are increasingly facing a double burden when attempting to establish quality relationships with their patients.

Although the literature on gender and the physician-patient relationship is consistent, it focuses disproportionately on primary care. In fact, one study on the link between communication and malpractice indicates that communication is linked to the odds of a lawsuit only for primary care physicians (Levinson et al. 1997). That is, the expectation that empathy should increase patient satisfaction and thus reduce the risk of lawsuits appears not to be borne out in the case of specialists. Furthermore, as mentioned earlier, many young women physicians, who might have chosen to pursue primary care in previous generations, are entering fields that do not take advantage of women's ostensibly unique capacity for communication, fields such as radiology, ophthalmology, anesthesiology, and dermatology (Lambert and Holomboe 2005).

Collectively this literature suggests that U.S.-born women probably will have an effect on the provision of health care by enhancing the doctor-patient relationship, but the extent of this effect will likely be more limited than many have suggested. Furthermore, these studies do not imply that such differences stem from biological differences between male and female providers. Finally, research indicates that with adequate intervention, gender differences may be eliminated and the communication skills of all physicians may be improved.

Physician Gender and Concerns about Time

We empirically examined physicians' concerns with the time allowed for patients during office visits because office visits are a critical facet of health care. They not only constitute the primary environment for the delivery of therapeutic health services but also offer key opportunities to build constructive and trusting provider-patient relationships. Under optimal conditions, clinicians can use office visits not simply to cure biomedical pathology but also to provide critical preventive and screening services, encourage healthful behavior, address psychosocial problems, offer basic health education, and ultimately avoid high-cost acute-care services.

Although office visits have great potential, providers cannot utilize them fully if they are curtailed prematurely or inappropriately limited. In other words, rushed office visits can reduce providers' capacity to provide high-quality health care. To begin with, limiting visits restricts the capacity of providers to offer a full menu of services. For example, Blumenthal and Chang (1999) found that, while the average U.S. adult primary care visit during 1991 and 1992 lasted sixteen minutes, visits that included three or more preventive screening tests lasted an average of twenty minutes, or 25 percent longer. Similarly, in a study of British general practitioners, Morrell et al. (1986) found that compared to physicians using consultations of seven and a half or ten minutes, doctors using five-minute consultation intervals identified fewer problems and were significantly less likely to record patients' blood pressure.

The rising demands of insurance companies and quality control agencies, along with the growing expectations of patients (Mechanic 2003), are making it increasingly difficult for physicians of both genders to provide humane care. There is a well-established negative relationship between professional satisfaction and certain facets of managed care. In particular, physicians in HMO practice and primary care physicians who must serve as gatekeepers feel significantly more time pressure and less career satisfaction than their colleagues in other forms of practice (Linzer et al. 2000; Sturm 2002). Evidence suggests that women primary care physicians feel an especially high degree of time pressure and experience a greater risk of burnout (McMurray et al. 2000), and this gap stems in large part from the structure of the practices in which women physicians tend to work. In fact, research indicates that women primary care physicians are allotted less time for new-patient examinations than their male counterparts (McMurray et al. 2000). In particular, female physicians reported being allotted thirty-three minutes for a new patient evaluation or consultation compared with thirty-seven minutes reported by male physicians. Female and male physicians were, for the most part, allotted equal amounts of time for routine follow-up appointments. Nevertheless, since female physicians reported treating more female patients and more patients with complex psychosocial problems than their male colleagues, though the same numbers of patients with complex medical problems, their need for time with patients was presumably greater. Not surprisingly, time pressure in ambulatory settings was more intense for women, who on average reported needing 36 percent more time than allotted to provide quality care for new patients or consultations, compared with 21 percent more time needed by men (McMurray et al. 2000). Thus, even if women physicians have a "natural" tendency to offer more collegial and/or empathic care, the evolving nature of the American health care system may prevent them from acting on this tendency, further limiting gender differences in practice.

We turned once again to the CTS data to assess physicians' attitudes about the time allotted to their patients. We found that although most doctors reported being either somewhat or strongly satisfied with the amount of time they spend with their patients, a significant minority indicated moderate or low satisfaction. Furthermore, male and female physicians differed notably in their degree of satisfaction. Among primary care physicians, 36.7 percent of women but only 27.3 percent of men were somewhat or strongly concerned about their time for patients (see Figure 7.2).

On its face, this evidence appears to support the notion that women are more committed to spending time with their patients. A closer examination reveals, however, that male and female physicians are seeing different types of patients. For example, among primary care physicians, we found that women providers were more likely to report that their patients' conditions were "complex" (41.7 percent for women versus 28.1 percent for men).[4] We also found that female primary care providers served as gatekeepers for a significantly larger proportion of their patient panels than did their male colleagues. Among specialists we found equally compelling differences. Here again what may at first appear to be a "natural" difference between men and women turns out to reflect, at least in part, the different circumstances that male and female physicians find themselves in.

We discovered a similar pattern among specialists. One third of female specialists (33.1 percent), versus one quarter of their male counterparts (24.4), expressed dissatisfaction with the amount of time they spend with patients. Here again, female physicians were more likely to indicate that the

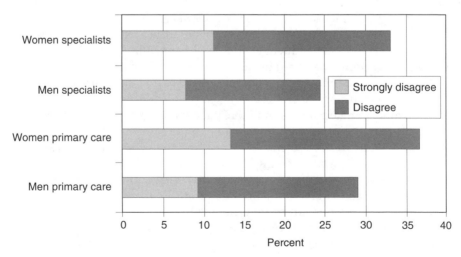

Figure 7.2. Physician Gender and Concerns Regarding Time with Patients. *Source:* 2004 CTS Survey.

complexity of patients' conditions on referral has increased over time and that the number of referrals they accrue has also grown.

We used multivariate regression models to estimate the difference in satisfaction with time for patients as measured on a five-point scale. Then we conducted parallel analyses of specialists and primary care physicians in order to assess how distinct practice pressures are influencing physicians' concerns about time for patients. (See Appendix Table 5 for a summary of the results, which consider primary care physicians and specialists separately.)[5]

Our results suggest that when female gender is the sole determinant of satisfaction with time for patients, there is a 0.29 point gap between female and male satisfaction among primary care physicians on a five-point scale. Physician characteristics explain a modest portion (14 percent) of this gap. Most of this decline is attributable to gender differences in physicians' age and years of work experience. Younger physicians are more likely to express these concerns, and women physicians are younger and less experienced on average than their male counterparts. Practice characteristics such as the percentage of revenue earned from managed care and the size of a practice explain only a small fraction of the gender gap (about 3 percent). The addition of community characteristics does not explain any of the primary care physician (PCP) gender gap in satisfaction with time for patients. Finally, in Model 5 we add physicians' assessments of patient panels. The addition of these variables, such as whether a physician must act as a gatekeeper and whether the physician feels that he or she must care for patients whose problems are inappropriately complex, narrows the gender gap another 16 percent to 0.19 point. Thus, taken together, physician characteristics, practice characteristics, community characteristics, and perceptions of patients account for approximately one third of the gender gap in satisfaction with time for patients among primary care physicians.

Our analysis of specialist physicians is more successful in explaining the gender gap in concern over time with patients. Female specialists are on average 0.26 of a point less satisfied with their time for patients than their male colleagues. Physician characteristics, including age, board certification, foreign medical graduate status, specialty, and work habits, account for 26 percent of the gender gap among specialists. Physician practice characteristics such as whether the practice is a solo, group, or HMO practice, and the amount of revenues earned from Medicare, Medicaid, and managed care, further narrow the gender gap among specialists an additional 19 percent to 0.14. Acknowledging community and geographic characteristics such as the number of people living in poverty and the population density of the area cause the gap to decline an additional 4 percent to 0.13. Finally, when we control for specialists' assessments of patients such as the complexity of their conditions at the time of referral, the gender gap declines to 0.09 and becomes statistically insignificant. Thus, among specialist physicians, practice, community, and patient characteristics explain the entire gender gap in satisfaction with their amount of time for patients.

Overall we find that women physicians are less satisfied than their male colleagues with their time for patients. Much of this difference, however, is attributable to differences in the personal characteristics of male and female physicians and differences in their practice locations. We also find that the satisfaction of female specialists and primary care practitioners with time for patients is disproportionately affected by practice conditions that limit physicians' capacity to provide holistic primary care services and force physicians to treat patients with increasingly complex medical conditions. We are able to explain the gender gap among specialists by statistically controlling for these factors. Still, we can account for only one third of the gender gap among primary care physicians.

We suspect that much if not all of the remaining gap in concerns about time stem from systematic differences in the types of patients seen by male and female primary care providers. As we noted earlier, female physicians see patients from different backgrounds and with different presentations from those seen by their male counterparts. As discussed earlier, research by McMurray and colleagues (2000) indicates that female primary care physicians routinely see patients with more complex psychosocial issues and equivalent numbers of patients with complex medical issues. Furthermore, as we suggested in chapter 1, research shows that a large proportion of the time differential between male and female primary care physicians stems from the fact that women physicians see more women patients, and women need time-consuming pelvic exams (Franks and Bertakis 2003). Much of the unexplainable gender gap in concern for time with patients is probably due to these factors, which remain uncontrolled in this analysis.

These results offer mixed support with regard to the hypothesis that women's unique nurturing tendencies are driving either their professional practice patterns or their professional concerns. There is an observable gender gap in concern for time with patients in the population of practicing physicians. But there is no gender gap among specialists once other relevant factors are taken into account, although much of the gender gap remains among primary care physicians. Most of the gap in concerns about time with patients is therefore clearly not explained by gender differences in nurturing. We suspect that the remaining unexplained gap among primary care physicians is also attributable to practice settings and patient attributes rather than essential gender differences in caring.

In this chapter we have examined the relationship between the provider's gender and the quality of health care. We began with a discussion of how gender relates to treatment patterns. Then we discussed the relationship between physicians' gender and their approach to patients. Finally, we examined how gender relates to concerns with time for seeing patients. The available evidence generally supports the view that, in most cases, treatment patterns do not appear to be affected by a physician's gender. Nevertheless, we demonstrate that there are some situations in which the provider's gender does appear to influence treatment. These special cases generally involve sexually sensitive conditions affecting personal privacy.

We offer multiple possible explanations for the observed relationships between the treatment of sexually sensitive conditions and provider gender, including differences in the experience and competences of male and female physicians, differences in the expectations that patients of both genders have for their physicians, and a tendency for male and female physicians to empathize more with patients of the same sex.

Our analysis of the 1996 Community Tracking Study physician survey corroborates the existence of a relationship between provider gender and treatment for sexually sensitive care. We attribute this gender effect to differences in how male and female physicians are trained and to their experience in and comfort with treating the sexually sensitive conditions of patients of the other sex. Overall, physicians are less aggressive in treating patients who share their gender. We suggest that this reflects greater familiarity and higher comfort levels on the part of physicians treating gender-concordant patients with sexually sensitive conditions. These results raise critical questions for medical educators about how to improve the training of medical students in matters surrounding patient sexuality.

This chapter also challenges the prevailing wisdom regarding physician gender and provider-patient relationships. While researchers have identified a small gender gap in empathy and communication skills, we emphasize that the gap is substantively small and has limited implications for practice. We suggest that the difference is best understood in a wider context. In particular, we highlight research indicating that both male and female physicians possess weak communication skills and that such skills can be acquired and enhanced through formal education. These studies imply that efforts should be made to improve the communication skills of all practitioners rather than focusing on the small differences between male and female physicians.

Most important, we wonder if the small differences in communication style between male and female physicians will ultimately affect the quality of patient care. As we suggest, the tremendous changes in the health care industry are limiting the numbers of young, domestically trained women physicians pursuing primary care, so in the absence of change, the women physicians who are most likely to possess superior communication skills will be less and less likely to practice in the fields where communication is most critical. At the same time, as a result of a heightened focus on productivity, those women physicians who do pursue primary care will be increasingly less able to provide the effective communication and empathy of which they are capable. Ultimately, the presence of women physicians should enhance communication, but because of structural changes, this effect should be limited. Ideally, reforms in the medical profession will further enhance the communication skills of both male and female physicians.

The final section of this chapter examined gender differences regarding concerns with time for patients. We used data from the CTS physician survey to assess how physicians' gender relates to perceptions of time with patients. Our results suggest that although women physicians are less satisfied with their time for patients, much of this difference is attributable to factors other than gender per se. In particular, the younger average age of female physicians explains much of the gender gap, because regardless of gender, younger physicians express these concerns more readily. In fact, all of the gender gap in concerns about time for patients among specialists stems from gender differences in age and gender differences in the practice settings where physicians work. While much of the gap among primary care physicians remains unexplained, we suspect that this residual difference stems from structural and social factors that we were unable to measure, such as differences in the characteristics of male and female physicians' patients. Ultimately these results cast significant doubt on the premise that women's disproportionate concerns about time for patients stem from their inherently greater tendency to nurture and care for their patients.

Taken in concert, these analyses suggest that although differences in practice styles between male and female physicians exist, their effects on patient care should be very limited. Social and structural factors will ultimately restrict such gender-linked differences. Ideally, interventions will be designed to ameliorate all physicians' weaknesses so that the highest quality of care can be provided consistently.

8

Medicine as a
Family-Friendly Profession?

Many have suggested that as the presence of women in medicine increases, the prevalence of family-friendly working conditions will also grow. For example, Levinson and Lurie maintain that "women are changing the profession itself. The effects can be seen in the work-family balance" (Levinson and Lurie 2004, 472; see also Croasdale 2002; Croasdale 2004b; and Wardrop 2004).

As we saw in chapter 6, women physicians remain unlikely to have stay-at-home husbands. As a result, these women rarely have the kind of family support system that allows some male physicians to work seventy or eighty hours per week. This type of single-minded devotion to a career is more challenging when both partners in a marriage are working full-time and are committed to their demanding careers. An exclusive focus on work can be even more challenging with the arrival of children. Consequently the time demands of their family lives are likely to lead many women physicians to be interested in opportunities that allow them to dovetail their professional goals with their personal lives. As the number of women in medicine increases, it is reasonable to expect an increase in interest in family-friendly career options.

Has the medical profession, which has historically presumed exceptionally high levels of professional commitment, been responsive? There is some evidence of change. There has been growth in the number of hospitals with maternity leave policies, and in the percentage of physicians working part-time. In particular, results from AAMC surveys conducted in 1989 and 1994 indicated that the number of teaching hospitals with specified maternity leave policies increased from 52 to 77 percent in that five-year period (Philibert and Bickel 1995). Furthermore, evidence from a survey conducted by the American Academy of Pediatrics indicates that the proportion of practicing pediatricians who defined their position as part-time increased from 11 percent in 1993 to 15 percent in 2000 (Cull et al. 2002). There is also increasing attention to the need for formalized reentry programs for physicians who take time off from medical work.[1]

In spite of the positive trends, we question the extent to which a family-friendly ethos has permeated the medical profession. In fact the medical profession has not evolved as much as the popular and medical press suggests. Changes are clearly occurring, but they are not keeping pace with the growth in the number of women physicians or the overall growth in demand for work-family balance. Furthermore, in certain instances, such as the flexible tenure clock, the ultimate meaning of the changes that have occurred is questionable. Moreover, the relative absence of reform in the medical profession does not stem from a lack of demand. Evidence from our research and others' suggests that physicians of both genders are overworked. It also indicates that those who work reduced hours have higher professional satisfaction.

Individual women and men are seeking a more meaningful work-family balance for themselves, but their ultimate capacity to create more manageable schedules is restricted by powerful countervailing pressures. These forces are evident at the macro-level environment and also in individual, or micro-level, decision making. That is, they permeate the broader institutional context of the profession, and they also operate through the cost-benefit calculus of individual physicians. Pressures from physicians' work environment, such as the need to pay for malpractice insurance and to meet productivity expectations, greatly limit opportunities for individual physicians and medical institutions to create work-family balance. Concerns such as mounting educational debt also deter many physicians from taking advantage of flexible schedules when they are available. In other words, reforms to date have fallen short because individuals' capacity to pursue family-friendly options are constrained.

At the same time, we suggest that many of the family-friendly reforms that are occurring in medicine stem from institutional developments that have little if anything to do with the representation of women in American medicine. One of the most obvious examples of such a change involves the relatively recent restrictions on resident work hours (Stanton 2007; Woodrow et al. 2006).

Family-friendly reforms in the medical profession have, by and large, not resulted from significant organized efforts by physicians of either gender to reform their workplace. Although the number of organizations designed to represent female physicians is growing, to date these groups have not pushed an aggressive agenda of family-friendly institutional reforms.

Policymakers and medical organizations are certainly aware of the increasing representation of women in the medical workforce, and many speculate about how women will change the profession.[2] Nonetheless, relatively few women in the medical community or elsewhere are actively lobbying to increase the family-friendly aspects of work environments for physicians, such as available child care.

Furthermore, family-friendly initiatives remain concentrated in a few corners of the profession. For example, primary care settings have made greater strides than other specialties, most notably surgery. These disparities reflect not only the number of women in a particular specialty or work environment but also broader institutional forces. If a unified group of female physicians mobilized around issues of changing the medical workplace, the medical profession could rapidly evolve in a much more family-friendly direction.

In this chapter we compare trends in part-time employment with interest in this type of flexible career option. We find that there is a sizable gap between interest in part-time work arrangements and the availability of part-time opportunities. Many physicians express interest in reducing their work schedules, while the extent of part-time work is not increasingly rapidly. We explore the reasons for this mismatch.

We ask how women and men in the medical profession are balancing their work and family life in light of their surprisingly unresponsive workplace. For the overwhelming majority of women physicians, the answer does not appear to involve either a rejection of parenting or a rejection of the medical workplace. Instead an increasing number of women and men in medicine are attempting to combine parenting with highly demanding professional commitments and inevitably enduring the stress that accompanies such a challenging and fast-paced lifestyle.

The Medical Workweek: Kinder and Gentler or Crazier Than Ever?

As we saw in chapter 6, although the data indicate that women physicians work less time on average than their male peers, they still typically work well in excess of forty hours in an average week, regardless of their personal status. The gender gap in the workweek exists only because male physicians work extremely long hours.

It may be useful to examine trends in the extremes of work schedules, not just the average. For example, Jacobs and Gerson (2004) show that while the average workweek in the United States has not changed substantially since the 1970s, more individuals are putting in long workweeks (50 hours or more). In recent years, professionals and managers have logged the longest workweeks.

Female physicians are more likely to log 50 hours per week on their jobs than was the case in 1980, while rates of long weeks have inched up for men as well. In 2000, over two thirds of male physicians (69 percent) reported working 50 or more hours per week, up slightly from 64 percent in 1980. Among female physicians, over half (52 percent) worked 50 or more hours per week in 2000, up from 38 percent in 1980. Thus the increased representation of women in the profession has not resulted in a general shift toward more limited work schedules. Rather, both men and women in medicine have a high likelihood of working a long week.[3]

At the other end of the spectrum, the fraction of physicians working part-time should be revealing as well. Although many believe that the part-time medical workforce is growing in the United States (Croasdale 2002 and 2004b), our findings from the U.S. Census suggest otherwise. In fact, census data suggest that rates of part-time work of 30 hours or less per week for women decreased slightly, from 18 to 15 percent, between 1980 and 2000. In contrast to the 15 percent of female physicians who worked part-time in 2000, only 6 percent of male physicians worked part-time, about the same as in 1980.[4] Clearly the vast majority of female physicians have been unable or unwilling to pursue part-time schedules.

Part-time employment is actually less common than it was during the 1970s, when few physicians were women. In 1970, 20 percent of women physicians worked fewer than 35 hours per week. Even more recent research on pediatricians indicates that although the absolute numbers of women pediatricians working part-time increased during the 1990s, between 1993 and 2000 there was no change in the tendency for women pediatricians to work part-time. Furthermore, growth in the percentage of pediatricians working reduced schedules stems entirely from growth in the representation of women in the specialty (Cull et al. 2002).[5]

Opportunities to pursue part-time work vary by specialty. Indeed, the growth in part-time schedules has been particularly evident in a few specialties. We compared data from the 1996 and 2004 Community Tracking Study Physician Surveys and found that in 1996, the percent of women working thirty or fewer hours in an average week varied from a high of 23 percent in psychiatry to a low of 6 percent in surgery. In 2004, the range was considerably greater, with a high of 34 percent in psychiatry to a low of 2 percent in surgery. In other words, between 1996 and 2004, the tendency for women psychiatrists to work part time increased by 11 percent while the tendency for women surgeons to work part time declined.

There is a similar although not as extreme variation in the tendency for men to work reduced schedules. According to our analysis of the CTS, in 1996, the tendency for men to work thirty or fewer hours ranged from a high of 6.8 percent in psychiatry to a low of 3.4 percent in surgery. In 2000, the tendency for men to work reduced schedules ranged from a high of 11.3 percent in psychiatry to a low of 3.7 percent in general internal medicine.

The relatively large increases in the percent of male and female psychiatrists working part time between 1996 and 2004 suggests that trends in part-time work among psychiatrists do not simply involve women's disproportionate desire for part-time work. Instead, it appears as if independent structural changes to the profession have increased the opportunity for reduced schedules. In fact, recent research suggests that over time psychiatrists are increasing the percent of direct patient care hours spent in publicly funded environments (Ranz et al. 2006). In particular, Ranz and colleagues found that between 1996 and 2002, the percent of direct patient care psychiatry hours in publicly funded settings increased from 40 to 50 percent for young psychiatrists and from 29 to 44 percent for mid-career psychiatrists. In 2002, the percent of direct patient care hours in publicly funded settings was higher than the percent in solo office practice. Since publicly funded settings are larger, such institutions are better equipped to absorb fixed costs like malpractice and offer part-time options. Regardless of its causes, however, it is important to recognize that only a small minority of physicians, 5 percent of men and 7 percent of women, practice psychiatry.

Over the last several decades the work effort of female physicians has come to resemble more closely the work effort of men who share their household composition. This trend is most pronounced for physicians over fifty. The trend toward parity, however, does not imply a trend toward greater work-family balance. The average work effort of female physicians is increasing, while the average workweek of male physicians has remained relatively constant at a very high level. Ultimately the trend is toward *less* work-family balance rather than more. This increase in work effort may signal increasing pressures on female physicians with regard to their lives outside of work.[6]

How do conditions in the medical profession compare to conditions in other occupations? While all employed non-resident male physicians worked an average of 52 hours per week, employed men overall work only 43.1 hours per week, and employed men in managerial and professional occupations work 45.6 hours per week (Jacobs and Gerson 2004, 34). The comparable numbers for employed women are 47 hours for women physicians, 37.1 hours for women overall, and 39.4 hours for women in managerial and professional occupations (Jacobs and Gerson 2004, 34).

Furthermore, in 2000, only 26.5 percent of all male workers reported more than 50 hours in their average workweek. The comparable number for all male professional, managerial, and technical workers was 37.2 percent. Since 64 percent of male physicians work at least 50 hours, on average male physicians are 1.7 times more likely than men in elite occupations overall to work long weeks.

Only 11.3 percent of the female workforce overall worked 50 or more hours. The comparable number for women in managerial, technical, and professional occupations was 17.1 percent in 2000. Since 48 percent of female physicians worked at least 50 hours, in 2000 employed women physicians were 2.8 times more likely to work a long week than other women employed in elite occupations. Even married physician mothers were 2.5 times more likely to work a long week than their female peers in other elite occupations.

Analysis of the 2000 Current Population Survey indicates, however, that rates of part-time work in medicine are not too different from rates in other elite occupations. In 2000, 14.8 percent of women and 5.8 percent of men working in managerial, professional, and technical fields logged fewer than 30 hours per week (Jacobs and Gerson 2004, 34). This pattern is broadly similar to the 15.1 percent of all employed female physicians and 7.8 percent of male physicians who work part-time.

Today's Physicians: Workaholics or Overworked?

The growth of long workweeks and the limited expansion of part-time work is surprising in light of evidence indicating that huge proportions of male and female physicians believe they work too much. While no doubt workaholics are well represented among physicians, there is a much larger and growing group that expresses interest in working fewer hours per week. For example, in the Survey of the Practice Patterns of Young Physicians, a nationally representative survey of physicians who finished training five years or fewer prior to the survey, revealed that in 1987, 43 percent of male respondents and 42 percent of female respondents wished they could work less than they were working at the time. In 1991, five years after the initial survey, respondents' dissatisfaction with work hours had increased in this population such that 53 percent of men and 46 percent of women wished they could work less than their current professional schedule. After accounting for the fact that men work longer hours, however, we find that the gender gap in the desire to work less disappears. The desire to work less or to pursue a part-time schedule has also been found in several studies of physicians in specific specialties including pediatrics and surgery (Fritz and Lantos 1991; Mayer et al. 2001). Interest in part-time opportunities goes well beyond physicians seeking more time for family. Many older physicians also seek reduced schedules. In fact, in 2005, 32 percent of physicians fifty to sixty-four years of age indicated that they were interested in part-time hours but did not have that option in their current position (Harris 2007).

In fact, dissatisfaction with work hours is significantly more pervasive among physicians than among the general population. This is not surprising, given the gap between physicians' work hours and those of their nonphysician peers. Jacobs and Gerson report that roughly one third of the workers in the U.S. labor force would prefer to work fewer hours per week (2004, 74).

The low rates of part-time work are even more surprising in light of recent research on the relationship between part-time work and physician satisfaction. According to analyses of the representative Physician Work Life Study, U.S. physicians of both genders who work part-time felt better able to control their work hours, work interruptions, and work hassles. Physicians working part-time were significantly more satisfied than full-time physicians with patient care issues, personal time, administrative issues, and their jobs overall, and they noted significantly less stress than full-time physicians (McMurray et al. 2005). A nationally representative study of members of the American Academy of Pediatrics found similar results: limiting work hours enhances pediatricians' sense of balance between work and personal life. Pediatricians working part-time were more satisfied with the time they had for their own children and other personal activities, and expressed similar or greater professional satisfaction (O'Connor et al. 2004). Additional research has shown that the strongest predictors of physician burnout involve how much control they have over their schedules and over the total number of hours worked in a week (*Medical News Today* 2007).

The relationship between work effort and professional well-being is not simply about access to part-time work. Recent research reveals that the strongest predictors of whether physicians of both genders will experience burnout and career dissatisfaction are how much control they have over the total number of hours they work in a week and their work schedules.

In other words, statistics suggest that physicians of both genders are not only working more but also feeling more overworked. Studies indicate that there is a growing belief that reducing work hours could address the problem. Such beliefs are grounded in reliable social research. Nevertheless, in spite of articles titled "Practices Must Cope as More Physicians Work Part-Time Hours" (Croasdale 2002) and "Women Physicians Find Ways to Make 'Part Time' Work" (Croasdale 2004b), a large-scale trend toward part-time work has yet to occur.

The Culture of Unfettered Professional Commitment

What we have seen is a mismatch between the preference on the part of many physicians for more manageable work schedules that is in tension with the increasingly long weeks many physicians regularly work. In seeking to understand the causes of this disconnect, it may be useful to put the dilemmas of today's physicians in historical context.

Before the large-scale entry of women, the traditional culture of the medical profession expected a high degree of professional commitment. In this context, physicians worked long hours because of a culture that assumed their total availability to patients (Adams 2004), because of a more established human connection between doctors and patients (Hobson 2005), because of a stronger association between work effort and reimbursement, because of a reluctance among physicians to rely on one another, and because of greater support at home from wives who did not work for pay outside the home. Even as late as 1980, most physicians generally worked alone or with one other partner (Kletke et al. 1996), so they did not enjoy economies of scale. The small size of the average practice meant that many physicians needed to work at night and on weekends. On-call hours have been greatly reduced as practice size has increased.

Similarly, community-based physicians in the 1980s and earlier often established long-standing relationships with their patients. They not only knew them in the office but also knew them in the community. This connection contributed to a larger incentive to create time for patients. The obstetrician who has known his patient since she was born (having attended her delivery) may make a greater effort to be available to deliver his pregnant patient's child than one who has only recently come to know his patient. Similarly, the pediatrician who sees his patients every time he goes to his child's sporting events will feel a unique personal connection to them. Research indicates that both physicians and patients enjoy greater satisfaction and trust when their relationship endures over time (Rodriguez et al. 2007). This enhanced satisfaction inevitably translated into greater availability and long hours for physicians.

Finally, physicians prior to the 1980s arrived in the office early and worked late in part because they had support at home to maintain this schedule. First, those with the support of a full-time homemaker spouse did not have to worry about being available for their children. Because many wives assumed responsibility for billing issues, they may also have had fewer concerns about the business aspects of their practices. And second, those with a homemaker spouse may have felt greater responsibility to provide income for the family, so they had an extra incentive to offer additional services. Even today, male physicians with stay-at-home wives work more hours per week than other physicians, although the difference is just a few hours.

Over time, although the factors keeping physicians' work effort high before 1980 have dissipated, other forces have emerged that have maintained the long workweek. Connections between physicians and patients have weakened. Turnover is higher for patients because of insurance restrictions and greater population mobility. Access to unique physicians is more limited because practices have grown, so even a patient who stays with one practice does not always see the same provider. Similarly, practice size has grown. As a result, physicians can share responsibilities. And since physicians' spouses have begun to work at higher rates, today's male medical professionals have somewhat less flexibility at home than in the past.

As the factors creating long weeks before 1980 dissipated, however, new structural forces have developed to take their place, and these new forces inevitably affect both male and female physicians. In particular, as health care technology and knowledge have improved and health care financing has evolved from a retrospective to a prospective model, the work of the average physician has become increasingly stressful and challenging (Schafermeyer and Asplin 2003). Charles Bosk, an astute observer of the medical scene, has stressed the role of the increasingly acute condition of patients in the growing demands on physicians:

> Many of the changes of managed care have in essence been the operational equivalent of speeding up the assembly line. If hospital stays are shorter and if service size is constant, then those patients being treated are sicker as a group than they were twenty years ago.... Sicker patients require more surveillance, more management, more worry, more coordination with nursing, more consulting with colleagues in other specialties, more scheduling of ancillary services and more communication with family members than do less sick ones. (2003, 250)

It is important to emphasize that this is occurring throughout the health care system rather than simply in the inpatient environment. Technological innovations have made it possible for patients with chronic illnesses such as diabetes to survive markedly longer than they once did. Most of these patients need significant medical attention throughout their lives. Caring for sicker patients inevitably takes more time.

Meanwhile, reimbursements for primary care physicians are declining, and administrative hassles are growing. A 2005 article in *U.S. News & World Report* titled "Doctors Vanish from View: Harried by the Bureaucracy of Medicine, Physicians Are Pulling Back from Patient Care" captured the sentiments of many in medicine. In particular, Carl Getto, associate dean for hospital affairs at the University of Wisconsin Medical School, spoke of "the hassle factors. Those rewards—including satisfying relationships, autonomy, high status, and comparably high pay—are increasingly outweighed by...reams of time-consuming paperwork, declining reimbursements...[and] a loss of autonomy" (Hobson 2005). Today, physicians must spend time seeking clearance to perform certain procedures and prescribe certain drugs. Since this time is not reimbursed, and since physicians' ability to set prices for their services has been severely restricted, these administrative hassles must either reduce physicians' pay or increase their work effort.

Furthermore, physicians' stress is not limited to the increasingly acute needs of their patients and the increased expectations of their bureaucracies. It also stems from the increasing demands and knowledge of their clientele. David Mechanic tracks changes in patients' expectations in his 2003 article "Physician Discontent: Challenges and Opportunities." He cites a 1957 study of ambulatory clinics that found patients to be poorly informed about their own illnesses and about common diseases and notes that they showed little evidence of demanding information. He then suggests that by the mid-1980s, as many as two fifths of persons studied were behaving to some extent in a consumerist manner—seeking information, exercising some independent judgment, showing cost consciousness, and demonstrating a reasonable level of knowledge. Those who demonstrated a consumerist orientation were on average better educated and reported less faith in and dependence on physicians (Roter and Hall 1992). Finally, Mechanic cites a Community Tracking Study by Tu and Hargraves (2003) which found that 38 percent of those surveyed in 2000–2001 had "looked for or obtained information about a personal health concern" from a source other than their physician. Those with a college education or higher were most likely to seek independent information and use the Internet. In addition to coping with better informed patients, physicians also find themselves treating a growing population of misinformed patients. Since 1998, when the FDA relaxed guidelines surrounding direct to consumer pharmaceutical advertising, doctors have had to confront a growing population of patients who seek specific prescriptions after seeing pharmaceutical advertisements on television. Physicians complain that they must either spend inordinate amounts of time negotiating with this population or provide the prescription inappropriately (Maguire 1999). Given changes in patients' knowledge and expectations, the average time a doctor spends per patient has actually been increasing (Mechanic et al. 2001). The increase in time per patient and the reductions in reimbursements together have contributed to the growing medical workweek (Mechanic 2003).

Do these current trends affect women as much as men? In general, the structural changes facing male physicians are also facing their female colleagues. One female physician we interviewed who had achieved tenure at an elite medical school reflected on how things had changed in medicine. She said that when she finished one of her rotations as a resident, the patients had held a going-away party for her. Such a party would be impossible today, she commented, because patients who are healthy enough to have a party are not in the hospital.

The increasing representation of women in specialty fields that demand long workweeks is another contributing factor. As we saw in chapter 4, the level of gender differentiation across specialties has remained roughly constant since 1985. Given the growing numbers of women in medicine, however, this means that the absolute numbers of women in fields such as general surgery which involve long and unpredictable hours are increasing (see also Croasdale 2007).

Ultimately the disconnect between the desire for work-family balance and the realities of the medical profession stems largely from structural pressures beyond the control of individual physicians. In some instances those forces reside in the general labor market. As we have suggested, our economy is constructed in a way that is increasing pressures on elite workers to work long weeks and limiting meaningful part-time opportunities. In others respects, medicine remains unique. Pressures on modern physicians are creating work environments that are increasingly difficult to manage. While technological advances such as personal computers, cell phones, and the Internet have inevitably heightened expectations for professional workers, we suggest that technological and financial change has been even more pronounced in medicine. Thus both male and female physicians endure longer weeks than their professional peers. Although female physicians are more likely to seek and find part-time positions, their ultimate effect on the availability of part-time work within the profession will be greatly restricted by independent trends in American medicine.

Obstacles to Part-Time Work

American women have entered a medical profession that initially took long workweeks for granted and now demands long weeks as a result of structural constraints. The pursuit of part-time opportunities runs counter to these historical patterns.

Overall there is a lack of viable part-time opportunities in many medical contexts. There are multiple barriers to part-time work in medicine. Some of these factors are unique to the profession, but others occur in many elite occupations. Part-time work is lacking in the United States for professionals in general. Furthermore, the part-time work that is available is clustered disproportionately in the lower tiers of most professions, including medicine.

Although barriers to part-time work include cultural and organizational obstacles, there are financial and patient-related factors that also limit demand for part-time medical work. Many physicians who would like to work less do not seek part-time schedules because such positions involve major financial sacrifices. Though many of the barriers to reduced schedules appear immutable, others can be removed or reduced.

Cultural and Organizational Factors

Women physicians seeking reduced work hours have often encountered superiors who are willing to reduce their salaries and rewards but are reluctant to reduce work-related expectations. This problem is evident throughout the profession, reflecting a long-standing view that devotion to medicine takes precedence over all other commitments (Adams 2004), but it is especially prominent in academic medicine. As the following observation quoted from the MomMD Web site suggests, those with authority in academic medicine can be reluctant to embrace part-time schedules for staff physicians and academic faculty:

> I have a similar experience in academic medicine (pathology). I asked my chair (a man) almost a year ago to be part-time. He was willing to cut my salary, but this did not come with a decrease in the work load. About a month ago, I informed him that I was not going to renew my contract as of July 1. I basically had to entirely quit my job to get more time for my family. There was no flexibility. (posted April 24, 2007, by doski)

Another woman concurs:

> I just have not figured out how to make it in my job only working 4 days. My boss has told me that in my area (mostly research) that women who "cut back" still wind up doing the same amount of work—they just get paid less for it. So she opposes part time or "less time." She thinks that is made up for by the amazing flexibility that my job provides. All she says is "I don't care when or where you work, just get the job done." But really, I would like to just do 80% of the job for 80% of the money. (posted August 24, 2006)

Conflicted Feelings

The failure to reduce work-related expectations for part-time workers co-exists with a trend toward increasing expectations for full-time professional workers that is in part responsible for increases in the average workweek of the highly educated labor force.

This pattern is evident for many professional women outside the medical context as well. In a qualitative study of highly educated women who were out of the labor force, Stone and Lovejoy find that "upon becoming mothers, about half of the women in our sample expressed a desire to cut back on their work hours and/or to increase the flexibility of their schedules" (2004, 68). Their efforts met with mixed results. One third of the study sample cited workplace inflexibility as a major factor in their decision to interrupt their careers. The authors note that women spoke repeatedly about having full-time responsibilities on a part-time schedule, of doing "a job and half" when they were supposed to be doing half a job.

The other side of this situation involves physicians who accept part-time positions and end up working full-time hours. One part-time internist we interviewed abandoned her position in favor of an oncology fellowship because she ultimately concluded that part-time work was not possible, and if she was going to work full-time, she preferred the type of work and the type of pay enjoyed by specialists.

Another critical problem limiting part-time employment among professional workers overall involves the uniquely high penalties that part-time workers in elite occupations must pay. Physicians report facing both short-term disapproval and longer-term career sacrifices for challenging time norms that demand they work more than forty hours a week so that they might spend time with their families.

Many physicians who seek a better work-family balance share these experiences. As the following remarks from the MomMD Web site suggest, part-timers often feel that they have to give up respect and a sense of professionalism:

> as a part timer, I have had to continually advocate for myself. (posted February 5, 2007 by kpzr/9145)
> I have been part-time for 5 years now, and am probably quitting, mostly due to the treatment I get as a part-timer. I get considered last for the work schedule, don't get my name on the group prescription pads, don't get invited to any company social functions—all due to my part-time status. I have no benefits at all. I made it clear to my employer that I was limited to part-time due to family but that I was planning to commit to working there for the future as I live in that area and would even consider going full-time there when my kids were older. I am getting no credit toward partnership for these years. (posted July 1, 2005, by Carole)

Physicians seeking a better work-family balance sacrifice more than professional rewards such as pay and promotion. They also incur the criticism of their colleagues. One survey of internal medicine specialists indicates that even in the Netherlands, where rates of part-time work are generally high, physicians view part-time colleagues with suspicion (Lugtenberg 2006). In *The Part-Time Paradox,* Cynthia Epstein and her colleagues report a similar pattern among lawyers who sought out part-time work (Epstein 1998). Furthermore, the available part-time work is clustered disproportionately in the less prestigious areas of the profession. According to the Physician Work Life Study, the highest proportions of part-time physicians were found in general pediatrics (20 percent) and in health maintenance organizations (22 percent). Although these results reflect in part the number of women in pediatrics and in HMOs, male pediatricians were significantly more likely than their family practice counterparts to choose part-time practice (16 percent versus 7 percent; $P = 0.05$) (McMurray et al. 2005). Here again, this pattern is reflected in other settings outside of medicine. Those professionals who do secure reduced schedules are often in the lower tiers of their industries (National Association of Legal Professionals 2006).[7]

One set of organizational constraints involves scheduling bottlenecks in hospital settings. Many physicians who desire flexible schedules must rely on hospitals and other institutions to provide their services. Hospitals have historically had problems allocating operating room time because assessing the length of an operation is very difficult (Jarnberg et al. 2001). In an effort to cut costs and maintain fiscal solvency, hospitals have been limiting staff anesthesiologists and operating room nurses, thus forcing surgeons and other providers who treat "add on" cases to wait until after the standard business day has ended in order to perform procedures that could theoretically be done during the regular workday if operating room staff were available (Mathias 1997). This is an especially prominent problem for cases that need prompt attention but are not life-threatening emergencies, such as kidney stones.

Economic Constraints

Many physicians who would like to work less do not attempt to negotiate or find a reduced workload because of the inevitable financial penalty that part-time work entails. Although physicians have high earnings prospects, there are several financial considerations that hit physicians harder than many other workers.

Like other Americans, physicians are increasingly too strapped financially to consider part-time work. Rising tuition costs often leave medical students with considerable debt. Median debt in 2003 was 4.5 times median debt in 1984. By 2003 the median debt was $100,000 for public medical school graduates and $135,000 for private medical school graduates (Croasdale 2004a).

As a result, part-time work is financially unrealistic for a growing proportion of newly minted physicians. Research on pediatricians indicates that loans are a major obstacle to part-time work (Cull et al. 2002). Financial barriers are especially pronounced if, like the author of this MomMD post, physicians attempt to start their own practice:

> As far as payback, it is tough. I always wanted to work part-time, but I can't see cutting back at all anytime in the next several years. Right now, between my husband and myself, we are just barely covering our expenses, living paycheck to paycheck. We have no savings at all and have significant credit card debt because of all of those "emergencies" that pop up—like the cars breaking down, etc. At the moment one of our cars may be broken beyond repair and if that happens we'll have to take out yet another loan to buy a new (used) one. I'm not sure where we will come up with the money for that. (posted December 5, 2006, by rydys)

It is misleading, however, to think that financial stress is limited to those in the initial stages of establishing a practice. As these posts from MomMD suggest, declining reimbursements and rising overhead are making it increasingly difficult to make ends meet in some specialties:

> "One Family Practice physician recently complained that her net take-home pay after all expenses (including malpractice and student loans) is

approximately $37,000 per year. Less than her husband's salary as a Chief Petty Officer in the Navy." Now I really want to be a Dr bcuz I want to help people and I am challenged and interested by the field but the money part is somewhat important too. I mean, 11 yrs of school and tons of work to make 37k/yr is ridiculous!! Is this realistic?!?!?! (posted April 7, 2007, by ALLALLY)

Yes, I personally know docs who have taken home less than 50K in a year. It has become extremely difficult to make a good living in private practice. (posted April 7, 2007, by *AnnaM*)

The same financial struggles are also seen in the general population. Although many people indicate that they want to work less in general, answers shift markedly when issues of wages are added. When options are posed as trade-offs between time and money, working less becomes less attractive.

The fixed costs associated with a medical practice tend to encourage long workweeks. If there are costs that are present no matter how much work is done, the physician must devote a considerable portion of the workweek to recouping these unavoidable expenses. Malpractice insurance is an example of a large and growing cost of practicing medicine that remains the same whether the physician is employed thirty hours per week or sixty.

The limited availability of part-time work in medicine reflects these types of pressures, especially in those areas of medicine where malpractice costs are high. The experience of one academic obstetrician captures this phenomenon:

Creative options for balancing work and family are few. The recent escalation in the cost of malpractice insurance coverage has largely precluded options for part-time practice; the physician who delivers one patient per month pays just as high a rate as everyone else. At my academic medical center, premiums in my department increased by 68% last year, which brought the base rate to $100,000 per physician per year. (Some of my colleagues were assessed twice that.) A number of senior men, but interestingly enough, none of the women, promptly gave up obstetrics altogether and switched to a predominantly surgical gynecology practice. When I asked to cut back to a 4-day work week, I was told I couldn't possibly generate enough revenue to cover the expense of keeping me, what with salary, overhead, and liability insurance. (Plante 2004, 840)

Although malpractice insurance is a particularly severe barrier for high-risk specialists wanting work-family balance, malpractice premiums present a significant obstacle to any physicians seeking part-time work (Walpert 2002).

Practice ownership similarly tends to induce proprietors to put in long workweeks. Incentives among self-employed professionals involve a trade-off between autonomy and control and the burden of fixed operating costs. On the one hand, the self-employed ostensibly have more control over their work lives and should therefore be better able to strike a satisfying balance between work and family. And there are instances when such control has actually helped women in medicine. For example, when Sandra Adamson Fryhofer, a general internist in Atlanta and a past president of the American College of Physicians, gave birth to her twins in the late 1980s, there was no maternity leave. But because she was in solo practice, she could choose not to schedule patients when she had a parent-teacher conference or another conflict between home and work. The result may have been that she earned less that day, but it was her choice (Gesenway 1999).

On the other hand, the self-employed in medicine and other professions encounter severe pressures to work long hours not only because they must personally shoulder all of the fixed costs associated with their businesses but also because they often reap the financial rewards of additional work more directly than their professional peers who work for others and are generally reimbursed with a fixed salary.

Ultimately the pressure to earn money and pay the bills appears to be winning out among physicians. Data from the 2000 U.S. Census indicate that both male and female employed physicians between thirty and fifty who are self-employed owners or co-owners of incorporated businesses work significantly longer hours than their peers. While women physicians work an average of 46.9 hours per week, self-employed women physicians with incorporated businesses work 51 hours per week. And while male physicians work an average of 55.1 hours per week, self-employed male physicians with incorporated businesses work 58 hours per week.

The pressures on self-employed physicians to work long hours are inevitably stronger when physicians are part-owners rather than sole proprietors. Physicians who have partners must balance their desire for flexible schedules with their need to pay their share of the overhead. Since changes in health care are making solo practice increasingly difficult and unprofitable, fewer physicians are considering it as an option (Cook 2007), and those who do attempt private practice may have less control than Dr. Fryhofer because of the increasing bureaucratic demands on private practice physicians. Thus, while her solo practice seems like an ideal situation for a working mother, it is increasingly unrealistic to expect physicians of either gender to pursue self-employment as an option (Cook 2007). Furthermore, as we discussed earlier, today's young medical graduates may simply be unable to make the choice that Dr. Fryhofer made because of a radically different financial horizon. The odds are that they have loans which she did not have, and the reality is that they will not be paid as well as she was (Dolan 2006).

In 2000, Sandra Fryhofer dropped all insurance contracts and now maintains a self-pay practice. Patients pay cash up front for services and then negotiate with insurance companies themselves (Bryant 2000). While the self-pay option might solve Dr. Fryhofer's needs, it cannot work for most physicians simply because most patients cannot afford to pay cash up front.

Practice Considerations

Cultural, organizational, and financial considerations are not the only barriers to flexible professional schedules. Physicians are often expected to be continuously available to their clients. While systematic data on client expectations are not readily available, we suspect that patients are even more likely than other types of clients to expect continuous access to services because of the essential nature of health problems. As this post on the MomMD Web site suggests, some patients, including physician patients, do not react well to part-time physicians:

> I know for one (and I hope that this does not piss anyone off) that if I had a pediatrician and my kid was sick and needed to see her/him and she was part-time and not available until X day…that would tick me off and we would chose someone else. I know this sounds bad and it is probably not the PC thing to say but it "is" how I feel for now. (posted August 27, 2005, by efex101)

In fact, studies of patient satisfaction with primary care suggest that it depends on access to care and care continuity (Anderson et al. 2007; Fan et al. 2005). Thus the perception that patients want their physicians to be constantly available is grounded in some degree of reality.

The need to be persistently available is equally present for specialists. For them, however, the issue often involves being available for referrals:

> I've been reading with interest about how physicians work part-time or job share, but I don't know how to cut back on my work hours. I am a general surgeon (with 2 young children) in a group practice, taking call every 4th weekend. Over the past 8 years, I have tried to limit my work hours and numbers of patients seen, but in a field where my business depends on *my availability for referrals* [emphasis added] as well as my desire to follow my patients postoperatively, I don't know how I can cut back any more without going out of business. I love surgery, especially the laparoscopy, and I want to "stay in the game" while still raising a family. (posted on MomMD)

The issue involved with "availability for referrals" involves more than the absolute number of hours a specialist works. Specialist physicians must court primary care physicians in order to maintain referrals. This networking is normally done in the off hours and thus conflicts with the needs of physicians seeking a more realistic family life.

Again, the need to be continuously available is a consideration not just for physicians but in many other professions as well. Cynthia Epstein et al.

found that clients "stigmatize part time lawyers by avoiding or refusing to work with them. Some attorneys reported that clients wanted to know why they have to work with someone who could be gone tomorrow" (1998, 32). Epstein's respondents reported being told that they needed to be available to take calls from clients on their day off.

A related problem that plagues many professionals seeking reduced schedules involves periods of high workload. As this MomMD post indicates, there is an expectation that part-time physicians will contribute additional time during periods of unanticipated high patient demand:

> I currently work part-time 2 days per week in a private pediatric office. My 2 days have been set for some time now, and I've therefore arranged my childcare around my schedule (don't have childcare on my off days). On multiple occasions over the past couple of years, my office mgr. has approached me to see if I could work "extra" days during busy winter months....I have firmly explained that I don't have childcare on those days, and that it would be impossible for me to add "extra" days....Now my office mgr. has approached me again to see if I could add a 3rd day because the other docs are feeling so "slammed" this winter. I am very frustrated. I told her, once again, that I am unable to do this, and reviewed the reasons why. I might also mention that my contract specifies my days and hours. I wouldn't give it another thought, but I know that my office mgr.'s requests are coming from the other docs in the office, and it creates an aura that feels like I'm not "pulling my weight." I already feel this way, being the only part-time doc in the office. Does anyone have any suggestions for how to prevent these requests from continuing? (posted December 12, 2006, by kiddoc)

The immediate response to this part-time worker was less than supportive:

> While I can certainly understand where you are coming from, I can understand the other docs' position as well. During the busy times of the year, everyone ends up working harder. For full time docs, that means staying later, working longer hours, and never having a day off. In the offices that I know the docs do not take vacation during holiday seasons and even if someone is usually off one day a week, they will often come in on that day to help out during the busiest weeks. There are a certain number of patients who need to be seen and the work just has to get done. During the busy seasons I often get out an hour or two later than usual and many docs I know will add extra evening hours.

The bottom line is that the part-time physician feels that since her hours are clearly stated in her contract, she should not have to work late. The respondent suggests that although full time is also clearly delineated, the expectation is that full-time physicians will work overtime to satisfy the need since they are professionals, so she reasons that a similar expectation should be placed on part-time professional workers. While this interaction may seem uniquely medical, we suggest that deadlines are common to many professional settings. A parallel situation inevitably exists, for example, for part-time accountants during tax season.

A final practice-related consideration concerns whether physicians working part-time can provide optimal care. The issues in this area differ for primary care and specialist physicians. Because primary care is often defined as continuous, coordinated, and comprehensive care (Safran 2003), some have inferred that continuous physician availability is important and that a traditional full-time work schedule is optimal for patient care (Parkerton et al. 2003).

Although the reasoning seems sound, some research calls the continuity-equals-quality theory into question. For example, one study on part-time primary care physicians suggests that rather than demonstrating lower performance, primary care physicians working fewer clinical hours were associated with both slightly higher cancer screening rates and better diabetic management, and with patient satisfaction and ambulatory costs similar to those of full-time physicians (Parkerton et al. 2003). Research also suggests that part-time primary care physicians in an academic environment are more productive than their full-time counterparts. Most of these clinicians worked full-time but limited their clinical responsibilities in order to attend to teaching and research (Warde 2001). Another study finds that although physicians working sixty-five hours or more a week provided higher continuity of care, they also had significantly lower professional satisfaction, which ultimately may compromise their capacity to offer quality health care services (Murray et al. 2000).[8] In other words, while the relationship between patient continuity and physician work effort is not debatable, the association between patient continuity and health care quality is.

In light of the relationship between continuity and patient satisfaction, how can we explain the comparable satisfaction ratings of part- and full-time primary care physicians discussed earlier? One possibility is that the patients of part-time physicians tolerate the lack of continuity because they believe that the higher quality of care provided by these physicians is worth the wait. This explanation jibes well with research which suggests that part-time physicians provide higher-quality care, and that although part-time medical work presents unique difficulties, they are not insurmountable.

The issue for specialists has to do with the idea that "practice makes perfect." Thus in some procedural areas there is an association between case volume or surgical experience and patient outcomes for a variety of procedures (Gordon et al. 1999; Migliore et al. 2007; Dimick et al. 2003; Hammond et al. 2003). In spite of this research, the leap between the volume-quality association and resistance to part-time surgical work may not follow as perfectly as it seems to. At the very least, part-time workers could avoid the problem by limiting the range of procedures they perform so that they can accrue sufficient volume. In fact, academic surgeons routinely specialize in this manner.

Furthermore, while the research documenting a volume-outcome association is consistent and accepted, until fairly recently it has been limited in scope. Little effort has been made to follow surgeons over the course of their careers and to assess how total experience rather than annual volume relates to outcomes. One study on radical prostatectomy suggests that total experience plays a major role in outcomes. In particular, five-year progression-free probabilities revealed a lifetime learning curve for the first 250–500 radical prostatectomies. This was true even after adjusting for positive surgical margins. The probability of recurrence decreased from 17.9 percent in the first ten cases to 10.7 percent after 250 prior cases. For every eleven men treated by an inexperienced urologist, one will relapse, compared to much lower relapse rates among those treated by an experienced surgeon (Vickers et al. 2007). If lifetime experience is a better proxy for skill than annual volume, the decision to funnel patients to high-volume surgeons should be rethought. Under such conditions, barriers to part-time surgical work might relax somewhat.

Furthermore, research suggests that although high-volume surgeons have better outcomes than low-volume surgeons, there is significant variation in outcomes among the high-volume population. These results suggest that volume may not entirely explain surgical outcomes. In fact it is now thought that volume differences are only a proxy for skill differences.[9] A better approach to quality enhancement for surgical patients involves continuing education for surgeons, certification by procedure, and more frequent evaluation of health outcomes. Such improvements in outcomes research and surgical quality maintenance could enhance opportunities for part-time work among truly qualified surgeons.

Residents and the Eighty-Hour-per-Week Rule

One major step toward making medical training more family-friendly has been the introduction of the eighty-hour rule for residents. As we will see, this development had less to do with women's entry into the profession than with concerns about patient safety. Nevertheless, research suggests that residents of both genders are taking as much advantage of the eighty-hour work rule as they can (Jones and Jones 2007; Arnold et al. 2005).

Until 2003 there was no official maximum on the number of hours per week that residents could spend in the hospital setting. Historically, residency training has been especially rigorous, with seventy hours of work per week required in even the most lenient specialties. Before these regulations, most surgical residents worked a thirty-six-hour shift every third night and routinely put in twelve-hour days on their "nights off."

Residents always worked Saturday mornings. They often worked all day on Saturday and routinely spent at least one Sunday a month in the hospital. Residents in other fields normally had somewhat less demanding schedules that involved thirty-six-hour shifts every fourth night and less time on Saturday mornings, but routinely required twelve-hour days.

The eighty-hour work rule was adopted primarily because of public concern about patient safety (Woodrow et al. 2006). Although the American Medical Student Association and the Council of Interns and Residents actively advocated for resident work hour restrictions, the well-being of residents of either gender was far from the major focus of the debates leading up to the adoption of work hour limits for U.S. resident physicians, and the status of physician parents was hardly mentioned in these discussions. The initial public recognition of resident overwork came after a patient in a New York hospital, Libby Zion, died in 1984 as a result of the inadequate care provided by overworked and undersupervised medical residents. Her father, a writer for the *New York Times,* strove to bring the issue to public attention (Kwan and Levy 2006).

The Libby Zion case led the New York State Department of Health to convene a committee to review the state's residency training system. The committee recommended a series of reforms that were adopted by New York State in 1989. The regulations, often referred to as the Bell Code, stated that residents must not work more than twenty-four consecutive hours and no more than eighty hours a week, among a number of other provisions designed to enhance patient safety. While the Bell Code represented a milestone with respect to the regulation of residency training programs, these regulations were not uniformly implemented. Since penalties for violations were limited, and oversight was nearly nonexistent, many hospitals simply ignored the regulations.

A 1998 inquiry conducted by the New York State Department of Health found that 60 percent of surgical residents were still working more than ninety-five hours per week (Kwan and Levy 2006). The investigation found violations at every single hospital it reviewed. As a result, the state dramatically increased financial penalties for work code violations and hired an independent firm to monitor its hospitals.

As New York began to ratchet up its controls on resident work hours, national attention was drawn to the issue. In November 1999 the Institute of Medicine released its report *To Err Is Human,* which suggested that 98,000 patient deaths and countless injuries every year result from medical errors. Although the report focused public attention on patient safety, it had relatively little to say about residents' work effort (Steinbrook 2002).

In April 2001 the American Medical Student Association, the Committee on Interns and Residents, and the nonprofit organization Public Citizen filed a petition with the Occupational Safety and Health Administration

(OSHA) requesting that it restrict residents' workload to eighty hours a week. The petitioners' main justification for their request involved the hazards faced by student physicians. In November 2001 Representative John Conyers of Michigan introduced the Patient and Physician Safety and Protection Act limiting resident work hours. The OSHA petition was denied, however, and the federal legislation did not pass. Instead, the Accreditation Council on Graduate Medical Education (ACGME) adopted its own regulations in July 2003. But unlike the OSHA petition, the major impetus involved efforts to improve patient care (Kwan and Levy 2006).

While the 2003 ACGME restrictions on resident work hours promised to limit the work effort of residents in the most challenging specialties, residency programs remain far from family-friendly. Residents who become parents and seek to be meaningfully engaged in their children's lives will continue to face serious challenges. Even if the reforms are implemented accurately—and evidence suggests that they are still defied frequently (Landrigan et al. 2006; AMA 2005)—residents still must work eighty hours a week and endure twenty-four straight hours of work periodically. Furthermore, the regulations leave a number of gray areas. In particular, at-home call is not subject to the same limitations as in-house call. Official regulations state that at-home call must not be "so frequent as to preclude reasonable rest and personal time." While the intent of the legislation is clear, there is ample room for interpretation and potential abuse. Ultimately, at-home call can be more dangerous for residents because it can require driving to and from the hospital multiple times in one night. And research suggests that call duties vary significantly by specialty. One study found that residents in general surgery took call once every 6.9 minutes, while residents in geriatric and general medicine took call once every five hours (Chiu et al. 2006).

As we noted earlier, changes in the technical content of American medicine are altering the nature of medical education. In particular, technological advances have increased the average morbidity of patients at all levels of care. Simply put, faced with more severe patient acuity, residents who are on call at night have more to do—more procedures to complete, more tests to order, and more information to evaluate—than was the case a generation ago. Residency programs remain very demanding physically and mentally, as well as in terms of time.

Not only are residency programs taxing, but also they can conflict with the peak period of family demands. Many, and perhaps most, female residents who become mothers do so during their residency training programs. Potee and colleagues (1999), who surveyed women who graduated from Yale University Medical School between 1922 and 1999, found that the overwhelming majority of these elite female physicians became mothers or intended to become mothers. The rate of having a first child during medical training was increasing for this group. Other studies confirm that more than half of female physicians have their first child during residency (Seltzer 1999).

Accompanying the growing trend toward childbearing during residency is increasing evidence of problem pregnancies for female physicians. Multiple studies show that pregnant residents suffer higher rates of preterm labor, restricted fetal growth, and preeclampsia than women of comparable age and socioeconomic status (Klebanoff et al. 1990; Gabbe et al. 2003).

Inadequate maternity leaves post-childbirth compound these problems. In separate studies of family practice and obstetrics-gynecology residents, the average length of maternity leave was between four and eight weeks, derived from multiple sources including vacation, sick leave, and home-based electives. In other words, although residents took time off after childbirth, most did not have a real maternity leave (Gjerdingen et al. 1995; Gabbe et al. 2003). Residents who returned to work so quickly usually did not do so in stages: between four and eight weeks after delivery, these women had the full responsibilities of a resident. So it is not surprising that many of them experienced difficulty arranging child care, guilt about being absent from their children, and difficulty continuing breast-feeding (Gjerdingen et al. 1995). In fact, recent research indicates that although many initiate breast-feeding, residents are often unable to continue because of their work schedules.[10]

Readers unacquainted with the specifics of medical training might find the results of these studies surprising, especially in light of the 1993 Family and Medical Leave Act (FMLA). This federal law requires that employees of firms with more than one hundred workers who have at least one year of firm-specific experience be given at least twelve weeks of unpaid maternity leave. Since most residents do not become pregnant during their first year, and since most hospitals have at least one hundred employees, residents should be eligible for twelve weeks of time off that does not count against their vacation or sick leave. Yet it appears that residents are not availing themselves of this opportunity.

This occurs, in part, because the status of residents is unclear. Since they are considered both employees and students, their eligibility for maternity leave under the Family and Medical Leave Act is debatable. In other words, if residents are considered students, they are not eligible under FMLA. Only if residents are considered workers do they become eligible for FMLA coverage.

Second, although the number of teaching hospitals with established maternity leaves is increasing (surveys by the Council of Teaching Hospitals confirm this trend), female residents know that much of the time they take before or after childbirth will have to be made up before they can graduate. They also know that other residents usually have to shoulder the additional workload whenever a resident takes any form of leave. Although practices may now be changing as a result of work hour restrictions, historically replacement workers were almost never used to cover resident absences. Third, because of their initially low salaries and high debt, residents are often not in a financial position to take unpaid maternity leave.

The obstacles are frequently logistical as well as financial. The structure of residency programs makes it very difficult to incorporate women or men who wish to make up their leave time, especially if these individuals need to receive compensation during their make-up period. Medicare pays hospitals for the residents they train and makes no allowance for temporary staff, so residents making up time and receiving pay are occupying the full-time slot of one of the potential next generation of residents. Needless to say, residency directors do not want to give up a training slot so that one student can work a few additional months.

Given these conditions, true flexibility for pregnant or nursing medical residents remains elusive. Systematic research on residents in pediatrics revealed that only 43 of the 6,609 pediatrics residents in 2003 completed all or some of their training on a part-time basis (Holmes et al. 2005).

In order to better assess the prevalence of family-friendly opportunities in residency programs, we conducted an analysis of the officially posted policies. We examined all of the family practice residency programs, on the grounds that this was one of the divisions of medicine most likely to have undertaken initiatives in this area. Data from the American Academy of Family Physicians Web site on family practice residency programs in the 2005–6 training year indicate that of the 459 residency programs listed, only 45 provide part-time or shared residency programs. If these opportunities are rare in family practice residencies, they are even less likely to exist in traditionally male residency programs such as surgery.

There is also some evidence that the female family practice residents are selecting those programs that offer family-friendly supports. We calculated the percentage of residents in each program who were women in the years 2003–4 through 2005–6. We then compared this three-year average for the programs with part-time options to the programs without such flexible work schedules. In fact, programs with part-time schedules averaged 56 percent female, while programs without part-time options averaged 50 percent female. This evidence suggests that residency programs with part-time opportunities are more attractive to female residents.

The difference is less pronounced for on-site child care. Programs with this option were, on average, 52 percent female, while programs without this option were 50 percent female. The existence of an on-site child care program, however, does not ensure that resident parents can meet their child care needs, since waiting lists frequently exist for these services, and they are generally not available before or after standard business hours, when residents are often working. As the number of female residents expands, these issues will become salient ones for growing numbers of newly minted MDs.

Development of the Eighty-Hour Work Rules

Although an eighty-hour maximum work rule offers some relief to physicians in training, the Bell Code and AGCME national rules that followed were not designed to make medicine more family-friendly. As suggested earlier, the principal impetus instead was patient safety. The residency training period remains a physically demanding one, especially for physicians who are pregnant or nursing. Organizational and cultural barriers continue to inhibit the adoption of work structures that are truly conducive to a meaningful balance between work and family. It is not surprising that institutions have failed to acknowledge the need for paternal involvement in the lives of residents' children. There is little evidence that residents themselves consider such issues. One newly hired attending reflected on surgical residents' reactions to work hour regulations:

> You might expect that, as residents, we'd stand up and rejoice that these regulations have been passed. But I'll tell you, if you're the chief resident on the GI service and a case comes up that you may have one or two opportunities to do during your entire residency—well, many of us have to be dragged kicking and screaming out of the hospital. (quoted in Gilbert and Miller 2004)

Although residents acknowledge that their lives are less stressed physically as a result of the regulations (Myers et al. 2006), many residents are critical of the regulations because the new policy can prevent them from gaining valuable experience or from getting to know their patients adequately (Cohen-Gadol et al. 2005).

The debate continues to center on whether eighty hours is enough time per week to expose residents to the range of cases necessary to give them thorough training, and whether such regulations ultimately improve patient outcomes. Research on the effect of the policy on residents' experiences is mixed. One study of internal medicine programs found that although hours allotted to inpatient clinical activity did not change, residents' attendance at morning conference, a key didactic aspect of residents' training, declined. Furthermore, residents' clinical elective time was reduced (Horwitz et al. 2006). Similarly, some studies suggest that operative experience did not change after work regulations were adopted (de Virgillio et al. 2006), while others suggest a different reality (Jarman et al. 2004). Still others suggest that the effect of regulations depends on the stage of the resident, with the fifth-year residents getting sufficient operative experience (Ferguson et al. 2005). There is also the contention that the quality of medical students' experiences may be harmed by resident work restrictions (White et al. 2006). Furthermore, studies of how the new policy influences patient outcomes have also yielded unclear results (Unger 2007; Fletcher et al. 2004).

Thus it appears that although the reforms were ultimately implemented, general resident well-being has not been prioritized in our health care system, and the well-being of resident parents is almost completely outside the purview of the public. Research indicates that resident well-being has improved since the implementation of work regulations, but there is no reason to believe that these reforms were spearheaded by the residents themselves. Nevertheless, the association between part-time residencies and the representation of women in family practice programs suggests that over time the collective power of women's individual choices might cause change in the profession. The change may be gradual, but it should occur because women's presence will ultimately be too significant to be overlooked.

Inflexibility in the Lives of Individual Male and Female Physicians

In light of the significant limitations on family-friendly reforms in the profession, we consider how individual male and female physicians and physician organizations are coping. As we have discussed, since part-time work is available for only a select few, and since the percentage of male physicians with full-time spouses at home is declining, physicians must consider alternative methods of achieving work-family balance.

Those who attempted to balance work and family during the late 1970s and early 1980s did so largely on their own and inevitably endured extremely high levels of stress. Bonita Stanton reflects on her experiences as a young physician and mother in 1978. She returned to work just weeks after her first daughter was born, including taking on-call responsibility every fourth night:

> My first night back on call was simply a disaster; I could not get back to my call room to nurse my hungry daughter. Patients kept arriving to be admitted and those already hospitalized demanded attention. As I hustled about, a cadre of students anxious for teaching were left as hungry as my child. Meanwhile, holed up in my hospital call room, my husband paged me repeatedly, eventually putting the phone next to our crying infant to emphasize the point that she was hungry. By the time I got to my room, my daughter was too overwrought to nurse. By the early light of day when a moment of quiet finally arrived, I was stunned with disappointment in the complete failure of my first foray into combining my roles as parent, physician, spouse, and teacher—and overwhelmed with the loneliness of the position in which I found myself. This was not how I had expected young motherhood to feel. (Stanton 2007)

While this episode may well represent an extreme case, other female physicians also struggled to raise children during that era.

In addition to severe physical stress, physician mothers of the 1970s and early 1980s suffered social isolation. They lacked support from a broader community of working professional women. Gail Jacoby, who graduated from Jefferson Medical College in 1972, had her first child during the third year of residency. She worked until the day her daughter was born and returned five weeks later. A month before she and her husband finished their residencies, they moved into a house. She was the only full-time working mother of an infant in the neighborhood. Similarly, Lori DePersia, a 1981 medical school graduate, reflected on her efforts to balance work and family in an issue of the Jefferson Medical College alumni bulletin:

> What was the climate like for working mothers at that time? Most of the working moms had jobs to make ends meet. Being a new mom and working was frowned upon by much of society....Most of the other mothers at the schools did not work. It is different now, but back then most professional women took a few years off or went super part time (one weekend a month or less) until their children were older. (20–21)

Inevitably, women physicians of this era withstood not only the grueling hours associated with medical work and the inevitable guilt associated with leaving young children but also the condemnation of their community.

In some respects, conditions have improved over time for mothers in medicine. Medical mothers not only encounter other physician mothers in the workplace but also are more likely to encounter professional mothers in their neighborhoods simply because more women work. So the sense of isolation that the early generation experienced has lessened.

Furthermore, as we suggested in chapter 5, in some specialties, opportunities to pursue reduced schedules have expanded, so that women in those fields now find relatively more family-friendly work opportunities than professional women overall. Laura Weinstein, a 1994 graduate of Jefferson, comments that she went part-time after her youngest child turned three. She says that she reduced her hours so she could spend more time with her children now that "they're interactive humans." Another woman we interviewed, a 1994 graduate of an elite medical school, dropped out of the labor force when her second child was born and then ultimately returned to work fifteen hours a week as the medical director of a public clinic.

Yet as we noted earlier, it would be premature to suggest that women entering the medical workforce today encounter a truly family-friendly environment. In many ways, the challenges that women physicians confront as they struggle to balance work and family closely parallel those experienced by all working mothers in two-career families. For example, physicians struggle to continue breast-feeding after returning to work. One physician mother comments:

> When I breastfed in the late 90's, I worked in a small medical research insti-
> tute. I am a physician. When I asked if there might be a private area where I
> may pump milk, I seemed to be looked at as if I had two heads. I was told no
> one there had ever pumped breast milk before, and though they did find me
> a nice quiet area, I felt as if I was causing a great disruption. Mind you, this
> is a medical research institute filled with pediatricians and internal medicine
> physicians. Even in such a place, at least as recently as a half-dozen years
> ago, breastfeeding was an anomaly. (Kantor 2006)

Another woman commented on the lack of breast-feeding space in a recently built Harvard Medical School building:

> I'm at Harvard Medical School working in one of the newest and most
> spacious buildings on the campus, the New Research Building. Given that
> many of the young scientists and physicians and support staff are beginning
> families, you might think this building would include a room for breast-
> pumping. But in our new multi-million dollar beautiful building our "pump
> room" is simply a bathroom stall. This is just one of several ways in which
> Harvard remains hostile to women. (Kantor 2006)

While these comments may seem surprising, the conditions they describe
are faced by many working women with infants. In this way, medicine is
not unique. Only a third of large companies provide a private, secure area
where women can express breast milk during the workday, and only 7 percent offer on-site or near-site child care, according to a 2005 national study
of employers by the nonprofit Families and Work Institute (Rabin 2006).
Thus for many women breast-feeding on the job involves breaking new
ground.

   Women in medicine, like other working women, endure criticism for pursuing paid work outside the home. One participant in the MomMD Web
site shared her surprise when she received this type of judgment from another physician:

> I recently had a strange email interaction with another mommy physician,
> and I am wondering if I will be in for more of it as I transition to my "first
> job." I belong to a local mother of twins group and we have an email group.
> One of the other moms noticed I was a physician, so she emailed, "Oh, how
> nice, another mommy who is a physician" type of email. I thought I had
> made a new friend. I replied to her and asked her if she had any tips on
> balancing career and family, and she replied, "I only moonlight occasionally
> on the weekend. I find that my twins' mental health is more important than
> fulfilling my own selfish goals of having a career." (posted June 25, 2007, by
> tsunami)

Another participant complained about missing her children during the day when they were most energetic and cheerful, only to interact with them later on when they were tired and cranky:

> I always felt guilty and disappointed about this, that I couldn't be with the kids when they were their brightest. Be glad you are part-time so can enjoy them on your other days. I think it's very real—that we are tired and that our young children are tired by 5:30, and that we need more flexibility in the workplace to help us with our exhaustion. (posted August 20, 2007, by sisriver).

Like other women with demanding careers, many women physicians cope with the demands of parenting and work by neglecting household duties. This can incur the judgment and disapproval of others and inevitably raises the stress of those struggling to balance. One woman described her domestic challenges in a post to the MomMD Web site:

> We get nasty notes in our mailbox about our yard not being mowed and some of my kids' friends' parents have stopped allowing their children to come to our house and play because our house is very lived-in and NEVER up to their standards. The only way to do it all is to give up doing some of it (the things that are least important). (posted August 11, 2006, by OBRN2MD)

Research on women physicians indicates that they spend almost no time gardening or doing yard work. This compares with three hours per week for women overall (Robinson and Godbey 1997).

Like other women in the workforce, physician mothers struggle to focus their limited energy on bonding with their children. One participant in the MomMD Web site commented on her experiences:

> It is MOST frustrating to get home "early" then spend time with unhappy kids/feeling guilty/exhausted. I agree with change of dinner plans if possible—kids will be much better off with cereal for dinner and attention from you in the long run. I also agree from personal experience that you need to eat before you play, too! My husband and I stock "healthy" cereal, snack bars, leftover salad to snack on if it's a "witching hour" night for the kids. For a while, I tried just making time to play before making dinner, but then the kids are tired by dinnertime and won't eat (even if happy). My husband's stomach also couldn't deal with the delay. (posted August 20, 2007, by ohiomomMD)

Furthermore, like other working mothers, women physicians with families struggle to achieve the ultimate efficiency. One physician mother, Teresa Cabot, recalls: "When the kids were little, they slept in their clothes so I could shovel them from the car to the sitter's door without arousing them" (quoted in Chin et al. 2002, 291). Dr. Cabot is not alone. In a survey of eight hundred academic physicians in departments of medicine around the country, respondents were asked to provide coping strategies used to balance work and family life. More than 50 percent cited efforts to improve efficiency (Levinson et al. 1992). Inevitably, however, efficiency can go only so far without infringing on family life. Clearly, Dr. Cabot was not seeing her children when they were awake in the morning.

Another similarity between women physicians with children and other professional mothers involves spousal support. In general, mothers in elite occupations often suggest that supportive husbands are key to their success. Mothers in medicine are no exception. One reported on MomMD:

> I am really happy, but I think it's for exactly the reasons that have been already listed...and [a] great husband who really IS involved and very supportive. I wonder if we did a survey and correlated "happiness" with "supportive husband who actively participates in child and house care" whether that would explain most of the variance? (posted March 14, 2003, by psych)

In reality, however, like other working women, physician mothers often assume the bulk of child care responsibilities. This is especially true for women physicians with physician spouses. One midlife female physician with a physician spouse complained that she often had to reject speaking opportunities during the early years of her career because she could not arrange adequate child care, but that her husband accepted speaking invitations without ensuring that child care was available. He simply assumed that the children would be handled by his wife. Another younger attending we interviewed complained that her husband can "clip an aneurysm without breaking a sweat, but a poopie diaper makes him cry like a baby."

Still, it appears that because of their earning potential and their increasing willingness to marry men outside of medicine, there is an increasing cadre of women physicians who honestly share household chores equally and/or who have more supportive spouses. Two MomMD participants shared their experiences. The first wrote:

> My husband had a very involved dad, and I think that has really shaped him in being a very involved dad himself. He took over as primary parent during my first 1 and 1/2 yrs of residency (when my son was 1) until my schedule got reasonable again. When I had my daughter, I stayed home for 8 months, but I went back to work 2 evenings and Sat afternoon from 2 months on, and guess who took care of the baby and our 5 year old? My husband! I am so glad we talked about all of this before we got married. (posted April 11, 2003, by psych)

The other reports:

> My call is endocrinology (my specialty) and medicine shared and is 1 in 10. When I am off, I am OFF. I work in the office 8:30 to 4:45 with Wednesday

afternoon off. My husband is home all day on Thursdays. We have evening meals together. My husband has a gourmet kitchen store. He can cook, clean, wipe babies at either end. He does windows, does my taxes, reviews my contracts, and is a consistent, persistent force in my life. I am so sorry there aren't any available brothers. (posted April 16, 2003, by enddoc)

One woman physician whom we interviewed admitted being seriously involved with a retina surgeon but ultimately ended the relationship because she knew that the marriage would have required her to sacrifice her career. The woman is now the head of a hospital department and the mother of two children. Her husband is a part-time chaplain at the hospital where she works. Increasingly, women physicians find themselves in more balanced marriages. Here again, their experiences parallel those of other high earners. Research by Julie Brines finds that "men tend to share more housework as their wives' incomes approach theirs" (cited in McNeil 2004). Another woman we interviewed has four children and a husband who stays at home to maintain her house and care for them. She commented that they made this decision because his earning potential as an engineer was ultimately lower and less stable than hers as a primary care physician.

Still, the essential nature of physicians' work makes the challenges faced by physician parents unique in this respect. Since it is not possible for many physicians to stay home with sick children, they have to make alternative arrangements. Of course, many of the physicians in this category earn enough to hire in-house child care. One anesthesiologist addressed this issue in her comments on the MomMD Web site:

I (anesthesiologist) will be going back to work in Jan 2008 for 2 days of the week—after taking a yr + off. My husband is returning from an Iraq deployment soon and is an ER doc. Our son will be 15 months old when we start work in Jan 2008. Between both of our jobs, I don't foresee either one of us being able to leave immediately or even soon to get him if he is in daycare— how do other people work this esp if no family is in the area? We don't live in a neighborhood with extremely friendly people—I think that is just part of living in DC—and everyone we know works full-time. Anyone been in this situation? We'd like to avoid paying an agency for back-up care esp as I only work 2 days per week. (posted October 7, 2007, by bpt)

This woman was quickly advised to seek in-home nanny care so that she would not have to confront the possibility of leaving work for a sick child, and the woman seemed very receptive to the idea, not mentioning the possibility that such services would be costly relative to two days' earnings.

Another discussion on the MomMD Web site involved the struggle to find housekeeping and child care services simultaneously. Prior research on working women physicians indicates that they typically spend about one half hour a day cooking and another half hour per day on housework (Frank et al. 2000). A nationally representative survey indicates that working women in general spend one hour and ten minutes per day on cooking and only forty minutes per day on housework (Robinson and Godbey 1997). Women physicians appear to make up the gap by relying more on domestic services. One woman participant on the MomMD Web site discussed how she solved her need for household help by hiring two nannies:

> But my experience and that of my friends who have worked with nannies in the past, it's difficult to find a nanny who wants to both take care of your child and do the housework and do the cooking. I started with one nanny for my twins at 8 weeks. All we asked of her was to prepare meals for the kids and pick up after them and do their laundry as needed (though we frequently did it ourselves). We also had someone come clean our house once a week for a few hours. As they got older and more mobile, she asked that we hire someone part-time to help her. Also, the nanny and housekeeper did not get along so we had to get rid of the housekeeper. Well, in the end, we have one full-time live-out nanny (7–6 PM M–F) and another nanny/housekeeper (9–6 M–F) who helps with the kids and picks up the house, cleans bathrooms, kitchens, etc. She's not the best housekeeper and we end up doing more stuff on the weekends ourselves, but it keeps our house from looking like a war zone and she's great with the kids and gets along with our primary nanny. (posted August 6, 2007, by pulpo)

Another couple we interviewed who were expecting their fourth child turned to the two-nanny solution when the wife decided to quit a part-time primary care internal medicine job and pursue an oncology fellowship. The wife commented that her entire fellowship salary would not cover their child care costs. While the two-nanny solution discussed in this post may seem extreme, it may be increasingly common throughout the medical workforce as the number of two-physician, two-career marriages grows. As we have seen, 95 percent of female physicians with physician spouses are in two-career marriages, and 50 percent of these couples work an average of one hundred hours or more collectively in an average week. So these couples are facing extreme pressures on their time, and increasingly they have significant additional income. Since many of these couples have children, they often seek more help. For some, two nannies is an attractive solution.

Although efforts to promote greater work-family balance remained limited, there is some evidence that the critical mass of women in medicine began having an effect on the structure of the profession during the 1980s and 1990s. One of the first major reforms that occurred involved the couples match. Prior to 1983, physician couples seeking residency spots had either to limit their selections to one city or rely on the poorly known and rarely used "option 7," which allowed physician couples to negotiate their residencies outside of the match system. Apparently the few who attempted to use option 7 encountered significant resistance from hospitals, which preferred single residents or residents with a supporting spouse. Nevertheless, the growing number of two-physician couples forced the system to evolve so that couples could match together (Belkin 1985). Since its inception, the number of two-physician couples taking advantage of the couples match increased markedly.

There is also limited evidence that conditions are improving for women in the medical education system. One woman we interviewed who graduated in 1985 told the story of a classmate who was pregnant with her first child during their first year in medical school. When the woman gave birth two days before her final exams, she was not granted an extension and was told that she would have to take the test or else get a zero grade. She took the test standing because she couldn't sit on account of her episiotomy. She received a D. Although this incident appears draconian, relatively little changed throughout the 1990s. This 2006 letter to the editor of the *New York Times* captures the experiences of one physician mother struggling to breast-feed:

> To the Editor:
> I am a mother of four and a pediatrician. My first child was born when I was in medical school, and my second and third during my residency. Returning to work after only 10 weeks (12 weeks was the maximum maternity allowed), I struggled to breast-feed my babies while working nights, weekends, 15-hour days and 24-hour shifts. I was forced to pump breast milk in bathrooms, call rooms, wherever I could find an outlet and a place to sit. I would struggle with engorgement through rounds that lasted for hours, or E.R. shifts that were too busy to take a break from. If the very profession that is supposed to be the largest supporter of breast-feeding treats its own mothers in this way, who are we to put such pressure, guilt and expectation on all new mothers? Until this society is structured to support and nurture those women who are lucky enough to be able to breast-feed, we can only expect any mother to do the best she can.
>
> Dr. Kimberly Fahey Brown
> Sands Point, N.Y.

By contrast, in 2007 a Massachusetts appeals court ruled in favor of a woman who requested additional break time while taking step 2 of the U.S. Medical Licensing Exam in order to pump milk for her infant.

It also appears that medical specialty societies such as the American Academy of Pediatrics and the American College of Physicians have acknowledged the increasing demand for flexible schedules. In particular, the American Academy of Pediatrics' Committee on the Pediatric Workforce has a section dedicated to women's issues. It has helped fund significant survey research to understand the scope of part-time work in the specialty and has drafted written resources for those in the field who are seeking flexible schedules.

Nevertheless, women physicians failed to unite even during the 1990s over work and family issues. Instead the growing number of women in medicine have largely continued to face motherhood alone. One woman obstetrician reflected on her experiences trying to combine work and family as a fellow during the 1990s:

> When, at age 37, I delivered my firstborn 1 week to the day after beginning a fellowship in high-risk pregnancy, I was devastated to have him admitted to the neonatal intensive care unit. On my way out the door, I ran into the senior fellow, who said to me, "Too bad about what happened. When can I put you back on the call schedule?" I seriously considered skipping my 4 allotted weeks of maternity leave, since if both my son and I were at the hospital, I could arrange to see him more. Little has changed since then: Our residents get a few weeks off for maternity leave, after which they must either resume their 12-hour days (and every third or fourth night in the hospital) or add extra time to their 4 years of residency training. (Plante 2004, 840)

The efforts that women physicians must make to balance work and family do not end when their children age out of infancy. They continue to make hard choices, and ultimately they severely limit their time for parenting. One woman surgeon we interviewed suggested that it was very possible to combine surgery and motherhood provided that the woman in question was comfortable being a part-time mother. While all women who work must restrict the time they allot to parenting, most do not face the drastic choices encountered by many women in medicine.

Although relatively little has been done to promote family-friendly work environments, we remain cautiously optimistic. The increasing numbers of women in all aspects of the medical profession will inevitably enhance the possibilities for meaningful change. Mary Lou Schmidt, an associate professor of pediatrics and a contributor to Eliza Chin's 2002 anthology on the experiences of women physicians, reflects on her friend Becca and "her six girlfriends who created their own private OB/GYN practice where everybody works four days a week, everybody has at least one or two kids, and everybody shares the profits equally" (280). And Becca is not alone; the number of all-female practices is inevitably increasing. The questions are whether a critical mass of women physicians will be able to take medicine in a new direction, and how many women it will take to create that critical mass.

9

Conclusion: A Prognosis for Gender and Medical Care

Since 1970 American medicine has been in a state of constant flux. As the overall size of the profession has grown, so too have its complexity, capacity, and diversity. Today's physicians have a much larger arsenal of treatments, and as a result, they spend more years in training and specialize more than their predecessors.

The funding and oversight of medical practice have also changed dramatically over the past generation. Today's physicians must assume a larger portion of the cost of their education, and they must justify their professional decisions more than at any other time in the profession's history. Cost, quality, and standards occupy an increasingly prominent place in the modern physician's mind as she practices her profession.

As American medicine has evolved, so too has American society. Since 1970 the presence of mothers in the workforce has expanded so that today more mothers with children at home participate in the labor force than not. At the same time, the average educational level of women in America has caught up to, and in some respects surpassed, that of men. Thus American women are now better prepared for paid work than at any other time in our history.

In spite of these changes, however, the norms surrounding gender remain entrenched in many aspects of American society. Americans generally support women's labor force participation but believe that mothers should stay home with young children. General support for fathers' involvement has grown, too, but resistance continues to greet individual fathers who want to spend less time at work in order to care for their children.

Like women's entry into the profession, women's status as physicians has been greatly affected by the dramatic, overarching changes occurring in the medical profession and the U.S. labor market as well as by the conflicting normative attitudes surrounding gender in American society. Although there has been tremendous growth in the number of women in all aspects of medicine, women physicians continue to cluster disproportionately in the lower tiers of the medical hierarchy. While individual choices and gender differences in priorities have contributed to the gender gap in the medical workforce, these choices have been greatly constrained by the failure of the profession to evolve in a way that more fully accommodates dual-career families.

Our research has repeatedly highlighted how women's entry into American medicine must be understood within the context of overall independent structural changes. On the one hand, when opportunities are available, women *choose* to take advantage of them. On the other hand, whenever medicine has become more restrictive, women, and other minorities in the profession, have suffered disproportionately.

The medical profession has changed in many ways and the rapid pace of change continues unabated. In this chapter we summarize the key developments discussed in the book. We conclude with our prognosis for the immediate future of women in medicine by focusing on four questions in particular: whether the feminization of medicine will continue; whether medicine will become a more caring, patient-centered endeavor; whether women will lead medicine in bold new directions; and whether women will bolster research on issues pertaining to women's health.

Why Did Medicine Feminize?

In contrast to one popular view and scholarly argument, we find that medicine did not feminize because it lost status. There have been obvious assaults on the standing of medicine, but the profession remains a high-status field and a highly respected one. The growing number of women medical students during the 1970s was accommodated by a dramatic growth in the capacity of U.S. medical schools. In other words, at least initially, increases in the number of women physicians did not reflect a decline in the profession, nor did it trigger declines in the number of male physicians. Moreover, the challenges to the medical profession do not correspond in time with declines in numbers of male applicants to medical school or increases in female applicants. In fact, the period in which the status of medicine suffered most greatly, the early 1990s, was also the period when applications to medical school rose precipitously for both young men and women.

Instead we suggest that women's presence in medicine expanded because of broader changes in women's roles in society and because of increased opportunities in medicine. These parallel developments produced a positive feedback loop which led to further interest in medicine and much wider preparation for medical careers on the part of young women. Attitudes toward employment and advanced education for women have evolved since the late 1960s so that the majority of Americans now support paid employment and equal educational opportunity for women. Sharp and sustained increases in women's labor force participation, the rise in the age of marriage, and the decline in the number of children per family combined to produce a shift in the landscape with respect to women's roles. The rapid growth in women's share of college degrees awarded also facilitated the advance of women in medicine. The organized activism of the women's movement secured legal reforms that barred gender discrimination in higher education admissions. Title IX represented a watershed in the demographics of modern medicine. Shortly after it took effect, there was a dramatic spike in female applications to U.S. medical schools and in the numbers of female medical students. In other words, women saw the opportunity created by legal reform and rushed to seize it.

These early advances by women helped in turn to stimulate further developments that broadened the pool of prospective women physicians. The jump in women's entry into medicine in the early 1970s no doubt contributed to greater awareness of and interest in medicine on the part of their younger college classmates. The visibility of medicine as a possible career rose to the point where at present, more women college freshmen express an interest in becoming a physician than do their male counterparts. The focus of women's professional interests has changed dramatically, causing striking declines in the number of women opting for the traditionally female fields of education and nursing. These declines have been matched by corresponding growth in the number of women studying biological science, business, and computer science. It was this feedback from initial advances to further interest and preparation for medical careers that led to the sustained advance of women into the profession.

Young women considering medicine, science, higher education, and professional employment probably encountered less discouragement from parents, teachers, and other relevant individuals than in previous generations, and they may even have begun to find increasingly common pockets of encouragement. Ultimately these changes in values and behavior sparked advances in education for women both overall and in the biological sciences. Furthermore, the initial advances eventually created role models for the next generation of women, which further fomented the growth of women in higher education generally and biological science and medicine more specifically.

As mentioned earlier, the second critical change leading to the feminization of U.S. medicine was a dramatic growth in the capacity of the medical education system at both the graduate and undergraduate levels. The number of women in medical training climbed at least in part because of dramatic growth in the number of seats in medical schools and residency programs. Growth in the number of female physicians, however, did not stem from changes in the persistence of women interested in medical careers. Historically, research has shown more attrition of women at each stage of the premedical pipeline, including maintaining an interest in medicine, taking the required premedical curriculum, applying to medical school, and receiving an acceptance. Our data suggest that the pipeline remains leaky, but the sheer volume of women's interest more than offsets the excess attrition of women at all stages of the process.

Gender Disparities within the Medical Profession

Although the presence of women in medicine has grown dramatically, complete integration remains elusive. In other words, medicine feminized incompletely and unevenly. There are signs that gender equality is growing slowly over time and in certain respects, but the pace of these improvements is slow, and in some areas of the profession such improvements are nearly nonexistent. The slow progress and lingering disadvantages are evident in both the personal and professional lives of women physicians.

On the one hand, the absolute number of women in the higher tiers of medicine is increasing. Today there are significantly more women in surgery, both generally and in obstetrics-gynecology specifically.[1] There are also more women physicians in research,[2] more women in academic medicine, and more women in administrative and academic leadership positions.

On the other hand, women physicians are not fully distributed across all medical specialties. As we saw in chapter 4, although the level of segregation across medical specialties declined through the mid-1980s, segregation by specialty has remained relatively constant since then. This stability implies that women's presence overall is growing in all segments of the profession, but the advances in male-dominated fields such as surgery are not great enough to overcome women's historical underrepresentation in these areas. The persistence of such work-based segregation stems in part from personal choices but also from the way those choices are structured. During the initial years of their entry into the profession, women clustered in certain specialties because of social and structural opportunities and obstacles. In other words, gender segregation initially arose because women physicians took advantage of the opportunities within medicine that were available to them, and those opportunities were not distributed equally across the profession. We believe that gender segregation is persisting at least in part because of its initial entrenchment.

Furthermore, although the number of women physicians in research has grown, women are still underrepresented in medical research relative to their presence in the profession overall. Indeed women physicians' share of research positions has declined since 1990 relative to their representation in medicine as a whole. We were able to trace some of the gap to men's and women's different experiences in medical school. Even after controlling for gender differences in interest in research among freshmen, we found that male medical students were far more likely than their female counterparts to have research experiences during medical school and to publish research with their advisers, despite the high levels of interest in academic careers on the part of female medical students.

In addition, although the desire to balance work and family accounts for a portion of the difference between male and female physicians' careers, the continued persistence of discrimination and harassment inevitably contributes to such disparities. While sexual harassment and gender discrimination are less tolerated today than they were a generation ago, the evidence indicates that such phenomena still present real problems for women attempting to enter the more prestigious tiers of the medical profession.

Moreover, many women physicians we talked with reported that more subtle gender discrimination still exists and, in fact, may be pervasive. Some women physicians sensed disparities but felt that they would be unable to pinpoint how significant this behavior had been in influencing their opportunities. Others cited more specific and dramatic examples of discrimination that they believed had negatively affected their career opportunities.

We have also demonstrated that the wage gap between employed male and female physicians has been closing over time. But we note that declines in the wage gap for physicians have clearly been uneven. Although the gap between the earnings of childless male and female physicians is closing, the gap between male and female physician parents is growing. Physician mothers also appear to be falling behind their childless female peers.

Our analysis of gender and physicians' personal lives yields similar conclusions. Disparities between male and female physicians are declining, but the pace is slow. Our findings indicate that female physicians are not as likely to sacrifice marriage and family formation as they once were. The gap in marriage and fertility rates of women physicians relative to other women has narrowed or been eliminated, but this has been principally because of delayed marriage and declining fertility in our society as a whole. Women physicians are still less likely than their male peers to marry and have children, but this gender disparity too is closing.

Similarly, there is good and bad news for equity in the personal lives of married male and female physicians. There is certainly increasing gender equality in the marriages of male physicians. Over time the wives of male physicians have become significantly more educated, more likely to hold paid employment, and more likely to work in a prestigious occupation. In particular, in 2000, for the first time, married male physicians were more likely to report that their spouse was also a physician than to report that their spouse was a nurse. The increasing educational level and occupational prestige of male physicians' wives has affected the work habits of both members of these unions. Because these women are more educated, they are more likely to work outside the home. These trends suggest that as the structure of married male physicians' personal lives changes, their work-related behavior is also likely to change. Perhaps those male physicians without a full-time supporting wife are less willing or able to dedicate themselves entirely to their profession. We suggest that it is possible that efforts to make the medical profession more family-friendly will accelerate as more male physicians reject the single-minded commitment to work that characterized their predecessors and instead seek a more balanced lifestyle.

The marriages of female physicians more closely approximate the ideal of partners making equal financial contributions. Female physicians' husbands are well educated and work full-time in prestigious occupations. Nonetheless, married female physicians respond to parenthood in a traditionally gendered fashion. According to our analysis of U.S. Census data, presented in chapter 6, on average married female physicians reduce their work effort once they have children, while their spouse's work hours either remain constant or increase. Nonetheless, there are some signs of increasing equity. Most notably, the extent to which female physicians restrict their work effort because of children depends on the occupation and earnings of their spouse. Female physicians with physician husbands assume a more traditionally female parenting role than those with a spouse outside the medical profession. And there is also a small increase in the percentage of married female physicians with a husband outside the paid workforce. Since this group of women doctors tend to enjoy relatively high earnings, we speculate that they represent a small but growing population who have elected to assume the traditionally masculine role of primary breadwinner.

Nevertheless, in spite of increases in labor force participation among male physicians' wives and fewer domestic compromises by female physicians, male and female physicians continue to confront dramatically different home environments. Even though male physicians are more likely to have an employed spouse than in the past, they still earn the lion's share of the family income while their wife normally assumes the bulk of the domestic responsibilities. The same is not true in the marriages of female physicians.

We suggest that the slow progress toward gender equity in the personal lives of married physicians stems at least in part from entrenched traditional values surrounding parenthood. Although most Americans believe that women should pursue higher education and work, many still support traditional roles within the home and expect women to assume the bulk of domestic responsibilities. And this conflict is reflected in current trends for physicians and current trends more generally. Recent research on marriage has suggested that highly accomplished women are more likely to marry than less accomplished women. We have also seen that female physicians have grown more likely than other women to marry. But other studies find that women in highly educated couples continue to be significantly more likely to restrict their work hours for the sake of their children than their spouses are (Moen 2003). We have seen a similar pattern for married physicians.

Nevertheless, trends within marriage suggest continued, if slow, evolution toward greater gender equality. Our research suggests that the increasing gap in education and status between female physicians and their husbands is reducing the tendency for these couples to respond to marriage and parenthood in a traditional fashion. Similar trends are evident among men.

Gender and the Practice of Medicine

Male and female providers treat sexually sensitive conditions differently, but provider gender plays little if any role in the treatment of gender-neutral complaints. Our results do not necessarily indicate that women provide more empathic or higher-quality care to women because they are themselves women. Indeed it was the male physicians who were more likely to recommend an office visit for the symptoms of vaginal itching discussed in chapter 7. We suggest that this gap comes at least in part from documented differences in how men and women physicians are trained. Female physicians in training receive significantly more exposure to, and practice with, female patients and uniquely female problems (Orzano and Cody 1995), and ultimately this determines how much comfort they have with procedures for treating these conditions (Lurie et al. 1997). The same pattern holds for men treating male patients in circumstances involving sexual privacy. We suggest that this training gap should either be addressed and ameliorated through appropriate training or acknowledged and accommodated through the encouragement of provider-patient gender concordance.

Until recently, women's growing presence in medicine has done relatively little to facilitate work-family balance. In fact, the profession is becoming more rather than less demanding. Over time the average workweek for female physicians has come to resemble more closely that of their male colleagues, but this gap has closed because women have increased their work effort while men have maintained theirs. Work effort is growing in spite of substantial evidence that physicians of both genders would prefer to work less.

As medicine has evolved, some changes have facilitated balance in certain specialties. Furthermore, recent regulations on resident work hours have eased conditions for the growing number of residents who choose to become parents. Yet with few exceptions these pro-family reforms had little if anything to do with the growing presence of women in the medical community.

Nevertheless, we are cautiously optimistic regarding the prospects for work-family reform. The potential for women to effect change may soon increase substantially, both because they now constitute a critical mass in the profession and because men are increasingly finding themselves in two-career families. Together these changes will inevitably increase the demand for flexibility and balance in medical work.

Prognosis for Change

The dizzying rate of change in the medical arena makes prognostication an especially hazardous undertaking. Nonetheless, we summarize recent trends and offer our appraisal of trends for the immediate future in several key areas. Will women continue to enter the profession in such large numbers? Will physicians continue to deliver primary care to patients? Will women increasingly occupy positions of leadership in the profession? Answering these questions speaks to whether the medical profession will soon become a more female-dominated and patient-centered institution.

We expect that in the coming years women will continue to pour into the medical profession, and their representation will continue to increase, passing the 50 percent mark. Women will also become increasingly prominent in leadership positions, although progress in this echelon may not be commensurate with women's overall presence in the profession. We are more skeptical, however, as to whether medicine will become a substantially more patient-centered, caring profession in the near future. The increasing departure of physicians from primary care settings, along with escalating cost pressures, will make it difficult for a caring agenda to prevail, whether championed by women or by others inside or outside of medicine. Finally, the prospects for continued progress in research on women's health issues, and gender differences in health processes more generally, appear to be quite bright.

Women's Representation in the Profession

We feel confident in predicting that women medical students will surpass parity with their male classmates and will soon represent a majority of incoming medical students. We make this claim despite of the fact that between 2003–2004 and 2006–2007 women's presence among applicants declined slightly from 50.8 percent to 49.3 percent (Magrane et al. 2007). Our prediction reflects a series of related developments that show no immediate signs of abating. Women's representation in college continues to increase. In 2006 the National Center for Education Statistics' *Digest of Education Statistics* projected that women will make up 60 percent of new college graduates within the next decade. Among women in this burgeoning group of college students, an increasing share are well prepared for medical school in terms of their high school and college-level course work. Furthermore, freshman women's interest in pursuing medicine continues to outpace that of men. In 2006, 6.7 percent of female college freshmen expressed an interest in pursing a career in medicine, compared with 5.3 percent of their male classmates (Sax et al. 2006). Although fewer women than men maintain this goal and actually persist to the point of applying to medical school, women's share of applicants to medical school will continue to rise. There would have to be a substantial drop in women's interest in medicine, or persistence rates, to change this pattern. Since the sluggish economy has contributed to the recent increases in medical school applications, we predict that male interest in the profession will decline once the economy improves.

One final important trend is that more women who have left college or graduate school return than do men. More students, and more women in particular, are taking time out before completing their studies. As students age into their late twenties and early thirties, the balance in favor of women increases (National Center for Education Statistics 2006c, Table 178). As medical schools draw from this pool of older and returning students, they will find more women in the pool of candidates.

We expect that women's presence in the population of practicing physicians will increase markedly in the near future as the first generations of physicians educated in the post-Medicare era, a largely male population, begin to retire. We cannot foresee where this trend toward the feminization of medicine will end. Given the trends just cited, however, it would not be surprising if in the next decade 55 or even 60 percent of medical students were women. It will take many years for these students to populate the profession fully. Nonetheless, the process of feminization has already been set in motion.

The Future of Primary Care

As we suggested in chapter 7, research studies routinely report that women physicians are more empathetic toward patients than are their male counterparts. If more doctors are women, and if women are more caring than men, is a more humanistic, patient-centered profession on the horizon?

We suggest that the ameliorative scenario envisioned by this line of reasoning will be relatively modest in scope. First, as we noted in chapter 7, the magnitude of the gender gap in empathy is small. Second, the evolving nature of American health care will inhibit any nascent trend toward more humanistic care. Productivity expectations will simply make it too difficult to engage in lengthy, multifaceted visits with patients. Finally, there are good reasons to believe that the first stage of patient encounters, the stage when humanism, communication, and collegiality have been shown to be most influential—namely, the delivery of primary care—will involve fewer and fewer physicians.

Primary care is declining as a specialty for both male and female graduates of U.S. medical schools. In 1997, 17.6 percent of medical school graduates expressed an interest in pursuing a career in family medicine. By 2007 that fraction had declined to 6.1 percent. A similar decline is evident in pediatrics: 5.7 percent of graduates in 2007 planned to pursue pediatrics, down from 12.6 percent in 1997 (AAMC 1997 and 2007).

Interest in primary care is declining at similar rates for both male and female graduates of U.S. allopathic medical schools (Lambert and Holomboe 2005). The medical profession's continued trend away from primary care delivery in favor of specialization will undermine whatever "natural" inclinations toward empathetic care women may possess.

We are by no means the first to note the precarious future of primary care. Lynne Kirk, the president of the American College of Physicians, declared in 2006 that primary care was in a state of "crisis." Similar alarms have been raised about family practice (Phillips and Starfield 2003) and general internal medicine (Kirk 2006).

The departure of many U.S.-trained physicians from the field has forced a number of primary care residency programs to rely on foreign-trained physicians. The trend is especially pronounced in family practice. During the 1990s, international medical graduates made up an increasing percentage of family practice residency programs, from 16.7 percent in 1996 to 47.9 percent in 2001 (Koehn et al. 2002). Between 2003 and 2007, around 58 percent of family practice residency spots were filled by international medical graduates (National Resident Matching Program 2007b).

Reliance on foreign medical graduates is less severe in internal medicine and pediatrics. From 2003 to 2007, approximately 44 percent of all internal medicine residency spots and 27 percent of all pediatric residency spots were filled by international medical graduates. These numbers are somewhat misleading, since many internal medicine and pediatric residents sub-specialize. The share of internists planning to pursue general internal medicine, as opposed to a subspecialty field, dropped from 54 percent to 20 percent between 1998 and 2005 (Garibaldi et al. 2005).

Recent trends reveal a significant decline in the number of foreigners planning to practice medicine in the United States. Historically, foreign physicians seeking to practice in this country were first required to pass step 1 and step 2 of the standardized medical licensing exams and score adequately on the Test of English as a Foreign Language. In 1998 another exam was added to list of prerequisites for foreign physicians wishing to practice in the United States, the Clinical Skills Assessment (CSA). The CSA requires that international medical graduates (IMGs) be able to elicit an appropriate patient history, properly perform a physical exam, demonstrate good interpersonal skills, and write an accurate account of the patient encounter. Administered in English only, the exam also requires that IMGs demonstrate proficiency in English.[3] While the other required exams are given at five hundred test centers across the world, the CSA exam is administered only in Philadelphia, the headquarters of the Educational Commission for Foreign Medical Graduates. Many foreigners cannot afford to make the trip to Philadelphia, and as a result, in the first years that the CSA was administered to foreigners, the number of IMGs registering for the test declined each year. The number of IMG registrations dropped from almost 67,000 in 1997, the year before the exam was instituted, to 27,000 in 2000 (Kupersanin 2001).

In the face of declining domestic and foreign interest, family practice residencies have been under increasing stress and have begun eliminating training spots. The number of family practice residency openings actually declined by 10 percent between 2003 and 2007. Although these declines are not surprising in light of declining interest, they raise significant questions about the future supply of physicians. A study conducted by the National Association of Community Health Centers and the American Academy of Family Physicians that was released in March 2007 suggests that already 56 million Americans, nearly one in five individuals, are medically disenfranchised, meaning they have inadequate or no access to primary care physicians because of the shortage of such practitioners (Arvantes 2007).

It appears that mid-level health care providers or nurse practitioners (NPs) and physician assistants (PAs) are beginning to fill some of the gap in the primary care workforce. The number of PAs and NPs has exploded since the early 1990s, and currently there are more NPs and PAs providing primary care than there are family physicians (McCann et al. 2005).

In 2007 the American Academy of Physician Assistants surveyed over seventy thousand practitioners, more than double the size of the field a decade earlier. In 2004 the Bureau of Labor Statistics projected more than 27 percent growth in the number of physician assistants by 2014, making it one of the fastest-growing occupations in the U.S. labor force. Analysis of the National Ambulatory Medical Care Survey indicates that in 2004, nearly one quarter (23 percent) of all primary care visits in the United States were provided by an "extender" rather than a physician, more than twice the share in the late 1990s (Hooker and Craig 2001). Research indicates that physician assistants are capable of providing care for 86 percent of the diagnoses seen in outpatient primary care settings and that patient acceptance of such practitioners is high (Hooker and Freeborn 1991). Analyses have also found that the cost of employing a physician assistant ranges from 25 to 53 percent that of a physician (Hooker and Freeborn 1991). Similarly, treatment costs 10 to 40 percent less when provided by a nurse practitioner instead of a physician (Vaughn 2006), and an increasing body of research indicates that nurse practitioners provide care that is of equal quality. So there is every reason to believe that the percentage of care provided by extenders will increase.

Since the greatest growth in non-physician clinicians involves those who provide primary care, it is reasonable to surmise that the percentage of all primary care visits handled by nurse practitioners and physician assistants will increase significantly (Cooper et al. 1998). There are also signs that potential physicians are being tempted by careers as non-physician clinicians. One premedical student enrolled in a baccalaureate nursing program expressed ambivalence about a career in medicine. She told us:

> One thing that I'm kind of struggling with is financial....Some nurse practitioners can make more than some doctors. I was thinking I'm going to go through med school for four years and owe a fortune. I could go to graduate school [in nursing] for two years. The hospital can pay for it and I'll make six figures. So, I guess I'm thinking, in my case, do I need to go to medical school to do what I want to do? Now, some doctors like general pediatricians make $90,000 a year. Some nurses make that without their masters.

In the present political environment, nurse practitioners and primary care physicians do not have equivalent privileges. Currently nurse practitioners are authorized to prescribe medication in all fifty states, but there is considerable variation in the extent of their authority to do so. In 2002, although 82 percent of nurse practitioners have some authority to prescribe, only 45 percent were authorized to prescribe controlled substances (Phillips et al. 2002). Nevertheless, in some areas the daily work lives of primary care nurse practitioners closely parallel those of primary care physicians. In twenty-six states, including Connecticut and New Jersey, nurse practitioners can practice without a link to a physician (Freudenheim 1997).

In the absence of significant and dramatic changes to our current health care financing system, there is every reason to believe that the role of physicians in the provision of primary care will decline. Today a physician entering practice has on average accumulated more than $100,000 in student debt. The median indebtedness of medical school students graduating in 2006 was expected to be $120,000 for students at public medical schools and $160,000 for students attending private medical schools. About 5 percent of all medical students graduated with debt of $200,000 or more (Arora 2006). Research suggests that returns on this educational investment are ultimately lower for primary care physicians than for procedure-based medicine, dentistry, law, or business (Weeks and Wallace 2002).

Many suggest that the solution to the declining interest in primary care involves increased reimbursements (Cross 2007). Few believe, however, that private companies will increase payments unless the federal government sets a new reimbursement standard. In the face of looming budget shortages and the prolonged involvement of the United States in the Iraq war, funding for additional health care expenses in the near future seems unlikely. Medicare pay rates for services have not kept up with inflation since 1997 (Glendinning 2007), and evidence suggests that total expenditures on Medicare will outpace overall economic growth even if physician reimbursements are cut dramatically. These increases will stem primarily from the medical needs of an increasingly chronically ill elderly population and from the increased capabilities of modern medicine (Glendinning 2007). In the absence of dramatic revisions in our health care system such as the adoption of universal health insurance, the prospects for increases in payment to primary care physicians appear dim.

The confluence of these trends suggests that women's capacity to humanize medical care will be rather limited. "In the future your doctor may be a nurse," said Sara Foer, a spokeswoman for the American Nurses Association (Freudenheim 1997). In the absence of significant change, responsibility for humanizing health care may well be assumed by an entirely distinct specialty.

Those providing direct patient care are likely to be women. Historically, the great majority of nurse practitioners have been women. In recent years the representation of women among physician assistants has grown, with women now making up roughly two thirds of PAs. These trends suggest that direct patient care will likely be in the hands of women, though the practitioners providing this care may not be physicians. Regardless of gender or specialty, however, there is every reason to believe that increasing efforts to control costs will limit primary care providers' ability to offer holistic and humane health care.

But even in the most dramatic scenario, primary care physicians will not be rendered irrelevant. While nurse practitioners have been lobbying for and slowly gaining the right to practice primary care independently, physician assistants have not generally aspired to independent practice. Thus, at the very least, primary care physicians will remain a critical part of the care delivered by physician assistants. Furthermore, it is politically unlikely that nurse practitioners will be granted universal rights to independent practice in the near future, and even if they are given such a scope of practice, it is likely that many will opt to continue working under physician supervision. A closely related scenario is one in which nurse practitioners and physician assistants work collaboratively with physicians in providing primary care to patients. While many NPs and PAs have pushed for a more independent status, a collaborative arrangement may be possible. In other words, one possible future for primary care is a teamwork model rather than the replacement of physicians with other kinds of medical practitioners.

What do we know about female physicians as team players? Hojat and colleagues (2001; 2003) found that physicians' gender does not influence attitudes toward collaboration with nurses in the United States and elsewhere, including Israel, Mexico, and Italy. In other words, male and female physicians indicated that they were equally willing to collaborate with nurses and to participate in training designed to enhance collaboration. Several studies indicate, however, that there is often a disconnect between physicians' and nurses' perceptions of collaboration, with male and female physicians uniformly perceiving more collaboration than either male or female nurses (Hojat et al. 2003). The finding persists in a variety of medical environments, including intensive care units (Thomas et al. 2003; Hamric and Blackhall 2007), operating rooms (Makary et al. 2006), and emergency departments (Hansen et al. 1999). It also persists in many countries, including the United States (Hojat et al. 2003), Australia (Copnell et al. 2004), and Mexico (Hojat et al. 2003).

Other studies provide a more troubling picture of the collaboration between female physicians and other medical practitioners. Research conducted in the United States and across the world indicates that nurses, a primarily female population, treat female physicians differently from male physicians (Brooks 1998; Gjerberg and Kjølsrød 2001; Zelek and Philips 2003; Wear and Keck-McNulty 2004; Cassell 1997). In particular, although nurses generally prefer communicating with female physicians and prefer the female managerial style, female physicians frequently report discriminatory treatment from nurses. More than 80 percent of female physicians feel that at some time in their careers they have experienced unequal treatment, more intense scrutiny, or a lack of respect from nurses because they (the doctors) were female (Wear and Keck-McNulty 2004). And survey research suggests that female physicians are not simply imagining this treatment. Although nurses expect both male and female physicians to remove needles on a suture tray, they are more willing to clean up after men and do so with less hostility (Zelek and Phillips 2003). In light of this unequal pressure, it is reasonable to suspect that women physicians approach subordinates more collegially primarily because the penalties for doing otherwise are more severe for them. In fact, in their survey of Norwegian physicians, Gjerberg and Kjølsrød (2001) find that female physicians commonly employed two strategies to cope with discriminatory treatment from nurses. Some did as much as they could on their own, and others actively befriended the nurses. Some female physicians' resentment of nurses, however, may limit the collegiality they will "offer" to nurses.

Finally, the potential for women to employ a more collegial relationship with other members of the health care team must be understood in terms of the broader changes in the U.S. health care system. Most important, the changing status of nurses and other health care workers may force physicians of both genders to change their behavior. Leonard Stein's classic article "The Doctor-Nurse Game" (1967) described the traditional relationship between doctors and nurses. Stein initially observed that by showing initiative and making important recommendations while appearing to defer passively to the doctor's authority, nurses have historically avoided usurping physicians' power and deflected open disagreement. But when Stein revisited the nurse-doctor game in 1990, he found that nurses had unilaterally decided to stop playing (Zelek and Phillips 2003). Stein suggested that the end of the game had occurred in large part because of the growing numbers of female physicians. The increasing status concordance between nurses and physicians may also have empowered nurses to take more initiative and act more assertively with all physicians regardless of gender.

Nurses' status and empowerment are also intimately intertwined with independent changes in the health care system. In particular, during the 1980s hospitals implemented primary nursing systems that associated each patient with a specific nurse. This management trend forced physicians to take individual nurses more seriously. Further, recent efforts to improve medical safety as delineated in the 2000 Institute of Medicine Report, *To Err Is Human,* have resulted in a greater tendency to view health delivery more coherently rather than to focus on individual players. The current focus on safety has also highlighted the need to "Develop a working culture in which communication flows freely regardless of authority gradient" (178). Such recommendations should ultimately enhance nurses' status throughout the hospital, especially when they are coupled with increased use of error reporting and assessment. Yet, they are largely independent of women's presence in medicine.

In another, related trend, the increasing employment of nurses' aides in hospitals threatens the professional status of nurses (Weinberg 2003, 49). The trend toward deprofessionalization of nursing at the hospital bedside coexists, however, with the increasing employment of nurse case managers for costly, chronically ill patients and of nurse utilization review by insurance companies. This trend translates into a dramatic new reality for medicine. Physicians increasingly have to "get permission" to perform procedures in the context of insurance company utilization review requirements, and nurses are not infrequently in the role of deciding whether to grant this permission.[4]

Thus it seems that the premise that women physicians are more "collegial" in the approach to other health care workers stems largely, if not entirely, from the distinct expectations of these workers rather than from innate differences in women's leadership style. Furthermore, since the status and expectations of nurses and other allied health professionals are intimately intertwined with independent changes in the health care system, it is not possible to predict how these relationships will evolve as the structure of American health care continues to change. If nurses continue to gain status, they may became increasingly unwilling to defer to physicians of either gender.

The future of primary care as a patient-centered enterprise is thus not a foregone conclusion but will instead depend very much on who is delivering this care and under what organizational and financial rubric. The feminization of medicine by itself will not humanize the profession, especially if the flight from primary care continues.

Women and Leadership

As we suggested in chapter 4, there has been tremendous absolute growth in the number of women in leadership positions within the medical arena. Nevertheless, the number of women physician leaders have not kept pace with women's entry into the profession overall, and women leaders remain segregated in the less prestigious, less well reimbursed areas of medicine. The persistence of segregation is especially obvious in academic medicine. Women have made up at least 30 percent of medical students since 1985 and have since become at least 50 percent of medical students. Yet by the early years of the twenty-first century, only 10 percent of department chairs in American medical schools were female (Carnes 2005). As we discussed in chapter 5, similar trends exist in the leadership of the AMA (Executive Women in Healthcare 2005; Gentry 2004). In the absence of significant change, we predict that more women physicians will lead, but women physicians will also cluster disproportionately at the bottom of the profession.

The growth of women in medical leadership will continue in part because, as we noted earlier, there is every reason to believe that women's entry into medicine will persist. As time goes on, momentum will inevitably push some of the growing numbers of women physicians up the organizational hierarchy.

Gender disparities in medical leadership will persist both because gendered norms of parenting persist in our society and because gender discrimination remains significant in the medical and scientific arenas. In other words, women physicians will continue to be doubly disadvantaged by a disproportionate share of domestic responsibilities and by substantially greater expectations and significantly reduced support from professional colleagues. In a representative survey of medical faculty, Foster and colleagues (2000) found that women physicians were four times as likely as their male colleagues to believe that they were being excluded from valuable informal networking opportunities (24 versus 6 percent). Moreover, evidence of discrimination is not restricted to individuals' perceptions. Trix and Psenka reviewed 312 letters of recommendation for medical faculty hired at a large U.S. medical school and found that letters for women were shorter and more likely to include doubt-raising comments (Trix and Psenka 2003).

Like our predictions regarding primary care, our assessment of women's influence on medical leadership conflicts with much of the existing literature. Policymakers and physicians have suggested that women's increasing presence in medicine will result in more collegial and collaborative leadership among physicians (Levinson and Lurie 2004). Some have assumed an essential difference in the management styles of men and women to support their claims (Regan and Brooks 1995; Eagly and Johnson 1990; Eagly et al. 2003). In their meta-analysis of more than 160 studies of sex-related differences, Eagly and Johnson (1990) found that women employed a more democratic leadership style grounded in a strong interpersonal approach, whereas men relied more on task-related behaviors, though these results were diminished in organizational settings and male-dominated environments. More recently a meta-analysis of forty-five studies of transformational, transactional, and laissez-faire leadership styles by Eagly and colleagues (2003) found that women demonstrated more transformational behaviors (e.g., clearly communicated values, motivation, optimism, willingness to consider new perspectives, and attention to individual needs) than their male counterparts. Women also demonstrated higher levels of contingent reward, or behaviors in which the leader rewards followers for the completion of tasks. Both transformational leadership and contingent reward behaviors have been identified as predictors of effectiveness (Lowe et al. 1996), which would suggest that women may possess a leadership advantage under this postindustrial paradigm (Dugan 2006). In particular, some researchers also claim that women's leadership involves more participation, motivation by inclusion, and power by charisma (Rutherford 2001, 329).

We are skeptical that incremental growth in the representation of women in leadership positions will dramatically change the direction of the medical profession. First, unlike the research on physician gender and communication, the research on gender and management is much less uniform and thus does not support the claim that women physicians will change the nature of medical leadership (Wajcman 1998; Hymowitz 2005). Second, the leadership styles of women physicians are inevitably circumscribed by the organizations in which they work, by the expectations of the people they supervise, and by independent structural change in their industry (Eagly and Johannesen-Schmidt 2001, 794). Like women physicians' potential to change primary care, women physicians' capacity to transform medical leadership is limited by structural constraints.

Even research which identifies a gender difference in leadership and management style often suggests that such differences are slight and that gender per se is not a decisive determinant of managers' approach to their jobs (Eagly et al. 2003). An AAMC report on women in academic medicine reached a similar conclusion: they maintain that women are as different from each other as men are, so generalizations in the area of leadership are precarious (Bickel et al. 1996). Furthermore, although some researchers believe that women employ more collaborative leadership, others question this premise (Wajcman 1998). One meta-analysis involving the research firm Catalyst analyzed forty studies of men and women leaders and found no real differences in leadership style (Hymowitz 2005).

Moreover, the leadership style of women physicians is influenced by the organizations that employ them (Ely 1995; Bickel et al. 1996). Since the highest tiers of medical management remain extremely male dominated, it is reasonable to suspect that women physicians' leadership style may be constrained by the demands of their superiors. One woman residency program director whom we interviewed recalled that she had worked for years to secure breast-feeding space for her residents in the hospital. Her ability to provide a humane environment was restricted by the leadership of her organization.

Like the potential for women to change primary care, the potential for women physician leaders also needs to be understood in an appropriate context. Although continued growth in the numbers of female physician leaders seems the most likely course, the role of the medical profession in the overall health care industry is increasingly challenged by other powerful contingents such as hospitals and insurance companies. So the ultimate potential for women physicians to change health care may be undercut by the declining influence of physicians overall. As we suggested earlier, hospitals are increasingly turning to physicians to assume management responsibilities; it is too soon to assess the effect of this trend. The ultimate influence of these medical managers, however, remains untested.

Another related factor worth considering involves the growing diversity in hospital leadership. According to the Association of Executive Women in Healthcare, there has been significant growth in the number of women leading America's hospitals. In 2005 there were approximately nine hundred female CEOs and twelve hundred women making up the C-suite (COOs, CAOs, CFOs, and CIOs) (Executive Women in Healthcare 2005). Since there are about 5,810 hospital members of the American Hospital Association, approximately 15 percent of American hospitals are led by women. Although health care administration remains very male dominated, there has been significant growth in the number of women with influence over America's hospitals.

Like their male colleagues, most of the women leading America's hospitals are not physicians. In contrast to the men, however, the new generation of female leaders has not been trained primarily in the business of health care. Instead they come to health care administration as non-physician clinicians. Nearly two thirds of the nine hundred women hospital CEOs have degrees in nursing. We can only speculate as to how leadership by female nurses will affect the work lives of women physicians (Executive Women in Healthcare 2005). In light of the documented tensions between women physicians and women nurses, however, it is reasonable to suspect that the growing presence of women among hospital executives will not necessarily make the unique needs of women in medicine a high priority. Nevertheless, the growing diversity in the topmost echelons of medical leadership should help women physicians in some respects.

Finally, the potential for women to employ a collaborative approach to leadership in the upper echelons of health care management is severely curtailed by the growing size and complexity of the health care industry. Individuals who lead hospitals and clinics must deal with the need to increase gross revenues and satisfy a growing number of interested parties, including health insurance companies and federal regulators. Furthermore, health care management must be accomplished in an increasingly stressed fiscal environment. It is difficult to employ collaborative leadership and consensus building under such conditions regardless of an individual's gender. There are simply too many competing parties.

Nevertheless, as we have seen, women physicians bring different values and goals with them into the medical profession. Thus they are more likely to lead physicians' unions and to support universal health care than are their male counterparts, and are more interested in helping people, at least at the start of their career.

Women physicians may well seek to lead the medical profession in new directions as they broaden their representation in leadership roles. We feel, however, that we should not expect dramatic immediate changes, especially in the area of management style, simply as a result of greater leadership roles on the part of women physicians.

Women Physicians and Women's Health Research

While we urge caution with regard to expecting too much from women in leadership, the recent research record provides more grounds for optimism. Since the early 1990s there has been an explosion in the quantity of women's health research. Without doubt, more women are now included in clinical trials, and many more studies focus on diseases that especially afflict women (Purnell et al. 2005). Even more important, however, the historically entrenched assumption that men and women are biologically equivalent apart from the process of reproduction is being systematically challenged in almost every way (Price 1997). This means that while the field of women's health historically was limited to issues surrounding reproduction, it now involves studies of all organ systems. One indication of the tremendous growth of research on women's health is the fact that the *Journal of the American Medical Association* received 412 submissions, a record high for *JAMA*, for its 2006 women's health theme issue (DeAngelis and Glass 2006).

Much of the recent literature on women's health stems directly from the Women's Health Initiative (WHI), a major effort funded by the National Institutes of Health designed to address the exclusion of women from several major studies, most of which focused on heart disease.[5] Launched in 1991, the WHI reflected increasing attention to women's health and a strong demand for reliable information to guide women's health care decisions. It was the first broad-scale examination of the major causes of disability and death among postmenopausal women, recruiting more than 161,000 volunteers in the United States between fifty and seventy-nine years of age. Clinical trials tested three interventions: hormone therapy to prevent coronary heart disease and osteoporotic fractures, a reduced-fat diet to prevent breast and colorectal cancers and coronary heart disease, and calcium and vitamin D supplementation to prevent fractures and colorectal cancer (Nabel 2006).

One of the most widely noted findings of the WHI was the discovery that hormone replacement therapy increases the risk of breast cancer and does not affect the risk of heart disease. At the time the WHI began, the standard of care was to put all women on female hormones from the time they reached menopause until the day they died. There was a widely accepted belief that hormones protected women against heart disease and other illnesses. In fact, one of the major concerns about the WHI study on hormones involved the ethical implications of denying some women what was assumed to be a therapeutic intervention. In 2002 the study was prematurely stopped in order to protect women from the negative effects of hormones (Marshall 2005). The decline in breast cancer incidence that followed has been attributed to the decline in hormone replacement therapy prompted by the WHI study (Kolata 2007).

Another major outcome from the WHI was an effort to redress the exclusion of women from the Physicians' Health Study, a study of the effects of aspirin therapy on the risk of heart attacks. In March 2005 researchers reported that overall women aspirin takers did not have a significantly lower risk of heart attack, but they did have a somewhat lower risk of stroke (Marshall 2005). The reverse is true in men (Kaiser 2005).

The WHI was a tremendous undertaking in its size, scope, and cost. Official estimates indicate that by 2007, the federal government had invested $725 million in the project. And the WHI was not the only NIH-initiated effort on women's health during the 1990s. By 1993, $75 million had been authorized for basic research on ovarian and other reproductive cancers, and three contraceptive and two infertility research centers had been initiated. Approximately $40 million had been allocated for research on osteoporosis and bone disorders (Auerbach and Figert 1995).

A significant portion of the current focus on women's issues also stems from independent grass-roots efforts by breast cancer survivors and political organizations such as the National Breast Cancer Coalition to encourage the government to increase attention to the condition. Activists focused on breast cancer rather than other female-specific conditions because it remains the most common non-skin cancer in women and is second only to lung cancer in its capacity to kill. About forty thousand women annually succumb to this disease in the United States alone.

Prior to the 1990s federal funding for breast cancer was relatively limited. In 1989 the U.S. government allotted only $74.5 million to the condition, less than 5 percent of what it had dedicated to AIDS at the time, although AIDS killed about half as many people on average (Lerner 2002). By recruiting representatives throughout the country, the National Breast Cancer Coalition obtained 2.6 million signatures in support of the National Action Plan on Breast Cancer in 1993. As a result of these efforts and others, the organization persuaded Congress to fund what it called a "war on breast cancer." Total annual funding for breast cancer research jumped to over $550 million by 1996 and totaled approximately $700 million in 1999 (Lerner 2002). And it is worth noting that several private organizations have contributed significant amounts to breast cancer research, education, and awareness. In particular, the Susan Komen Foundation, Yoplait yogurt, and the Avon Foundation are major contributors to breast cancer research and advocacy. Since its inception the Komen Foundation has collected more than $180 million for breast cancer research and significantly more for breast cancer outreach and care (Arnst 2005a).[6]

Much of the breast cancer funding was dedicated to basic science. One of the most valuable accomplishments of these funds was the discovery that the overexpression of the gene ERBB2 promotes aggressive growth in more than 25 percent of breast cancers. The subsequent development of the antibody Herceptin, which inhibits ERBB2 growth, represents a significant advancement in breast cancer therapy (Lerner 2002). And Herceptin is not the only major advance that the war on breast cancer produced. A group of estrogen-blocking drugs called aromatase inhibitors have proven effective in preventing breast cancer from recurring after surgery (Arnst 2005b).

The tremendous growth in funding for women's health has not only made research efforts possible but also broadened the focus and awareness of medical researchers more generally so that sex differences are now more firmly within the general scope of research questions. In other words, as suggested earlier, the assumption that men and women are basically the same physiologically and biochemically apart from the reproductive function is no longer pervasive. In particular, analyses by the Food and Drug Administration of adverse drug reactions during the 1990s revealed that at least nine drugs on the market posed unique hazards for women. By 2001 the FDA had pulled four of these drugs off the market, including Seldane, a popular antihistamine. Although no effort has been made to analyze the effects of these drugs on mortality, researchers believe that women died disproportionately from heart arrhythmias while these medications were on the market (Kaiser 2005).

In fact, the new awareness of gender may ultimately improve the care of both genders. For example, according to research stemming from the new perspective, the female brain has more intercellular connections, which may be why women are twice as likely to recover the ability to speak after a stroke. The male brain, by contrast, produces more depression-fighting serotonin, which helps explain why men are far less likely to suffer depression (Yellin 2004). The positive implications for men and women have caused some to refer to these trends as the development of gender-specific medicine rather than the more limited term "women's health."

In spite of the tremendous growth in funding and attention, however, gaps remain in women's health research. In particular, although women are now being included in clinical trials, and there is a growing appreciation of a new paradigm with respect to gender, health, and medicine, research specifically assessing differences in how men and women react to clinical treatments continues to represent a small sliver of the health research pie. In 2005 the Society for the Advancement of Women's Health Research reported that between 2000 and 2003, the National Institutes of Health awarded an average of 3 percent of their grants per year for research on sex differences, while the total percentage of grants awarded during the same period increased by 20 percent (Simon 2005).

In addition to the relative lack of attention to sex differences, there also appears to be a distribution problem in the efforts to advance women's health research and treatment. In particular, the striking increase in breast cancer funding has raised concerns among some activists, policymakers, and providers that the highly effective political tactics of breast cancer activists have resulted in too great a focus on one women's disease and, correspondingly, too little focus on others diseases that also kill large numbers of women. In 1997, National Cancer Institute funding per death from breast cancer was four times its funding per death from lung cancer, even though lung cancer kills four times as many people (Lerner 2002).

It is difficult to track the dramatic trends in women's health research without wondering why and how such a significant change in national research efforts occurred in such a relatively short period of time. The evidence suggests that although the process was relative rapid, it had multiple determinants and took place in discrete stages. Throughout these twists and turns, women physicians and researchers have played a major role in advancing this agenda (Riska 2001, 124).

In fact women physicians were not only a central part of the community of women's health researchers; they also played a major role in the initial effort to focus public attention and resources on women's health. Furthermore, women physicians were instrumental in creating the organizational structure that allowed massive amounts of women's health research to occur. Nevertheless, the efforts of women physicians to promote and conduct research on women's health must be understood within a broader context. Women physicians were only one of several groups who contributed to this dramatic change. The increased research on women's health could not have occurred without the help of female leaders in the private sector, female leaders in Congress, the efforts of many grass-roots women's health activists, and the support of many male leaders throughout the medical community and the broader society.

Previous research has repeatedly suggested that the origins of the Women's Health Initiative can be traced to the publication of a report by the Public Health Service Task Force on Women's Health in 1985. The commissioning and publication of this report was due in large part to grass-roots women's health movements of the 1970s (Auerbach and Figert 1995). Although individual female physicians inevitably participated in the women's health movements of the 1970s and early 1980s, women physicians as a group did not play a major role in these efforts and generally did not distinguish themselves as leaders of the initial movement (Riska 2001, 121–22).[7]

The 1985 report called for expanded biomedical and behavioral research on women and increased representation of women in study populations of federally funded research (Pinn and Chunko 1999). As a result of the report, the NIH issued a new policy in 1986, which became effective in 1987, to encourage the inclusion of women in clinical scientific trials. Once the report was issued, however, influential women physicians and women scientists began to play a more central role in the advancement of women's health research. In particular, a meeting was held in 1988 where major female leaders in biomedicine as well as feminist attorneys and lobbyists decided to "change the climate of thinking" about women's health research. Part of the plan involved initiating a study to demonstrate funding problems with women's health research and a media campaign to raise awareness. Eventually, in 1990 these leaders formed the Society for the Advancement of Women's Health Research, a formal organization dedicated to implementing the initial plans developed at the 1988 meeting (Auerbach and Figert 1995).

In fact the establishment of the NIH Office of Research on Women's Health and the initiation of the Women's Health Initiative can be traced directly to one woman physician who attended the original 1988 meeting. Florence Haseltine, an obstetrician-gynecologist and cofounder of the Society for the

Advancement of Women's Health Research, used her own money to hire a lobbying firm to promote the priorities of the 1988 meeting shortly after the 1988 gathering occurred (Marshall 2005). Had Dr. Haseltine not dedicated her personal resources to this goal, it would not have been realized in as complete or as timely a fashion.

The Haseltine-funded pro–women's health lobbying efforts raised awareness among members of the Congressional Caucus for Women's Issues (CCWI) and contributed to the decision by Representatives Olympia Snowe, Patricia Schroeder, and Henry Waxman in December 1989 to request that the Government Accounting Office conduct an analysis of the extent to which the NIH was implementing its 1987 policy regarding women's issues. The completion of this report led to a pivotal congressional hearing on June 18, 1990, when Congressman Waxman asked each of the NIH institute directors what they were doing to enforce the three-year-old mandate to include more women in clinical trials. At the time, none of the directors had a great deal to report (Marshall 2005).

While Dr. Haseltine's efforts catapulted women's health issues into the popular press and onto the priority list of national leaders, they could not have succeeded without the support of the primarily female members of the Congressional Caucus for Women's Issues (CCWI). Thus the initial efforts of women physicians and other professionals to raise awareness about women's health depended critically on the advancement of women, not only in medicine and science but in other aspects of national life as well.

Since the congressional hearing in 1990, Congress, the NIH, and researchers and advocates have worked together to develop a range of solutions to the systematic exclusion of women from key medical investigations. Almost immediately after the critical congressional hearing, the NIH created the Office of Research on Women's Health (ORWH).[8] Although it was the primarily male leaders of the NIH who ultimately created the ORWH, the idea for such an entity initially emerged in the Women's Health Equity Act, an omnibus legislative package introduced by the CCWI (Auerbach and Figert 1995).

Regardless of its origins, the ORWH has served as a launching pad for the explosion of research described earlier and the incremental establishment of women's health organizations throughout the federal government (Pinn and Chunko 1999). Dr. Vivian Pinn, a female physician, served as director of the office from shortly after its creation, overseeing the introduction and implementation of multiple programs designed to advance women's health research and to promote women physicians as leaders within the broader field of women's health. Shortly after the NIH established the ORWH, the U.S. Public Health Service created its own Office on Women's Health. Its stated mission was to stimulate the development and implementation of effective research on women's health programs, to strengthen and sustain a broad range of research on the diseases and conditions that affect women, and to promote comprehensive and culturally appropriate health promotion and treatment services for women across the lifespan (Pinn and Chunko 1999).

One of the biggest contributions of the Public Health Service Office on Women's Health was the establishment of fifteen National Centers of Excellence in Women's Health. These centers, founded in medical schools across the country, have multiple goals, including furthering women's health research by providing culturally appropriate, high-quality women's health care and nurturing the careers of women physicians and women scientists. They are all directed by women physicians but employ significant numbers of male providers and researchers.[9] Like the ORWH, the Public Health Service Office on Women's Health was also led by a woman, although not a physician. Wanda Jones, the deputy assistant secretary for health and director of the office, has a doctoral degree in public health.

While Drs. Haseltine, Pinn, and Jones deserve tremendous credit for generating and maintaining the momentum of the women's health revolution, it was another female physician, Bernadine Healy, who directed and implemented the Women's Health Initiative. From the moment she became the first woman director of the National Institutes of Health, Dr. Healy made the Women's Health Initiative a priority. Reports indicate that she encountered significant resistance to the project throughout her entire tenure as leader of the NIH.[10] Without her commitment and skill, the revolution in women's health research would not have occurred as completely or as quickly as it has.

The efforts of the scientists and physicians who ultimately led the WHI must also be recognized. Like the administrative and organizational leaders, women are well represented in this group. In 2007, of the twelve members of the women's health initiative writing group, three quarters were female.

The story of the breast cancer movement and breast cancer research roughly parallels the evolution of support for women's health at the NIH and across the federal government. Most notably, one woman physician, the breast surgeon Susan Love, played a critical role in the breast cancer movement by raising initial awareness, helping to organize the National Breast Cancer Coalition, and continuing to participate in fund-raising efforts. Yet like Florence Haseltine, Vivian Pinn, and Bernadine Healy, Dr. Love could not have been successful without the support of other female and male leaders as well as multiple grass-roots activists.

Although many women physicians and scientists have been active in women's health research, so too have men. In 1993 the ORWH collaborated with the National Cancer Institute to fund nine women's health grants. Of those, only two were issued to female investigators. In 2004 the NCI issued six women's health grants, three of which went to women (Office of Women's Health Research 2004). On October 20, 2007, the American Association for Cancer Research sponsored a conference titled "Advances in Breast Cancer Research." Of the thirty-three lectures listed on the program, two thirds were to be given by male researchers and one third by female scientists.[11]

Since the 1970s, policymakers have speculated about how women's increasing presence in medicine in the United States will affect the profession. As we suggested earlier in this book, there are many reasons to suspect that women not only will change the way medicine is practiced on a daily level but also will influence the structure of the profession and the health care industry more broadly. Much of the editorializing on how women physicians will influence medicine is based on these assumptions.

Collectively, gender differences in work habits, interests, ambitions, and priorities lead some women physicians to form different expectations for their work lives and to have different levels of satisfaction. For example, they may lead women to trade pay willingly for more family-friendly work schedules and support systems such as on-site child care, parental leave, and breast-pumping space.

Our analysis of how women physicians will change the profession highlights the role of social pressures and independent structural change. Women physicians are different in some respects from their male colleagues, but their capacity to act on these differences is limited by their circumstances. We believe that ultimately women physicians will change the profession, but the extent of this change in the years to come will be incremental. Research will focus more on women's issues, care will be more collegial, and physicians will be more attentive to female-specific tests and procedures. Yet the dramatic change in the willingness to support a meaningful work-family balance will emerge only incrementally; the desire of women to offer collegial care will be greatly limited by changes in the context in which ambulatory care is delivered; and the capacity of women physicians to implement changes in medical leadership will be restricted by the large-scale aggregation of health systems and the specialization of health care functions.

The most optimistic scenario is that women in leadership positions and throughout medicine will soon form a critical mass that will enable them to take bolder steps toward change than have been evident to date. We remain cautiously optimistic.

Appendix

The data used in this book are drawn from a variety of sources. Given our multiple objectives and the historical scope of this project, no single data set by itself is sufficient to provide answers to all of our questions. Rather than be constrained by insights afforded by a single source of data, we have chosen the strategy of weaving together as comprehensive an account as possible, drawing on a wide range of data sources. We obtained data from literally millions of individuals—on virtually all U.S. allopathic medical school students as they entered and left medical school, on the incomes of tens of thousands of physicians, on the career plans of hundreds of thousands of college freshmen. Whenever possible we sought data that covered one, two, or three decades in order to understand more fully the evolution of women's roles in the medical profession. We also drew on dozens of informal interviews with physicians from leaders to those in the trenches, focus groups with physicians and aspiring physicians, and formal interviews with twenty-seven female physicians at varying stages of their careers.

In this appendix we describe these data sources and explain their strengths and weaknesses. In a number of cases we report aggregate statistics from published data sources. In other cases we conducted our own analyses of micro-level data sets. We describe the latter group in more detail.

1. Data on the Composition of the Medical Profession

The first portion of the book describes and seeks to explain the growth of women's representation in the medical profession since 1970. We drew on data concerning the status of the profession, male and female applicants to medical school, and the pool of premedical students from which these applicants were drawn.

Data on the number of practicing physicians are derived from the Physician Masterfile, a database compiled and maintained by the American Medical Association. It includes current and historical data on nearly all physicians, including AMA members and nonmembers, and graduates of foreign medical schools who reside in the United States and who have met the educational and credentialing requirements necessary for recognition as physicians. Data on international medical graduates (IMGs), a group comprising graduates of foreign medical schools residing in the United States, are included in the AMA Physician Masterfile when IMGs enter residency programs accredited by the Accreditation Council on Graduate Medical Education (ACGME). The AMA Physician Masterfile also includes data on IMGs who are licensed to practice medicine but who have not entered ACGME-accredited programs, and on physicians licensed to practice medicine in the United States but who are temporarily located abroad. Although the Physician Masterfile attempts to track all practicing physicians, there is some small but unknown rate of error in the data. A description of the AMA Masterfile is available at http:// www.ama-assn.org/ama/pub/category/2673.html.

We drew on data pertaining to applications to medical school compiled by the Association of American Medical Colleges (AAMC). We also employed data from the National Center for Education Statistics (NCES) documenting trends in recipients of the Medical Doctor degree by gender. Data from the AAMC and the NCES are based on the annual reports provided by each institution. Because these statistics include the entire relevant population, there are no associated confidence intervals or response rates. Each source is available on-line. The AAMC posts trends on applications to medical school at http://www.aamc.org/data/facts/. Data on recipients of the Medical Doctor degree can be found at http://nces.ed.gov/programs/digest/d05/tables/dt05_256.asp.

We compare the United States to thirty-four other countries drawing on data from the Organization for Economic Cooperation and Development (http://datalib.ed.ac.uk/EUDL/oecd_healthdata.html). The OECD data come in handy for a second reason, namely, to shed light on the gender composition of graduates of foreign medical schools.

2. The Status of the Medical Profession

The relationship between the status of the profession and women's entry is the main focus of chapter 2 and continues into chapter 3. Here we drew on data pertaining to the economic status of physicians as well as the reputation of the medical profession in society at large.

Trends in physicians' earnings play a key role in our analysis of the status of the profession. Our goal was to document trends in the average physician's income. We conducted analyses of physicians' earnings using data from the decennial U.S. censuses. In chapter 2 we report on physicians' incomes from the 1970, 1980, 1990, and 2000 U.S. Census samples. The 1970 estimates are based on a 1 percent sample. The 1980, 1990, and 2000 estimates are based on 5 percent samples. These data sources are publicly accessible via the IPUMS-USA (Integrated Public Use Microdata Series) Web site, http://webapp.icpsr. umich.edu/cocoon/ICPSR-STUDY/04295.xml. This data archive is maintained by the University of Minnesota. Technical information on the sample design is available under the heading IPUMS documentation at http://usa. ipums.org/usa/doc.shtml.

The strength of the census data is that there are large and consistent samples covering a long period of time. The census data also allow us to examine a range of questions regarding the families of physicians. The main weakness of the census data is that they include no information on physicians' specialties or other important practice characteristics. To address more detailed issues regarding the earnings of physicians, we drew on the Community Tracking Study physician surveys and the Survey of the Practice Patterns of Young Physicians. These data sources are described in more detail in Appendix Table 6.

In addition to these objective indicators of physicians' social standing, we also drew on surveys of the respect for medicine. One valuable source of such information is the General Social Survey (GSS), which was started in 1972 and completed its twenty-sixth round in 2006. This is a nationally representative sample which solicits responses on a wide range of social and political issues. We report trends in the respect for medicine along with trends for other notable institutions, such as science, banks, and other corporations.

We also report Gallup data on career advice for young people. In April 2005 the Gallup Organization posed two open-ended questions asking respondents to name the kind of work or career they would recommend if a young man or young woman came to them for advice. Trends in responses to this question since 1950 are displayed in Figure 1.1. Career advice specifically for young women was included in the 1950 administration of the survey but was unfortunately not repeated again until 1985. More details on this data series can be obtained from the Gallup Organization at http://www.gallup. com/poll/16048/Be-Doctor-Most-Common-Career-Advice.aspx.

3. Data on the Pre–Medical School Pipeline

Since the expansion of women's education is an important part of our story, we draw on a variety of educational statistics to document the dramatic growth in women's educational investments. The National Center for

Education Statistics (NCES) provides estimates of the number of women college graduates and the number of women pursuing the relevant coursework for medical school, including the number of women enrolled in high school advanced placement classes in math and biology. These data series are described further in the Digest of Higher Education Statistics, which can be accessed at http://nces.ed.gov/programs/digest/.

We track trends in the population of aspiring physicians from the point when they enter college. Our data on the career interests of college freshmen comes from a uniquely rich source, the College Freshmen National Norms Survey, administered by the Higher Education Research Institute (HERI) at the University of Los Angeles. The National Norms data include information on over 400,000 entering college students surveyed annually during orientation or registration. The HERI staff were kind enough to provide us with special tabulations of the college freshman data for the years 1978, 1982, 1987, 1992, 1997, and 2002. Technical details of the survey are described on the HERI Web site, http://www.gseis.ucla.edu/heri/cirpoverview.php.

We combine estimates published in the American freshman reports with original analyses of these data. Specifically, we examined trends in the stated importance of "helping people" and "earning money" for students interested in medicine over time, and then compared these to trends in the general student population.

We supplement our analysis of gender differences in interests among aspiring medical students by presenting data from the premedical questionnaire (PMQ). This data source captures trends in the interests, ambitions, and experiences of students who register to take the Medical College Admission Test, the exam required for acceptance to allopathic medical schools. Students interested in taking the MCAT are asked to complete the premedical questionnaire as a part of the MCAT registration process. Nearly all students who register complete the questionnaire, so response rates are very high. Nevertheless, the characteristics of PMQ respondents differ slightly from the characteristics of medical school applicants because some MCAT takers do not ultimately apply to medical school. Some apply to podiatric or veterinary programs, and some change their career plans.

In chapter 3 we sought to assess gender differences in persistence among aspiring medical students. We consult three data sources in this analysis. Figure 3.7 is derived from two of these three sources. We used data from the AAMC on medical school applicants described previously and data from the Cooperative Institutional Research Program (CIRP) survey to create a proxy for persistence among premedical students. Figure 3.7 presents the ratio of medical school applicants to the number of freshmen interested in medicine four years earlier.

The third data source used in our analysis of persistence is the Baccalaureate and Beyond survey (B&B). This is a nationally representative survey of recent college graduates that is administered by the National Center for Education Statistics. The B&B survey is particularly valuable for us because it follows the same students over time. We analyzed the sample that graduated from college in 1993. Technical details about the Baccalaureate and Beyond survey are described on-line at the NCES Web site, http://nces. ed.gov/surveys/b&b/.

4. The Medical School Experience

We sought to understand the role of the medical school experience in shaping the career prospects of physicians. We did so primarily by using a unique data source from the AAMC. The file includes students who took both the 1998 Matriculating Student Questionnaire (MSQ), a survey administered to all first-year allopathic medical students, and the 2001 Graduating Student Questionnaire, a survey administered to all graduating allopathic medical students shortly before they receive their Medical Doctor degree. Both surveys measure a full menu of experiences, interests, and ambitions. Response rates to both surveys are generally very high: in 2003, 75 percent of all students responded to the MSQ. The Medical School Graduation Questionnaire (GQ) is a national questionnaire administered by the AAMC. It has been administered annually since 1978 to graduating medical students in the United States. Response rates are generally over 90 percent for this survey. Technical details of the administration process for both the MSQ and the GQ are available at http://www.aamc.org/data/msq/start.htm http://www.aamc.org/data/gq/.

Together these data measure students' demographic characteristics, including race, family income, maternal education and occupation, paternal education and occupation, and educational debt. In addition, they tap a wide range of student experiences before and during medical school, including job experience, academic courses, and participation in MCAT preparation programs as well as participation in elective medical clerkships and research rotations. These surveys also ask freshman students many questions about their motivations for studying medicine and the factors that most influenced their decision to seek acceptance to medical school. Graduating students are asked about their satisfaction with most aspects of their medical education and their career goals and interests. For example, these data allow us to determine whether those graduates who chose surgery were those who initially expressed interest in surgery.

5. Gender Differences in Physicians' Status

Chapter 4 includes a detailed description of current gender differences in status and discusses how these differences have evolved. Annual data on medical specialties since 1970 were obtained from the AMA Physician Masterfile. We were able to provide information on the attributes of physicians' patients by using data from the Community Tracking Study (CTS). Sponsored by the Robert Wood Johnson Foundation, the CTS is a large-scale investigation of changes in the American health care system and their effects on people. The CTS physician survey has been conducted several times (1996, 2000, and 2004). It is a nationally representative longitudinal study of physicians who provide direct patient care for at least twenty hours per week. It was designed primarily to assess how changes in the structure and financing of medical care in the United States are affecting relevant health outcomes; it includes no measure of physicians' personal lives outside of gender and race. Technical details of the Community Tracking Study physician survey are described on-line at the ICPSR Inter-University Consortium for Political and Social Research) Web site, http://webapp.icpsr.umich. edu/cocoon/HMCA-STUDY/04584.xml. The survey is available for analysis through the ICPSR.

We draw on the CTS data to answer a number of other questions as well, including a multivariate analysis of physicians' earnings in chapter 4. We return to the CTS in our analysis of how physicians practice medicine. To delve more deeply into questions regarding the representation of women on medical school faculties, we took advantage of data from the Association of American Medical Colleges on allopathic medical school faculty. The AAMC maintains the Faculty Roster System (FRS), a database that tracks allopathic medical faculty. Like many of the other data sources, it includes the entire population. Technical details of the FRS are described on-line at http://www.aamc.org/data/facultyroster/start.htm.

6. Physicians' Earnings

As mentioned earlier, we drew on data from the U.S. decennial censuses to examine the earnings of physicians relative to others in the U.S. labor force to investigate historical trends. The census data are very useful for this purpose because they provide largely comparable measures over time. They also allow us to examine variation by age as well as marital and parental status. The sample sizes are generally quite large, including over twenty thousand physicians in 1980 and over thirty thousand physicians in 2000.

As noted earlier, the main limitation of the census data is that there is little information about specialty and other important practice characteristics. Thus a complete analysis of earnings requires supplementing the census data with information from other sources. We draw on the 2004 CTS data set because it is a recent survey of a large sample with an extensive list of potential determinants of income. The CTS is also limited, however, by its failure to measure physicians' personal characteristics, including data on marriage and parenthood.

In order to assess how these qualities contribute to gender differences in earnings, and in order to track those trends over time, we turned to the survey of the Practice Patterns of Young Physicians, a.k.a. the Young Physicians Survey. This survey measures aspects of physicians' personal lives, including their marital status at multiple points as well as the occupation of their spouse. We use the 1991 and 1997 waves of the survey to assess the determinants of earned income. The 1991 sample includes 5,733 physicians who were initially surveyed in 1987. The initial sample included physicians born in 1952 or later who completed their medical training between 1986 and 1989. Minority physicians were overrepresented in both of the samples. The 1997 follow-up was restricted to physicians living in the seventy-five largest metropolitan areas, and had a response rate of 70.7 percent.

Both versions of the Young Physician Survey are available on-line from the ICPSR. Technical details of the 1991 sample are summarized in the relevant ICPSR codebook, which can be downloaded from ICPSR under the title cb6145.all.pdf. Technical details about the 1997 survey are described in the relevant codebook under the title cb2829.pdf.

7. Physicians' Work and Parenting Schedules

As we have seen, competing interpretations of women's experience in the medical profession hinge on issues related to the challenges of balancing work and family. Consequently, we devote considerable attention to work schedules and family attributes. Unfortunately, some of the best data for examining physicians' work experiences (e.g., the CTS data set) lack information on whether a physician is married or is a parent. Again, we overcame this lacuna by drawing on various sources of data.

The main source is the U.S. decennial census. We created a couples file by matching spouses to heads of households, following the procedure used by Jacobs and Labov (2002). This enabled us to examine the earnings and work experiences of physicians in the context of their family lives. For example, we can examine whether a physician is the sole earner in the family or if the physician is part of a dual-career marriage. Because the census provides information on the occupations of both partners, we can ask whether a physician is married to another physician.

Data from the AMA socioeconomic monitoring system and patient care physician surveys, reported in chapter 5, provide insight on how the work schedules of physicians in specific specialties have changed since the 1970s. In particular, these data allow us to track trends in the length of the workweek by specialty. These are nationally representative surveys of practicing physicians administered by the AMA and based on the AMA Masterfile as a sampling frame. They are published in a periodical series titled Socio-economic Characteristics of Medical Practice (Center for Health Policy Research 1983–1998 and 1999–2005).

8. Gender and Medical Practice

In order to assess if and when gender might affect the care given to individual patients, we again drew on data from the CTS survey. In the 1996 wave of the CTS, information was solicited concerning physicians' attitudes about the amount of time they spend with their patients. Specifically, they were asked to agree or disagree with the statement "I am satisfied with the time I spend with my patients." This question was asked in order to assess whether managed care was creating conditions in which physicians felt rushed and were unable to give their patients adequate time and attention. We examined whether there are gender differences in responses to this question. Since the CTS includes extensive information about physicians as well as their practice settings, we were in a good position to assess whether any observed gender disparities regarding time with patients is due to gender per se or is due instead to physicians' individual attributes such as their age, the attributes of their patients, or attributes of their practice setting, for instance, whether they are employed in a managed care setting.

In another component of the 1996 CTS survey, primary care physicians were asked to respond to six vignettes of model patients with presentations designed to have multiple appropriate treatment plans. In other words, physicians were presented with a hypothetical patient with a specified set of symptoms and asked whether they would follow a specified path of treatment for that patient. Following the same approach as in the case of concerns with time for patients, we examined whether any observed gender disparities in responses to these model patients were due to gender per se or instead to physicians' individual attributes or attributes of their practice setting.

9. Qualitative Data

In an effort to supplement our quantitative data, especially with respect to how work-family issues and situations potentially involving discrimination are experienced by physicians, we collected four types of qualitative data. We conducted informal interviews with dozens of practicing physicians, medical students, health policy analysts, and leaders in health care policy. We conducted formal interviews with twenty-seven female physicians at various stages of their careers and in various aspects of the profession. Interview participants included one woman who attended medical school in the 1960s and had recently retired from active practice, two department heads, one assistant department head, one past president of a county medical society, three mid-career female surgeons, and three women who had completed residency within the past fifteen years, among others.

We also monitored two medical Web sites, MomMD, a site for female physicians, and the student physician Web site, a site for physicians in training. Observations occurred at multiple points over a period of six months and totaled more than twenty-four hours. We read hundreds of postings and engaged in on-line exchanges with dozens of participants. Discussions on these sites provided a window into the struggles of women and men who are attempting to balance work and family. We also conducted a focus group at the University of Pennsylvania of advanced premedical students who were in various stages of applying to medical school. Drawing on these many sources allowed us to examine diverse aspects of gender and medicine and enabled us to examine trends in the profession since 1970.

Tables

Appendix Table 1. Nested Models Predicting the Log of Earnings in an Average Week and Hours in Patient Care

Predictor	Earnings 1996		Earnings Gap in Dollars	Earnings 2004		Earnings Gap in Dollars
	B	Std. Err.		B	Std. Err.	
Gender	−0.41	0.01***	$33,537	−0.39	0.02	$32,058
	ADJ R² = .08			ADJ R² = .06		
Demographics	−0.45	0.01305***	$35,051	−0.38	0.02	$31,666
	ADJ R² = 0.11			ADJ R² = .08		
Specialty	−0.37	0.01312***	$30,366	−0.31	0.02	$26,589
	ADJ R² = 0.20			ADJ R² = .15		
Ownership	−0.33	0.01	$28,293	−0.29	0.02	$24,944
	ADJ R² = 0.23			ADJ R² = .17		
Practice structure	−0.33	0.01	$27,875	−0.28	0.02	$24,393
	ADJ R² = 0.24			ADJ R² = .18		
Revenue source	−0.32	0.01	$27,690	−0.27	0.02	$23,914
	ADJ R² = 0.25			ADJ R² = .18		
Work effort	−0.28	0.01	$24,095	−0.23	0.02	$20,341
	ADJ R² = 0.28			ADJ R² = .20		

Note: ***$p < .01$.

Appendix Table 1. Young Physicians' Survey, 1991 and 1997

	1991		1997	
	B	Std. Err.	B	Std. Err.
Married parents				
Gross gender gap with no controls	−0.49	0.02***	−0.45	0.05
Net gender gap after all variables are controlled	−0.30	0.02***	−0.30	0.05
Adding practice structure				
		$R^2 = .3638$		$R^2 = .2042$
		n = 4132		n = 1007
Married non-parents				
Gross gender gap with no controls	−0.24	0.04***	−0.31	0.05
Net gender gap after all variables are controlled	−0.13	0.04***	−0.20	0.11
Adding practice structure				
		$R^2 = 0.2744$		$R^2 = .2086$
		n = 695		n = 83
Single, childless physicians				
Gross gender gap with no controls	−0.28	0.04***	−0.26	0.10
Net gender gap after all variables are controlled	−0.24	0.04***	−0.25	0.10
Adding practice structure				
		$R^2 = 0.2026$		$R^2 = .2086$
		n = 758		n = 113

Note: #p < .1 *p < .05 **p < .01 ***p < .001.

Appendix Table 2. Determinants of Interest in Surgery and Primary Care Pediatrics for Students Graduating in 2001

	B	Std. Err.	Odds Ratio	ADJ R^2
A. Surgery				
Gender	−1.16	0.06***	0.31	0.06
Demographic	−1.17	0.06***	0.31	0.07
Specialty interest as freshman	−1.17	0.06***	0.31	0.07
Medical school experiences	−1.09	0.06	0.34	0.12
Interests	−0.88	0.06***	0.42	0.12
Opinions regarding work, family	−0.86	0.07***	0.42	0.13
Med school experiences	−0.82	0.07***	0.44	0.18
Satisfaction with rotations	−0.85	0.07	0.43	0.24
Satisfaction with rotations	−1.10	0.06	0.33	0.19
Mistreatment	−1.09	0.06	0.34	0.19
Interests	−0.85	0.06	0.43	0.22
Medicine and family	−0.86	0.06	0.42	0.22
B. Primary care pediatrics				
Gender	1.45	0.08	4.25	0.07
Demographic	1.44	0.08	4.22	0.08
Specialty interest as freshman	1.44	0.08	4.22	0.08
Medical school experiences	1.38	0.08	3.98	0.09
Satisfaction with rotations				
Satisfaction with rotations	1.33	0.09	3.78	0.15
Mistreatment	1.34	0.09	3.83	0.15
Interests	1.18	0.09	3.26	0.16
Medicine and family	1.18	0.09	3.26	0.17

Note: ***p < .01. Demographics include age, age squared, years experience, years experience squared, board certification, and foreign medical graduate variables.

Appendix Table 3. Gender Differences in Intention to Pursue Full-Time Academics and Research

	Intent to Pursue Academics			Intent to Pursue Research		
		Odds Ratio	Std. Err.		Odds Ratio	Std. Err.
Bivariate models	0.03	1.03	0.04	−0.47	0.63	0.05***
Demographic characteristics	0.05	1.05	0.04	−0.45	0.64	0.06***
College and Precollege experiences	0.01	1.01	0.04	−0.44	0.64	0.06***
Motivations to study medicine	0.07	1.07	0.04#	−0.25	0.78	0.06***
Medical school characteristics	0.07	1.07	0.04#	−0.25	0.78	0.06***
Medical school experiences	0.14	1.16	0.04*	−0.13	0.87	0.06***
Medical school educational debt	0.14	1.16	0.04**	−0.14	0.87	0.07***
Specialty choice at graduation	0.24	1.28	0.05***	−0.06	0.94	0.07

Note: Fully adjusted, adjusted R2 for Model 1 = .1861.
Fully adjusted, adjusted R2 for Model 1 = .3061.
In the fully adjusted models, 135 out of 14,240 are lost due to missing values.
#p < .1, *p < .05 **p < .01 ***p < .001.

Appendix Table 4. Summary of Vignette Multivariate Analyses

Gender Effect Controls	Vignette 1: Referral to Cardiologist B	Vignette 2: MRI for Back Pain B	Vignette 3: PSA Test B	Vignette 4: Cholesterol Lowering Medication B	Vignette 5: Office Visit for Vaginal Discharge B	Vignette 6: Urology Referral B
None	1.18	-1.7***	-8.03***	-3.73*	-10.42**	13.12**
Physician characteristics	0.7	-3.05	-1.99	-1.94	-6.44**	14.17**
Physician and practice characteristics	-0.2	-4.43	-1.84	-0.29	-6.11**	13.55**
Physician, practice, and community characteristics	-0.2	-5.39	-1.75	-0.24	1.71**	13.34**
Physician, practice, and community characteristics and referral patterns	-0.32	1.7	1.7			

Note: ***p < .001, **p < .01 *p < .05 #p < .1.
Source: 1996 CTS data.

Appendix Table 5. Summary of Regression Analysis of Satisfaction with Time for Patients

Gender Effect Controls	Primary Care Physicians			Specialist Physicians		
	B	Std. Err.	R^2	B	Std. Err.	R^2
None	0.619	0.019**	0.011	−0.260	0.052**	0.01
Physician characteristics	0.895	0.155**	0.069	−0.174	0.055**	0.04
Working time	1.480	0.169**	0.097	−0.137	0.055**	0.61
Practice characteristics	1.561	0.300**	0.099	−0.130	0.055**	0.65
Patient demographics and referral patterns	1.644	0.305**	0.128	−0.091	0.056**	0.082

Appendix Table 6. Data Sources

Data Set	Source	Cost	Population Covered	Years Available	Description
Baccalaureate and Beyond Longitudinal Study (B&B)	National Center for Educational Statistics	Free	Two nationally representative longitudinal studies of students receiving bachelor's degrees.	Cohort 1 was surveyed in 1993, 1997, and 2003. Cohort 2 was surveyed in 2000 and 2001.	The Baccalaureate and Beyond Longitudinal Study (B&B) provides information concerning education and work experiences after completion of bachelor's degrees. B&B provides both cross-sectional information one year after bachelor's degree completion, and longitudinal data concerning entry into and progress through graduate-level education and the workforce.
Cooperative Institutional Research Program (CIRP) Freshmen Survey	Higher Education Research Institute	$5 per analysis	A nationally representative survey of college freshmen administered annually.	1977, 1982, 1987, 1992, 1997, 2002	The four page instrument covers a broad array of issues including demographic characteristics, expectations about the college experience, secondary school experiences, degree goals and career plans, college finances, attitudes, values, and life goals.
Pre-Medical Questionnaire (PMQ)	Association of American Medical Colleges	$200 per year	All students taking the Medical College Admission test. The test is required for admission to all U.S. medical schools.	1990–2000	In addition to a series of questions about why students' decided to become physicians, the survey includes questions about students' college-level educational experiences such as the courses they took and their extracurricular activities.

Name	Source	Cost	Sample	Years	Description
Matriculating Student Questionnaire (MSQ)	Association of American Medical Colleges	$100 per year	A survey of all first-year students at U.S. medical schools.	1987–2000	In addition to assessing student demographic and financial characteristics, the Matriculating Student Questionnaire includes: (1) an assessment of the college-level courses students take and why they take them, (2) an assessment of the activities students participated in during college, (3) the importance of different personal influences on students' decision to go to medical school, and (4) the reasons students decided to pursue medicine.
Graduating Student Questionnaire (GSQ)	Association of American Medical Colleges	$200 per year	A survey of all fourth-year students at U.S. medical schools.	1978–1999	In addition to assessing student demographic and financial characteristics, the GSQ assesses students' perceptions of: (1) their medical school curriculum and (2) student services offered at their medical school. It also asks students what types of elective academic and nonacademic activities they participated in while in medical school. The GSQ includes measures of perceived mistreatment and assesses student choice of specialty. In addition, selected years of the GSQ assess student motivations for choosing their specialty, and all years ask student perceptions of the state of health care.
U.S. Decennial Census (5% sample)	IPUMS	Free	This is a sample of people from the Census who self identify as physicians and indicate that they have professional level education.	1970, 1980, 1990, 2000	The Census is unique in its identification of a portion of the population of physicians outside of the labor force. In order to be identified as a doctor, a person must report having worked as a physician in the past five years. The Census allows analysts to match the records of family members. This will enable us to examine the potential affect of spouses and children on physicians' work effort.

Data Set	Source	Cost	Population Covered	Years Available	Description
Practice Patterns of Young Physicians	Inter-University Consortium for Political and Social Research (ICPSR)	Free	A random sample of physicians who were under age forty in 1986, the original survey year, and who had recently completed graduate medical training.	1987, 1991, 1997	A subset of the physicians interviewed in 1987 were reinterviewed in 1991, and all physicians interviewed in 1991 were reinterviewed in 1997, allowing for longitudinal analysis between 1987 and 1991 and between 1991 and 1997. Physicians were asked about "their graduate training, their perceptions of the medical profession, current practice arrangements, career decisions, family background, patient care activities, and current income and expenses. The survey allows us to measure job satisfaction. A 1999 article in *health services research* links incentives to reduce services to job satisfaction, but did not examine how gender and familial characteristics relate to or interact with job satisfaction.
Community Tracking Study Physician Survey	ICPSR	Free	A nationally representative longitudinal sample of physicians practicing at least twenty hours per week.	1996-1997, 1998–1999, 2000–2001	The survey instrument collects information on physician practice arrangements, physician time allocation, sources of practice revenue, level and determinants of physician compensation, provision of charity care, career satisfaction, physicians' perceptions of their ability to deliver care, effects of care management strategies and various other aspects of the practice of medicine.

Notes

1. Introduction

1. The question was worded as follows: "Supposing a young woman (or man) came to you for advice on choosing a line of work or career. What kind of work or career would you recommend?" During the 1980s, medicine fell behind computers as the top field recommended for young men (Saad 2005). Mazzuca (2003) reports that 11 percent of teenage girls and 6 percent of teenage boys want to be physicians.

2. Authors' calculations based on the 2000 U.S. decennial census.

3. The relationships between nurses and doctors needs to be understood from both sides of this professional divide (Gordon 2005). We discuss the issues of collaboration and conflict in more detail in chapter 9.

2. Feminization of an Evolving Profession

1. Reskin and Roos's theory is rich and multifaceted, and this discussion focuses on only one aspect of their theory. For example, they also discuss the role of occupational growth in contributing to shortages of men, which is consistent with the expansion of the medical profession during the 1970s.

2. Male and female applicants have been accepted at similar rates throughout the period discussed in this chapter. In most years the gap has been less than a few percentage points. Thus the number of applications is the key driver of changes in the gender composition of medical school classes.

3. Without the rise of information technology and an increased interest among academics and policymakers in the systematic evaluation of medicine, the adoption of DRGs would not have been possible (Stevens 1989, 324).

4. How can the costs go up so much when work effort increased only modestly? The difference is due to the significant increase in the number of physicians during this period. The number of physicians whose primary activity was patient care increased from 115 per 100,000 in 1970 to 182 per 100,000 in 1990 (Reinhardt 1997).

3. Applying for Change

1. The faster feminization of osteopaths stems in part from the faster growth of this population. In 2004 women were 27.9 percent of all osteopathic physicians and 26.6 percent of all allopaths. Between 1990 and 2004 the population of active osteopaths grew 43 percent, while the population of allopaths grew only 30 percent (American Osteopathic Association 2006).

2. See Riska 2001 for a comparative analysis of women's entry into medicine.

3. For more on foreign-born physicians, including a discussion of the implications of this immigration pattern as part of a "brain drain" for developing countries, see Astor et al. 2005, Mullan 2005 and 2006, and AMA 2006, although none of these focuses on gender.

4. Tracking changes in race and ethnicity over time with U.S. Census data can be challenging as a result of changes in classification. Comparing race and ethnicity across age groups at one point in time provides a reasonable approximation of the time trend, given the low rates of attrition from this profession.

5. Hall and colleagues (2001) examined the relationship between the percentage of male college graduates majoring in biology and the percentage of male college graduates applying to medical school. They show a strong connection between these two trends over time.

6. The AB calculus test covers only one semester of college-level math, while the BC test involves a full year of college-level calculus.

7. For more information on the CIRP freshman survey, see the discussion in the Appendix.

8. Linda Sax and William S. Korn graciously provided us with these tabulations.

9. For more information on the National Center for Education Statistics' Baccalaureate and Beyond longitudinal study, see the discussion in the Appendix.

10. What about those students who do not declare an interest in medicine? Are women more likely to be late aspirants than men? Here again, men have a slight relative advantage: 1.1 percent of 1994 non-medical male aspirants and 0.7 percent of non-medical female aspirants responded in 1997 that they wanted to be medical practice professionals.

11. Attrition from medical school has always been low but climbed between 1973 and 1992 from 4.8 to 10.4 percent for women and from 2.5 to 6.3 percent for men.

12. MCAT scores are also related to performance on step 1 of the National Licensing Examination, a major factor in residency decisions. Research suggests that MCAT scores are a stronger predictor of step 1 scores than college science GPA (Veloski et al. 2000; see also Huff and Fang 1999). Other research, however, indicates that MCAT scores do not predict performance in clinical clerkships (Silver et al. 1997).

4. The Gendered Map of Contemporary Medicine

1. We examined whether this trend was influenced by the composition of fast-growing or slow-growing fields by calculating a size-standardized index of segregation. Since both indexes exhibit a similar pattern of movement over time, there is no overall pattern of more rapid growth in more or less segregated specialties.

2. In 1996, 81 percent of men and 79 percent of women were board certified in their primary specialty.

3. SCHIP represented the single largest expansion in coverage for children since Medicaid was created in 1965. SCHIP supported work for low-income parents since it covered children in families with incomes up to, or exceeding, twice the federal poverty level. These families may have trouble affording private coverage (Kenney and Cook 2007). The expansion of SCHIP was being debated by Congress as this book was being completed.

4. These results are not presented here in a table owing to space constraints but are available from the authors.

5. Women physicians are also underrepresented in rural areas. In 2000, 11.8 percent of female and 16.2 percent of male physicians lived outside a metropolitan area. Much of this gap, however, is due to demographic differences, specifically age and minority representation.

Because younger physicians of both genders are significantly less likely to locate outside a metropolitan area, and women physicians are younger on average than men, women are less likely to be found outside metropolitan regions. Similarly, because racial minorities and immigrant physicians are less likely to locate outside metropolitan areas, and women physicians are more likely to be racial minorities or immigrants, they are less likely to be found in rural locales.

6. Phyllis Kopriva, American Medical Association, personal communication.

7. A survey of level 1 trauma center directors revealed that no women were involved in this type of medical management (Tran et al. 2002).

8. By comparison, the median female lawyer earns 73 percent of what the median male lawyer earns. The median female engineering manager earns 94 percent of what the median male engineering manager earns. The median female chemical engineer earns 80 percent of what the median male chemical engineer earns (Weinberg 2004, 12).

9. The results for the full regression models are available on the Web site at http://www.ssc.upenn.edu/soc/People/jacobsjerry.html. Web site supplement Table 1 presents results for the CTS data, and Web site supplement Table 2 presents results for the Young Physicians data.

10. We do not report results for unmarried parents because of the small number of observations.

5. Gender, Sorting, and Tracking

1. Only 13 percent characterized the harassment as severe. Nevertheless, Frank and colleagues document an association between reported harassment and poor mental health outcomes. These estimates are lower than those from the AAMC graduating student questionnaire, which indicates that in 2004 only 14 percent of medical students indicated that they had been mistreated during medical school (Yamagata et al. 2006). In the same survey, however, 30 percent of medical students indicated that they had reported incidents of mistreatment to faculty and staff.

2. As far as female-dominated specialties are concerned, the growing presence of women may make these fields even less welcoming to men. Male students have reported gender discrimination in pediatrics and obstetrics with respect to mentoring, educational opportunities, and general encouragement to enter the field (Stratton et al. 2005). If such trends are not addressed then we can expect the numbers of men opting for pediatrics to decline in the future. Research indicates, however, that such pressures can be addressed.

3. In particular, research on obstetrics and gynecology residency programs, a specialty with a large representation of women, suggests that even in this female-dominated area, many programs require other residents to cover for residents on leave.

4. Web site supplement Table 3 presents descriptive data on the students by gender.

5. The years 1993 and 1999 are missing from Figure 5.3 because the graduation questionnaire did not ask students about their intended involvement in research in either of those years.

6. Gender differences in the means of the covariates are presented in Web site supplement Table 3. The full results for the final models in Appendix Table 2 are presented in Web site supplement Table 4.

7. We constructed three scales to capture physicians' attitudes toward the practice of medicine. These are the "primary care" scale, the "altruism" scale, and the "technical" scale. These were constructed through the use of factor analysis. The basis for these scales is presented in Web site supplement Table 5.

6. Work, Family, Marriage, and Generational Change

1. The dramatic increase in women's presence in the workforce has created an impression that the traditional family is extremely rare. While it is certainly true that the traditional breadwinner-caregiver family is not as common as it once was, there are still tremendous

gender differences in how adult men and women approach paid work. Adult males are still significantly more likely to be employed and to work longer hours than employed adult women. Although more than half of all married women with children now work for pay, in 2004, 41 percent of mothers with one infant child worked full-time and 31 percent of mothers with at least one infant and one other child worked full-time. The majority of mothers with children under six years of age were not employed full-time (Dye 2005).

2. Extensive additional analyses of different age groups were conducted. These results, too detailed to be presented here, are available from the authors.

3. Data from the AMA Masterfile even suggest that employment rates for female physicians are rising. In 1989, 4.1 percent of female physicians between thirty-five and forty-four, prime child-rearing years, were listed as inactive in the AMA Masterfile. The comparable number for men was 1 percent. By 1992, only 3.9 percent of women and 1 percent of men in the prime child-rearing years were inactive. By 1997, 1.8 percent of women and 1 percent of men between thirty-five and forty-four were inactive.

4. Kanter (1977) examined demanding jobs held by men that presumed a full-time, stay-at-home partner to manage the house and family, and to entertain co-workers and clients. Blair-Loy (2003) develops the notion of work orientation as representing a type of professional "devotion." As women without full-time stay-at-home husbands hold more of these positions, the traditional expectations of these positions become hard to sustain over the course of a career.

5. Data from the 1980 census come from work by Uhlenberg and Cooney (1990). The age groups presented are designed to match those presented by Uhlenberg and Cooney.

6. http://discuss.prb.org/content/interview/detail/1172/.

7. Women Physicians Caring for Patients

1. Unfortunately we are unable to compare treatment of comparable male and female patients needing cholesterol-lowering drugs because physicians were not asked to evaluate a female model patient with high cholesterol. Indeed, five of the six vignettes in the CTS study involve hypothetical male patients.

2. Detailed regression analysis results for all vignettes are presented in Web site supplement Table 6.

3. Although all physicians respond to communication skills training, it appears that female physicians gain proportionately more from these experiences than their male peers (Roter and Hall 2004).

4. Full descriptive results by gender are displayed in Web site supplement Table 7.

5. Full results for the nested models presented in Appendix Table 4 can be found in Web site supplement Table 8a. Web site supplement Table 8b compares the final model for primary care and specialist physicians.

8. Medicine as a Family-Friendly Profession?

1. The Federal Office on Women's Health convened the National Task Force on Reentry into Clinical Practice for Health Professionals in 2000 (Mark and Gupta 2002). This effort led to recommendations for a national reentry policy and to an updated compendium of physician retraining initiatives (U.S. Department of Health 2001). The national task force was followed by the convening of an American Academy of Pediatrics–sponsored Physician Reentry into the Workforce Project, a collaborative effort that includes many medical institutions, among them the AMA, the Veterans Health Administration, the American Board of Medical Specialties, the American Academy of Family Physicians, the American Board of Surgeons, and the Council on Graduate Medical Education (Mark and Gupta 2002).

2. In fact the increasing relative and absolute presence of women in pediatrics was listed as the second-most-critical concern for the American Academy of Pediatrics' Committee on Workforce Issues (Committee on the Pediatric Workforce 2004).

3. Data from the Community Tracking Study physician surveys indicate that in 1996, 75 percent of men and 51 percent of women worked long weeks. By 2004, only 69.9 percent of men and 48.4 percent of women worked long weeks.

4. Data from the 2004 CTS physician survey indicate that 16 percent of women and 6 percent of men physicians work fewer than thirty-one hours in a normal week. Between the 1996 and the 2004 CTS surveys, rates of part-time work increased slightly, from 14.6 to 15.7 percent for women and from 4.1 to 5.9 percent for men. In contrast, between the 1990 and 2000 censuses, the frequency of part-time work among women declined from 16 to 15 percent. The CTS survey involves only physicians who provide direct patient care at least twenty hours per week and excludes radiologists, pathologists, and anesthesiologists. It also involves a survey of cities rather than a survey of the entire U.S. population. Regardless of the data source, however, rates of part-time work for female physicians are remarkably stable.

5. Data from the Physician Work Life Study indicates that 22 percent of U.S. women respondents and 9 percent of U.S. men respondents worked part-time (McMurray et al. 2005). Note, however, that this survey defines part-time as fewer than forty hours per week rather than thirty hours. See also Steinhauer 1999.

6. Long work weeks vary significantly by specialty. For example, 73 percent of female surgeons work fifty or more hours per week versus 29 percent for female psychiatrists (based on CTS data). Thus, depending on their specialty, female physicians range between 1.5 and 4.3 times more likely than the average female professional to work a long week.

7. In 2006 nearly all offices, 96 percent, allowed part-time schedules, either as an affirmative policy or on a case-by-case basis, but as has been the case since the National Association for Law Placement first compiled this information in 1994, very few lawyers were working on a part-time basis—just 5 percent overall. Associates are more likely to be working part-time (4.7 percent) than partners (2.8 percent), but other lawyers, such as of counsel and staff attorneys, show the highest rate of part-time work—over 16 percent (NALP 2006).

8. Research on the relationship between continuity of care and health outcomes for diabetes patients is mixed. Some studies fail to find an association (Gulliford et al. 2007), while others suggest that an association exists.

9. For example, evidence is mounting that surgeons can extend the survival of cancer patients by ensuring negative margins on their resections (Lange and Lin 2004). The theory is that the positive relationship between higher volume and outcomes for cancer surgery patients stems from the fact that surgeons who perform the procedure more often are more likely to ensure negative margins.

10. Healthy People goals suggest that 50 percent of mothers of six-month-olds should be breast-feeding. The rate for residents was only 15 percent. Residency work schedule was the most common reason cited for discontinuing breast-feeding (Miller et al. 1996).

9. Conclusion: A Prognosis for Gender and Medical Care

1. In 1970 there were 311 female general surgeons. In 2001, 3,754 women identified general surgery as their primary specialty. Between 1970 and 2001 the number of women in obstetrics-gynecology grew from 1,337 to 12,532.

2. The number of women in research increased from 743 to 2,702 between 1970 and 2001.

3. http://pn.psychiatryonline.org/cgi/content/full/36/7/28.

4. The increasing status of nurses in the everyday work lives of physicians is coupled with growing political pressure from nurses for official recognition and greater discretion in their everyday work, especially for those nurses with advanced practice certifications (Guadagnino 1999). Primary care physicians are increasingly forced to view advanced practice nurses as colleagues and competitors rather than subordinates.

5. It is worth noting that the pre-1990s bias against women in clinical trials did not stem directly or overtly from anti-female sentiment. Much of the reluctance to include women in such trials came from the thalidomide disaster. This drug, given to pregnant women to stop

nausea in the 1950s and early 1960s, caused thousands of birth defects. After it was with-drawn, regulatory agencies directed that young women should be kept out of clinical trials to protect fetuses they might be carrying. That attitude lived on into the 1980s—long after new tests and testing methods had made it easy to identify early pregnancy and avoid risks (Marshall 2005). While the longevity of the policy toward women in clinical trials may have stemmed in part from anti-female sentiment, it inevitably also resulted from the inertia and momentum that characterize public processes.

6. http://www.businessweek.com/magazine/content/05_42/b3955043.htm.

7. The women's health movement of the 1970s originated in a 1969 conference on health that led to the creation of the book *Our Bodies Ourselves* and the book collective of the same name. The members of these initial groups largely viewed the established medical profession as a part of the problem with women's health (Riska 2001).

8. While the NIH Office of Research on Women's Health lacks direct funding authority, it is charged by Congress with a threefold mandate: (1) to strengthen, develop, and increase research into diseases, disorders, and conditions that affect women; to determine gaps in knowledge about such conditions and diseases; and to establish a research agenda for the NIH; (2) to ensure that women are appropriately represented in NIH-funded biomedical and biobehavioral research studies, especially clinical trials; and (3) to create and direct initiatives to increase the number of women in biomedical careers and facilitate their advancement (Pinn and Chunko 1999).

9. In 2002 a comprehensive evaluation of the centers was published. It concluded that the centers have reinforced credibility for women's health at the host institutions. They have contributed to a greater focus on women's health than existed previously both in local re-search and in the local medical school curricula and have aided in the mentoring of women scientists and physicians.

10. From the start the WHI caught flak, Healy recalls. Critics said that it wouldn't work because it was too complex and poorly designed; they also feared that not enough women would enroll. Healy battled "relentlessly" to get money for it, she says, adding that she helped get it entrenched by committing money to forty study centers before she left NIH. She also says that she helped fend off a move to end the trial in the 1990s during the Clinton administration (Marshall 2005).

11. http://www.aacr.org/home/scientists/meetings-workshops/special-conferences/advances-in-breast-cancer-research/program.aspx.

Bibliography

AAMC. 1997. "Graduating Questionnaire: All Schools Final Summary Report." Washington, D.C.: Association of American Medical Colleges. http://www.aamc.org/data/gq/allschoolsreports/1997.pdf.

——. 2003. *AAMC Data Book: Medical Schools and Teaching Hospitals by the Numbers.* Washington, D.C.: Association of American Medical Colleges.

——. 2005. "Cultural Competence Education for Medical Students." Washington, D.C.: Association of American Medical Colleges. http://www.aamc.org/meded/tacct/culturalcomped.pdf.

——. 2006. "Women in U.S. Academic Medicine Statistics and Medical School Benchmarking, 2005–2006." Washington, D.C.: Association of American Medical Colleges. http://www.aamc.org/members/wim/wimguide/wim6.pdf.

——. 2007. "Graduating Questionnaire: All Schools Final Summary Report." Washington, D.C.: Association of American Medical Colleges. http://www.aamc.org/data/gq/allschoolsreports/2007.pdf.

AAMC Data Book. 2007. "Table B7 Archive of U.S. Medical School Total Enrollment by Race and Ethnicity." Washington, D.C.: Association of American Medical Colleges. http://www.aamc.org/data/databook/dbtoc.htm.

AAP Committee on Pediatric Workforce. 2006. "Women Leaders in Pediatrics." Vol. 2007. Chicago: American Academy of Pediatrics. http://www.aap.org/womenpeds/.

Aaron, Henry. 1991. *Serious and Unstable Condition.* Washington, D.C.: Brookings Institution.

Abbott, Andrew D. 1988. *The System of Professions: An Essay on the Division of Expert Labor.* Chicago: University of Chicago Press.

Abel, T. 1992. "Women to Have Positive Influence on the Practice of Medicine." *Michigan Medical Journal* 91 (12): 28–29.

Adams, Damon. 2002. "Physicians Are Working More, Enjoying It Less." *AMA News,* June 3.

——. 2004. "Generation Gripe: Young Doctors Less Dedicated, Hardworking?" *AMA News,* February 2.

Alexander, S. C., S. A. Keitz, R. Sloane, and J. A. Tulsky. 2006. "A Controlled Trial of a Short Course to Improve Residents' Communication with Patients at the End of Life." *Academic Medicine* 81: 1008–12.

American Academy of Family Practice. 2000. "Managed Care Backlash May Boost Patient Care." *Family Practice Report*, March 4.

American Association for Cancer Research. 2007. "Advances in Breast Cancer Research: Genetics Biology and Clinical Applications." Conference Program.

American Association of University Women. 2006. "Drawing the Line: Sexual Harassment on Campus." Press kit. Washington, D.C. http://www.aauw.org/About/newsroom/presskits/DTLpressconf.cfm.

American Medical Association (AMA). 2005. "Are Duty Hour Restrictions Defied?" November 21. http://www.ama-assn.org/ama/pub/category/211.html.

——. 2006. "IMGs in the United States." American Medical Association. http://www.ama-assn.org/ama/pub/category/211.html.

American Medical Association Task Force on Medical Student Debt. 2003. "Final Report Draft." American Medical Association, Medical Student Section. http://www.amaassn.org/ama1/pub/upload/mm/15/debt_report.pdf.

American Osteopathic Association. 2006. "Fact Sheet 2006." http://www.osteopathic.org/pdf/ost_factsheet.pdf.

Andersen, M., and N. Urban. 1997. "Physician Gender and Screening: Do Patient Differences Account for Differences in Mammography Use?" *Women & Health* 26 (1): 29–39.

Anderson, R., A. Barbara, and S. Feldman. 2007. "What Patients Want: A Content Analysis of Key Qualities That Influence Patient Satisfaction." *Journal of Medical Practice Management* 22: 255–61.

Andrews, Nancy C. 2002. "The Other Physician-Scientist Problem: Where Have All the Young Girls Gone?" *Nature Medicine* 8: 439–41.

Antony, James Soto. 1998. "Exploring the Factors That Influence Men and Women to Form Medical Career Aspirations." *Journal of College Student Development* 39: 417–26.

Arnold, M. W., A. F. Patterson, and A. S. Tang. 2005. "Has Implementation of the 80-Hour Work Week Made a Career in Surgery More Appealing to Medical Students?" *American Journal of Surgery* 189 (2): 129–33.

Arora, Vineet. 2005. "The Impact of Physician Payment Cuts on Access to Primary Care," November 17. http://www.acponline.org/advocacy/where_we_stand/medicare/med_pay1105.pdf.

Arora, V., T. B. Wetterneck et al. 2006. "Effect of the Inpatient General Medicine Rotation on Student Pursuit of a Generalist Career." *Journal of General Internal Medicine* 21: 471–75.

Arnst, Catherine. 2005a. "Nancy Brinker: Promise Keeper." *Business Week.* October 17.

Arnst, Catherine. 2005b. "If It Works for Breast Cancer." *Business Week.* May 23.

Arvantes, James. 2007. "Primary Care Physician Shortage Creates Medically Disenfranchised Population." *AAFP (American Academy of Family Practice) News.* http://www.aafp.org/online/en/home/publications/news/news-now/professional-issues/20070322disenfranchised.html.

Ash, A. S., P. L. Carr, R. Goldstein, and R. H. Friedman. 2004. "Compensation and Advancement of Women in Academic Medicine: Is There Equity?" *Annals of Internal Medicine* 141: 238–40.

Astin, Alexander W. 1998. "The Changing American College Student: Thirty-Year Trends, 1966–1996." *Review of Higher Education* 21: 115–35.

Astor, A., T. Akhtar et al. 2005. "Physician Migration: Views from Professionals in Colombia, Nigeria, India, Pakistan, and the Philippines." *Social Science Medicine* 61: 2492–3000.

Auerbach, Judith D., and Anne E. Figert. 1995. "Women's Health Research: Public Policy and Sociology." *Journal of Health and Social Behavior* 35: 115–31.

Babbott D., D. C. Baldwin, Jr., et al. 1988. "The Stability of Early Specialty Preferences among US Medical School Graduates in 1983." *JAMA: Journal of the American Medical Association* 259: 1970–75.

Baker, Laurence C. 1996. "Differences in Earnings between Male and Female Physicians." *New England Journal of Medicine* 334 (15): 982–83.

Baldwin, D. C., S. R. Daugherty, and E. J. Eckenfels. 1991. "Students' Perceptions of Mistreatment and Harassment during Medical School." *Western Journal of Medicine* 155: 140–55.

Balsa, Ana I., Naomi Seiler, Thomas G. McGuire, and M. Gregg Bloche. 2003. "Clinical Uncertainty and Healthcare Disparities." *American Journal of Law and Medicine* 29 (2/3): 203–19.

Barchi, R. L., and B. J. Lowery. 2000. "Scholarship in the Medical Faculty from the University Perspective: Retaining Academic Values." *Academic Medicine* 75: 899–905.

Barnsley, J., A. Williams, R. Cockerill, and J. Tanner. 1999. "Physician Characteristics and the Physician-Patient Relationship: Impact of Sex, Year of Graduation, and Specialty." *Canadian Family Physician* 45: 935–42.

Barzansky, B., and S. L. Etzel. 2003. "Educational Programs in U.S. Medical Schools, 2002–2003." *Journal of the American Medical Association* 290: 1190–96.

Batz, Jeannette. 1998. "The Doctor Is Out: Sickened by the Shift to Managed Care, More Physicians Are Claiming Disability, Moving into Administration, or Leaving Medicine Altogether." *Riverfront Times*, December 23. http://www.riverfronttimes.com/Issues/1998–12–23/news/feature.html.

Baxter, N., R. Cohen et al. 1996. "The Impact of Gender on the Choice of Surgery as a Career." *American Journal of Surgery* 172 (4): 373–76.

Belkin, Lisa. 1985. " A Group for Dual-Doctor Families." *New York Times*, June 16.

Belkin, Lisa. 2003. "The Opt-out Revolution." *New York Times*, October 26.

Bensing, J. M., A. van den Brink-Muinen, and D. H. de Bakker. 1993. "Gender Differences in Practice Style: A Dutch Study of General Practitioners." *Medical Care* 31 (3): 219–29.

Bensing, J. M., F. Tromp et al. 2006. "Shifts in Doctor-Patient Communication between 1986 and 2002: A Study of Videotaped General Practice Consultations with Hypertension Patients." *BMC Family Practice* 7: 62. http://www.biomedcentral.com/1471-2296/7/62.

Bergen, P. C., R. H. Turnage, and C. J. Carrico. 1998. "Gender-Related Attrition in a General Surgery Training Program." *Journal of Surgical Research* 77: 59–62.

Bernard, D. B., and D. J. Shulkin. 1998. "The Media vs. Managed Health Care: Are We Seeing a Full Court Press?" *Archives of Internal Medicine* 158: 2109–11.

Bertakis, K., P. Franks, and R. Azari. 2003. "Effect of Physician Gender on Patient Satisfaction." *Journal of the American Medical Women's Association* 58 (2): 69–75.

Bickel, Janet. 2000. *Women in Medicine: Getting In, Growing, and Advancing.* Thousand Oaks, Calif.: Sage.

Bickel, Janet, and Ann J. Brown. 2005. "Generation X: Implications for Faculty Recruitment and Development in Academic Health Centers." *Academic Medicine* 80 (3): 205–10.

Bickel, Janet, Valerie Clark, and Hisashi Yamagata. 2002. "Women in U.S. Academic Medicine Statistics, 2001–2002." AAMC. http://www.aamc.org/members/wim/statistics/stats02/start.htm.

Bickel, J., K. Croft, and R. Marshall. 1996. *Enhancing the Environment for Women in Academic Medicine.* Washington, D.C.: AAMC.

Bickel, J., and A. Ruffin. 1995. "Gender-Associated Differences in Matriculating and Graduating Medical Students." *Academic Medicine* 70 (6): 552–59.

Bird, Chloe E. 1990. "High Finance, Small Change: Women's Increased Representation in Bank Management." In *Job Queues, Gender Queues*, ed. Barbara Reskin and Patricia Roos, 145–67. Philadelphia: Temple University Press.

Bix, Amy Sue. 1997. "Diseases Chasing Money and Power: Breast Cancer and AIDS Activism Challenging Authority." *Journal of Policy History* 9: 5–32.

Blair-Loy, Mary. 2003. *Competing Devotions: Career and Family among Women Executives.* Cambridge: Harvard University Press.

Bluestone, N. R. 1978. "The Future Impact of Women Physicians on American Medicine." *American Journal of Public Health* 68 (8): 760–63.

Blumenthal, David. 2004. "New Steam from an Old Cauldron: The Physician-Supply Debate." *New England Journal of Medicine* 350: 1780–87.

Blumenthal, N. C., and Y. Chang. 1999. "The Duration of Ambulatory Visits to Physicians." *Journal of Family Practice* 48 (4): 264–71.

Bolzendahl, Catherine, and Daniel Myers. 2004. "Feminist Attitudes and Support for Gender Equality: Opinion Change in Women and Men, 1974–1998." *Social Forces* 83: 759–89.

Bosk, Charles. 2003. *Forgive and Remember: Managing Medical Failure.* 2nd ed. Chicago: University of Chicago Press.

Bouchard, L., and Marc Renaud. 1997. "Female and Male Physicians' Attitudes toward Prenatal Diagnosis: A Pan-Canadian Survey." *Social Science and Medicine* 44 (3): 381–92.

Bowman, Marjorie, Erica Frank, and Deborah Allen. 2002. *Women in Medicine: Career and Life Management.* New York: Springer.

Bowman, M., and S. Gehlbach. 1980. "Sex of Physician as a Determinant of Psychosocial Problem Recognition." *Journal of Family Practice* 10 (4): 655–59.

Briscoe, Forrest. 2006. "Temporal Flexibility and Careers: The Role of Large-scale Organizations for Physicians." *Industrial and Labor Relations Review* 60 (1): 67–83.

——. 2007. "From Iron Cage to Iron Shield? How Bureaucracy Enables Temporal Flexibility for Professional Service Workers." *Organization Science* 18 (2): 297–314.

Britt, H., A. Bhasale et al. 1996. "The Sex of the General Practitioner: A Comparison of Characteristics, Patients, and Medical Conditions Managed." *Medical Care* 34 (5): 403–15.

Brooks, Clem, and Catherine Bolzendahl. 2004. "The Transformation of U.S. Gender Role Attitudes: Cohort Replacement, Social-Structural Change, and Ideological Learning." *Social Science Research* 33: 106–33.

Brooks, F. 1998. "Women in General Practice: Responding to the Sexual Division of Labour?" *Social Science and Medicine* 47: 181–93.

Brotherton, S. E., and S. A. LeBailly. 1992. "The Effect of Family on the Work Lives of Married Physicians." *Journal of the American Medical Women's Association* 48: 175–81.

Brown, Kimberly Fahey. 2006. "To the Editor." *New York Times*, June 20.

Bryant, Julie. 2000. "More Docs Turning to Self-Pay Practices." *Business Courier of Cincinatti*, December 8. http://www.bizjournals.com/cincinnati/stories/2000/12/11/focus2.html.

Buchbinder, Sharon, Modena Wilson, Clifford Melick, and Neil Powe. 2001. "Primary Care Physician Turnover." *American Journal of Managed Care* 7: 701–13.

Buchmann, Claudia, and Thomas A. DiPrete. 2006. "The Growing Female Advantage in College Completion: The Role of Family Background and Academic Achievement." *American Sociological Review* 71 (4): 515–41.

Bunton, Sarah A., and William T. Mallon. 2007. "The Continued Evolution of Faculty Appointment and Tenure Policies at U.S. Medical Schools." *Academic Medicine* 82: 281–89.

Burgoon, M., T. S. Birk, and J. R. Hall. 1991. "Compliance and Satisfaction with Physician-Patient Communication: An Expectancy Theory Interpretation of Gender Differences." *Human Communication Research* 18: 177–208.

Burnside, J. W. 1989. "Are We to Blame for Our Own Unhappiness with Medicine?" *Texas Medicine* 85: 4.

Bylund, C., and G. Makoul. 2002. "Empathic Communication and Gender in the Physician-Patient Encounter." *Patient Education and Counseling* 48 (3): 207–16.

Carnes, Molly. 2005. "Women Physicians and Leadership." Power point presentation. www.ama assn.org/ama1/pub/upload/mm/19/mollycarnes.ppt.

Case, S., R. Hatala et al. 1999. "Does Sex Make a Difference? Sometimes It Does and Sometimes It Doesn't." *Academic Medicine* 74: 37–40.

Cassard, S., C. Weisman et al. 1997. "Physician Gender and Women's Preventive Services." *Journal of Women's Health* 6 (2): 199–207.

Cassell, Joan. 1997. "Doing Gender, Doing Surgery: Women Surgeons in a Man's Profession." *Human Organization* 56: 47.

———. 1998. *The Woman in the Surgeon's Body.* Cambridge: Harvard University Press.

Cejka Search. 2005. "Survey Reveals Emphasis on Tying Pay to Quality: Physician Executive Pay Increase Holds Steady Near 7 Percent." http://www.cejkasearch.com/about_cejka_search/history&profile.htm.

Center for Health Policy Research. 1983–1998. *Socioeconomic Characteristics of Medical Practice.* Chicago: Center for Health Policy Research, American Medical Association.

———. 1999–2005. *Physician Socioeconomic Statistics.* Chicago: American Medical Association.

Center for Studying Health System Change. 1996–1997; 2000–2001; 2004–2005. Community Tracking Study Physician Survey. Washington, D.C.: Center for Studying Health System Change.

Chin, E., ed. 2002. *This Side of Doctoring: Reflections from Women in Medicine.* Thousand Oaks, Calif.: Sage.

China Ministry of Health. 2004. *China Health Statistics Yearbook, 2004.* In Chinese. Electronic edition, http://www.moh.gov.cn/open/statistics/year2004/p23.htm.

Chiu, Tin, Andrew Old, Gill Naden, and Stephen Child. 2006. "Frequency of Calls to "On-Call" House Officer Pagers at Auckland City Hospital, New Zealand." *New Zealand Medical Journal* 119. http://www.nzma.org.nz/journal/119-1231/1913/.

Cochran, A., S. Melby, H. M. Foy, M. K. Wallack, and L. A. Neumayer. 2002. "The State of General Surgery Residency in the United States: Program Director Perspectives, 2001." *Archives of Surgery* 137: 1262–65.

Coffin, S., and D. Babbott. 1989. "Early and Final Preferences for Pediatrics as a Specialty: A Study of U.S. Medical Graduates in 1983." *Academic Medicine* 70: 552–59.

Cohany, Sharon, and Emy Sok. 2007. "Trends in Labor Force Participation of Married Mothers of Infants." *Monthly Labor Review* (February).

Cohen-Gadol, A. A., D. G. Piepgras, S. Krishnamurthy, and R. D. Fessler. 2005. "Resident Duty Hours Reform: Results of a National Survey of the Program Directors and Residents in Neurosurgery Training Programs." *Neurosurgery* 56: 398–403.

Cohn, Samuel. 1985. *The Process of Occupational Sex-Typing: The Feminization of Clerical Labor in Great Britain.* Philadelphia: Temple University Press.

Collins, Karen Scott, Cathy A. Schoen, and Firuzeh Khoransanizadeh. 1997. "Practice Satisfaction and Experiences of Women Physicians in an Era of Managed Care." *Journal of the American Medical Women's Association* 52 (2): 52–59.

Committee on Pediatric Workforce of the American Academy of Pediatrics. 2005. "Pediatrician Workforce Statement." *Pediatrics* 116: 263–69.

Conley, Frances. 1998. *Walking Out on the Boys.* New York: Farrar Straus and Giroux.

Conrad, C. 1998. "Physician Income in the 1990s: Problems and Disappointments." *Internet Medical Journal* 2. http://www.medjournal.com/forum/showthread.php? threadid=10.

Cook, Bob. 2007. "Finances Driving Physicians out of Solo Practice." amednews.com.

Cooper, R. A. 2003. "Impact of Trends in Primary, Secondary, and Postsecondary Education on Applications to Medical School. I: Gender Considerations." *Academic Medicine* 78: 855–63.

Cooper, Richard A., Prakash Laud, and Craig L. Dietrich. 1998. "Current and Projected Workforce of Nonphysician Clinicians." *JAMA: Journal of the American Medical Association* 20: 788–94.

Cooper-Patrick, Lisa, et al. 1999. "Race, Gender, and Partnership in the Patient-Physician Relationship." *JAMA: Journal of the American Medical Association* 282 (6): 583–89.

Cooter, Raelynn, James B. Erdmann et al. 2004. "Economic Diversity in Medical Education." *Evaluation and the Health Professions* 27: 252–64.

Copnell, B., L. Johnston et al. 2004. "Doctors' and Nurses' Perceptions of Interdisciplinary Collaboration in the NICU, and the Impact of a Neonatal Nurse Practitioner Model of Practice." *Journal of Clinical Nursing* 13: 105–13.

Cotter, Patrick S. 1986. "An Analysis of the Changing Patterns in Physician Employment Status, 1983 to 1985." Chicago: Center for Health Policy Research, American Medical Association.

Crandall, S. J., R. J. Volk, and V. Loemker. 1993. "Medical Students' Attitudes toward Providing Care for the Underserved: Are We Training Socially Responsible Physicians?" *JAMA: Journal of the American Medical Association* 269: 2519–23.

Croasdale, Myrle. 2002. "Practices Must Cope as More Physicians Work Part-Time Hours." amednews.com, October 21. http://www.ama-assn.org/amednews/2002/10/21/prl21021.htm.

——. 2004a. "High Medical School Debt Steers Life Choices for Young Doctors." amednews.com, May 17. http://www.ama-assn.org/amednews/2004/05/17/prsd0517.htm.

——. 2004b. "Women Physicians Find Ways to Make "Part Time" Work: The Trend toward Fewer Hours Is Gaining Momentum as Men Join In." amednews.com, November 15. http://www.ama-assn.org/amednews/2004/11/15/prl21115.htm.

——. 2007. "More Women Choosing Surgical Residencies." amednews.com, September 17. http://www.ama-assn.org/amednews/2007/09/17/prsc0917.htm.

Cross, Margaret Ann. 2007. "What the Primary Care Physician Shortage Means for Health Plans." *Managed Care*, June. http://www.managedcaremag.com/archives/0706/0706.shortage.html.

Culbertson, Richard, and Philip Lee. 1996. "Medicare and Physician Autonomy." *Health Care Financing Review* 18: 115–30.

Cull, W. L., H. J. Mulvey et al. 2002. "Pediatricians Working Part-Time: Past, Present, and Future." *Pediatrics* 109: 1015–1102.

Cunningham, P. J., J. M. Grossman, R. F. St. Peter, and C. S. Lesser. 1999. "Managed Care and Physicians' Provision of Charity Care." *JAMA: Journal of the American Medical Association* 281: 1087–92.

Cutler, David, and Jonathan Gruber. 2001. "Health Policy in the Clinton Era: Once Bitten Twice Shy." Pp. 825–874 in *American Economic Policy in the 1990s*, ed. Jeffrey Frankel and Peter Orszag. Cambridge: MIT Press.

Cyran, E. M., L. A. Crane, and L. Palmer. 2001. "Physician Sex and Other Factors Associated with Type of Breast Cancer Surgery in Older Women." *Archives of Surgery* 136 (2): 185–91.

Davis, P., B. Gribben, A. Scott, and R. Lay-Yee. 2000. "The 'Supply Hypothesis' and Medical Practice Variation in Primary Care: Testing Economic and Clinical Models of Inter-Practitioner Variation." *Social Science and Medicine* 50 (3): 407–18.

DeAngelis, Catherine D., and Richard M. Glass. 2006. "Women's Health—Advances in Knowledge and Understanding." *JAMA: Journal of the American Medical Association* 295: 1448–50.

Derose, K. P., R. D. Hays, D. F. McCaffrey, and D. W. Baker. 2001. "Does Physician Gender Affect Satisfaction of Men and Women Visiting the Emergency Department?" *Journal of General Internal Medicine* 16: 218–26.

Detsky, A. 1995. "Regional Variation in Medical Care." *New England Journal of Medicine* 333: 589–90.

de Virgilio, C., A. Yaghoubian et al. 2006. "The Eighty-Hour Resident Workweek Does Not Adversely Affect Patient Outcomes or Resident Education." *Current Surgery* 63: 435–39.

Dimick, J. B., J. A. Cowan Jr., J. C. Stanley, P. K. Henke, P. J. Pronovost, and G. R. Upchurch. 2003. "Surgeon Specialty and Provider Volumes Are Related to Outcome of Intact Abdominal Aortic Aneurysm Repair in the United States." *Journal of Vascular Surgery* 38: 739–44.

Doescher, M., K. Ellsbury, and L. G. Hart. 1997. "The Distribution of Rural Female Generalist Physicians in the United States." *Abstract Book/Association for Health Services Research* 15 (93). http://gateway.nlm.nih.gov/MeetingAbstracts/ma?f=102234172.html.

Dolan, P. L. 2006. "MGMA: Doctors on 'Unsustainable Course.'" amednews.com, November 6. http://www.ama-assn.org/amednews/2006/11/06/bisd1106.htm.

Dorschner, John. 2003. "Growing Number of Female Doctors Changing Medical Profession." *Standard Times*, March 25.

Dorsey, E. R., D. Jarjoura, and G. W. Ruteki. 2005. "The Influence of Controllable Lifestyle and Sex on the Specialty Choices of Graduating Medical Students." *Academic Medicine* 80: 791–96.

Drago, Robert S., et al. 2006. "The Avoidance of Bias against Caregiving." *American Behavioral Scientist* 49 (9): 1222–47.

Dresler, C., D. L. Padgett, S. E. MacKinnon, and G. A. Patterson. 1996. "Experiences of Women in Cardiothoracic Surgery: A Gender Comparison." *Archives of Surgery* 131 (11): 1128–34.

Ducker, D. G. 1978. "Believed Suitability of Medical Specialties for Women Physicians." *Journal of the American Medical Women's Association* 33: 25–32.

Dudley, R. Adams, and Harold S. Luft. 2001. "Managed Care in Transition." *New England Journal of Medicine* 344: 1087–92.

Dugan, J. P. 2006. "Explorations Using the Social Change Model: Leadership Development among College Men and Women." *Journal of College Student Development* 47: 217–55.

Dulmen, A. V., and J. Bensing. 2000. "Gender Differences in Gynecologist Communication." *Women and Health* 30: 49–61.

Dunn, Marvin, and Rebecca Miller. 1997. "U.S. Graduate Medical Education, 1996–1997." *JAMA: Journal of the American Medical Association* 278: 751–54.

Dye, Jane Lawler. 2005. "Fertility of American Women: June 2004." Washington, D.C.: U.S. Department of Commerce, U.S. Bureau of the Census. http://www.census.gov/prod/2005pubs/p20–555.pdf.

Eagly, Alice, and Mary Johannesen-Schmidt. 2001. "The Leadership Styles of Women and Men." *Journal of Social Issues* 57: 781–97.

Eagly, A. H., M. C. Johannesen-Schmidt, and M. van Engen. 2003. "Transformational, Transactional, and Laissez-Faire Leadership Styles: A Meta-Analysis Comparing Women and Men." *Psychological Bulletin* 95: 569–91.

Eagly, Alice, and Blair Johnson. 1990. "Gender and Leadership Style: A Meta-Analysis." *Psychological Bulletin* 108: 233–56.

Edlefsen, K. L., M. T. Mandelson et al. 1999. "Prostate-Specific Antigen for Prostate Cancer Screening: Do Physician Characteristics Affect Its Use?" *American Journal of Preventive Medicine* 17: 87–90.

Elder, Glen H. 1974. *Children of the Great Depression: Social Change in Life Experience.* Chicago: University of Chicago Press.

Ely, Robin. 1995. "The Power in Demography: Women's Social Construction of Gender Identity at Work." *Academy of Management Journal* 38: 589–634.

Emmons, S., et al. 2004. "The Impact of Perceived Gender Bias on Obstetrics and Gynecology Skills Acquisition by Third-Year Medical Students." *Academic Medicine* 79 (4): 326–32.

England, Paula, Paul Allison, and Yuxiao Wuc. 2007. "Does Bad Pay Cause Occupations to Feminize, Does Feminization Reduce Pay, and How Can We Tell with Longitudinal Data?" *Social Science Research* 36: 1237–56.

Epstein, Cynthia, Carroll Seron et al. 1998. *The Part-Time Paradox: Time Norms, Professional Life, Family, and Gender.* New York: Routledge.

Executive Women in Healthcare. 2005. "Executive Briefing." Vol. 2005. http://www.lemastergroup.com/news/ewih071105.pdf.

Fadem, Barbara. 1995. "The Relationship between Parental Income and Academic Performance of Medical Students." *Academic Medicine* 70: 1142–44.

Fan, V. S., M. Burman, M. B. McDonell, and S. D. Fihn. 2005. "Continuity of Care and Other Determinants of Patient Satisfaction with Primary Care." *Journal of General Internal Medicine* 20: 226–33.

Fang, Margaret, Ellen McCarthy, and Daniel Singer. 2004. "Are Patients More Likely to See Physicians of the Same Sex? Recent National Trends in Primary Care." *American Journal of Medicine* 117: 575–81.

Ferguson, C. M., K. C. Kellogg, M. M. Hutter, and A. L. Warshaw. 2005. "Effect of Work-Hour Reforms on Operative Case Volume of Surgical Residents." *Current Surgery* 62: 535–38.

Field, Mark. 1988. "Turf Battles on Medicine Avenue." *Society* 25: 12–16.

Fiorentine, Robert, and Stephen Cole. 1992. "Why Fewer Women Become Physicians: Explaining the Premed Persistence Gap." *Sociological Forum* 7.

Fishman, D. B. and C. N. Zimet. 1972. "Specialty Choice and Beliefs about Specialties among Freshmen Medical Students." *Journal of Medical Education* 47: 524–33.

Fitzpatrick, Kevin M., and Marilyn P. Wright. 1995. "Gender Differences in Medical School Attrition Rates, 1973–1992." *Journal of the American Medical Women's Association* 50: 204–6.

Fletcher, Kathlyn E., Steven Q. Davis, Willie Underwood, Rajesh S. Mangrulkar, Laurence F. McMahon, and Sanjay Saint. 2004. "Systematic Review: Effects of Resident Work Hours on Patient Safety." *Annals of Internal Medicine* 141: 851–57.

Flocke, S., and V. Gilchrist. 2005. "Physician and Patient Gender Concordance and the Delivery of Comprehensive Clinical Preventive Services." *Medical Care* 43 (5): 486–92.

Foster, S. W., J. E. McMurray, M. Linzer, J. W. Leavitt, M. Rosenberg, and M. Carnes. 2000. "Results of a Gender Climate and Work Environment Survey at a Midwestern Academic Health Center." *Academic Medicine* 75: 653–60.

Fox, N. J. 1992. *The Social Meaning of Surgery:* Birmingham, U.K.: Open University Press.

Frank, Erica, Donna Brogan, and Melissa Schiffman. 1998. "Prevalence and Correlates of Harassment among U.S. Women Physicians." *Archives of Internal Medicine* 158: 352–58.

Frank, Erica, Jennifer S. Carrera et al. 2006. "Experiences of Belittlement and Harassment and Their Correlates among Medical Students in the United States: Longitudinal Survey." *British Medical Journal* 333: 682–84.

Frank, E., and L. K. Harvey. 1996. "Prevention Advice Rates of Women and Men Physicians." *Archives of Family Medicine* 5 (4): 215–19.

Frank, E., L. Harvey, and L. Elon. 2000. "Family Responsibilities and Domestic Activities of U.S. Women Physicians." *Archives of Family Medicine* 9: 134–40.

Franks, P., and K. Bertakis. 2003. "Physician Gender, Patient Gender, and Primary Care." *Journal of Women's Health* 12 (1): 73–80.

Franks, P., and C. Clancy. 1993. "Physician Gender Bias in Clinical Decision Making: Screening for Cancer in Primary Care." *Medical Care* 31: 213.

Freeman, Catherine E. 2004. "Trends in Educational Equity of Girls and Women, 2004." *Education Statistics Quarterly* 6 (4). http://nces.ed.gov/programs/quarterly/vol_6/6_4/8_1.asp#2.

Freidson, Eliot. 1994. *Professionalism Reborn: Theory, Prophecy, and Policy.* Chicago: University of Chicago Press.

Freidson, Eliot. 2001. *Professionalism: The Third Logic.* Chicago, IL: University of Chicago Press.

Freudenheim, Milt. 1997. "As Nurses Take on Primary Care, Physicians Are Sounding Alarms." *New York Times,* September 30.

Friedan, Betty. 1963. *The Feminine Mystique.* New York: W. W. Norton.

Frishman, W. H. 2001. "Student Research Projects and Theses: Should They Be a Requirement for Medical School Graduation?" *Heart Disease* 3: 140–44.

Fritz, N. E., and J. D. Lantos. 1991. "Pediatrician's Practice Choices: Differences between Part-Time and Full-Time Practice." *Pediatrics* 88: 764–69.

Gabbe, S. G., M. A. Morgan et al. 2003. "Duty Hours and Pregnancy Outcome among Residents in Obstetrics and Gynecology." *Obstetrics and Gynecology* 102.

Gabel, Jon, Larry Levitt et al. 2002. "Job-Based Health Benefits in 2002." *Health Affairs* 21 (5): 143–51.

Garibaldi, Richard A., Carol Popkave, and Wayne Bylsma. 2005. "Career Plans for Trainees in Internal Medicine Residency Programs." Academic Medicine 80: 507–12.

Gentry, Suzanne. 2004 "Defining Women as Hospital Administrators: PHNS Survey Reveals Lifestyle, Attitudes of Women Hospital Leadership." *Business Wire,* December 9.

Gesensway, Deborah. 1999. "Changes in Medicine's Mommy Track." *American College of Physicians Observer* (December). http://www.acponline.org/clinical_information/journals_publications/acp_internist/dec99/mommy.htm.

Gilbert, Patrick, and Mary Ellen Miller. 2004. "Out of Time." Hopkins Medicine Winter on-line edition. http://esgweb1.nts.jhu.edu/hmn/W04/top.cfm.

Gilligan, Carol. 1982. *In a Different Voice: Psychological Theory and Women's Development.* Cambridge: Harvard University Press.

Gjerberg, E., and L. Kjlsrd. 2001. "The Doctor-Nurse Relationship: How Easy Is It to Be a Female Doctor Co-operating with a Female Nurse?" *Social Science and Medicine* 52 (2): 189–202.

Gjerdingen, D. K., K. M. Chaloner, and J. A. Vanderscoff. 1995. "Family Practice Residents' Maternity Leave Experiences and Benefits." *Family Medicine* 27: 512–18.

Glendinning, David. 2007. "Medical Trends behind Jump in Medicare Physician Spending." amednews.com, July 2. http://www.ama-assn.org/amednews/2007/07/02/gvsb0702.htm.

Goldin, Claudia. 1997. "Career and Family: College Women Look to the Past." In *Gender and Family Issues in the Workplace,* ed. Francine Blau and Ronald Ehrenberg, 20–58. New York: Russell Sage Foundation.

———. 2004. "The Long Road to the Fast Track: Career and Family." *Annals of the American Academy of Political and Social Science* 596: 20–35.

Gordon, Suzanne. 2005. *Nursing against the Odds: How Health Care Cost Cutting, Media Stereotypes, and Medical Hubris Undermine Nurses and Patient Care.* Ithaca: Cornell University Press.

Gordon, T. A., et al. 1999. "Complex Gastrointestinal Surgery: Impact of Provider Experience on Clinical and Economic Outcomes." *Journal of the American College of Surgeons.* 189: 46–56.

Gorman, E. H. 1999. "Bringing Home the Bacon: Marital Allocation of Income-Earning Responsibility, Job Shifts, and Men's Wages." *Journal of Marriage and the Family* 61 (1): 110–12.

Grandis, J. R., W. E. Gooding et al. 2004. "The Gender Gap in a Surgical Subspecialty: Analysis of Career and Lifestyle Factors." *Archives of Otolaryngology—Head and Neck Surgery* 130: 695–702.

Grant, Linda, Layne A. Simpson, Xue Lan Rong, and Holly Peters-Golden. 1990. "Gender, Parenthood, and Work Hours of Physicians." *Journal of Marriage and the Family* 52 (1): 39–49.

Greenfield, Teresa Arámbula. 1998. "Gender- and Grade-level Differences in Science Interest and Participation." *Science Education* 81: 259–76.

Guadagnino, Christopher. 1999. "Advancing the Battle for Nursing Autonomy." *Physicians News Digest,* June 5.

Guelich, Jill, Burton Singer, Marcia Castro, and Leon Rosenberg. 2002. "A Gender Gap in the Next Generation of Physician Scientists." *Journal of Investigative Medicine* 50: 412–18.

Gulliford, M.C., S. Naithani, and M. Morgan. 2007. "Continuity of Care and Intermediate Outcomes of Type 2 Diabetes Mellitus." *Family Practice* 24 (3): 245–51.

Haas, J., K. Phillips et al. 2002. "Effect of Managed Care Insurance on the Use of Preventive Care for Specific Ethnic Groups in the United States." *Medical Care* 40 (9): 743–51.

Hafferty, Frederic, and Donald Light. 1995. "Professional Dynamics and the Changing Nature of Medical Work." *Journal of Health and Social Behavior,* extra issue: 132–53.

Hager, Mary, ed. 2007. *Women and Medicine: Proceedings of a Confernece Chaired by Catherine D. DeAngeles.* New York: Josiah Macy Foundation.

Hall, Carl T. 1995. "Younger Doctors Disheartened: Many Complain of Growing Intrusion of the Bottom Line." *San Francisco Chronicle,* November 18.

Hall, Celia. 2004. "Influx of Women Doctors 'Will Harm Medicine.'" *Telegraph,* March 8.

Hall, Frances, et al. 2001. "Longitudinal Trends in the Applicant Pool for U.S. Medical Schools, 1974–1999." *Academic Medicine* 76 (8): 829–34.

Hall, Frances, Collins Mikesell et al. 2001. "Longitudinal Trends in the Applicant Pool for U.S. Medical Schools, 1974–1999." *Academic Medicine* 76: 829–33.

Hall, Judith A., Julie T. Irish et al. 1994. "Satisfaction, Gender, and Communication in Medical Visits." *Medical Care* 32 (12): 1216–31.

Hammond, J. W., W. S. Queale, T. K. Kim, and E. G. McFarland. 2003. "Surgeon Experience and Clinical and Economic Outcomes for Shoulder Arthroplasty." *Journal of Bone and Joint Surgery* 85A: 2318–24.

Hamric, A. B., and L. J. Blackhall. 2007. "Nurse-Physician Perspectives on the Care of Dying Patients in Intensive Care Units: Collaboration, Moral Distress, and Ethical Climate." *Critical Care Medicine* 35 (2): 422–29.

Handler, Arden, Deborah Rosenberg, Kristiana Raube, and Michele A. Kelley. 1998. "Health Care Characteristics Associated with Women's Satisfaction with Prenatal Care." *Medical Care* 36 (5): 679–94.

Hansen, H. E., M. H. Biros, N. M. Delaney, and V. L. Schug. 1999. "Research Utilization and Interdisciplinary Collaboration in Emergency Care." *Academic Emergency Medicine* 6: 271–79.

Harris Interactive. 2004. "Doctors at Peak of Prestigious Jobs List." *AMA News*, October 18.

Harris, L., F. Luft, D. W. Rudy, and W. M. Tierney. 1995. "Correlates of Health Care Satisfaction in Inner-City Patients with Hypertension and Chronic Renal Insufficiency." *Social Science and Medicine* 41 (12): 1639–45.

Harris, Scott. 2007. "Solutions Sought on Predicted Oncologist Shortage." *AAMC Reporter* (April). http://www.aamc.org/newsroom/reporter/april07/shortage.htm.

Haug, M. R. 1973. "Deprofessionalization: An Alternate Hypothesis for the Future." *Sociological Review Monograph* 20: 195–211.

Hayes, M. 1981. "The Impact of Women Physicians on Social Change in Medicine: The Evolution of Humane Health Care Delivery Systems." *Journal of the American Medical Women's Association* 36 (2): 82–84.

Health Resources and Services Administration, Bureau of Health Professions. 1999. *Area Resource File (ARF) System.* Fairfax, Va.: Quality Resource Systems. February.

Heaton, C., and Marquez, J. 1990. "Patient Preferences for Physician Gender in the Male Genital/Rectal Exam." *Family Practice Research Journal* 10 (2): 105–15.

Henderson, J., and C. Weisman. 2001. "Physician Gender Effects on Preventive Screening and Counseling: An Analysis of Male and Female Patients' Health Care Experiences." *Medical Care* 39 (12): 1281–92.

Henrich, J. B. 2004. "Women's Health Education Initiatives: Why Have They Stalled?" *Academic Medicine* 79 (4): 283–88.

Hill, L., et al. 2001. "Obstetrician-Gynecologists' Attitudes towards Premenstrual Dysphoric Disorder and Major Depressive Disorder." *Journal of Psychosomatic Obstetrics and Gynecology* 22 (4): 241–50.

Hinze, Susan W. 1999. "Gender and the Body of Medicine or at Least Some Body Parts: (Re)Constructing the Prestige Hierarchy of Medical Specialties." *Sociological Quarterly* 40 (2): 217–39.

——. 2000. "Inside Medical Marriages: The Effect of Gender on Income." *Work and Occupations* 27: 464–99.

——. 2004. "Women, Men, Career, and Family in the U.S. Young Physician Labor Force." *Research in the Sociology of Work* 14: 185–217.

Hinze, Susan W., Heidi T. Chirayath et al. 1997. "MD2 Couples in the Nineties: The His and Hers of Medical Marriages." Presentation at the American Sociological Association Meetings.

Hobson, Katherine. 2005. "Doctors Vanish from View: Harried by the Bureaucracy of Medicine, Physicians Are Pulling Back from Patient Care." USNews.com, January 31.

Hoff, T. J. 2004. "Doing the Same and Earning Less: Male and Female Physicians in a New Medical Specialty." *Inquiry* 41: 301–15.

Hojat, Mohammadreza, Joseph S. Gonnella et al. 2003. "Comparisons of American, Israeli, Italian, and Mexican Physicians and Nurses on the Total and Factor Scores of the Jefferson Scale of Attitudes toward Physician–Nurse Collaborative Relationships." *International Journal of Nursing Studies* 40: 427–35.

Hojat, M., T. J. Nasca et al. 2001. "Attitudes toward Physician-Nurse Collaboration: A Cross-Cultural Study of Male and Female Physicians and Nurses in the United States and Mexico." *Nursing Research* 50: 123–28.

Holmes, A. V., W. L. Cull, and R. R. Socolar. 2005. "Part-Time Residency in Pediatrics: Description of Current Practice." *Pediatrics* 116: 32–37.

Hooker, Roderick, and Linda Craig. 2001. "Use of Physician Assistants and Nurse Practitioners in Primary Care." *Health Affairs* 20: 231–38.

Hooker, R. S., and D. K. Freeborn. 1991. "Use of Physician Assistants in Managed Health Care Systems." *Public Health Reports* 106: 90–94.

Horwitz, L. I., H. M. Krumholz, S. J. Huot, and M. L. Green. 2006. "Internal Medicine Residents' Clinical and Didactic Experiences after Work Hour Regulation: A Survey of Chief Residents." *Journal of General Internal Medicine* 21: 961–65.

Hosmer, D., and S. Lemeshow. 1989. *Applied Logistic Regression.* New York: John Wiley and Sons.

Hueston, William J. 1998. "Family Physicians' Satisfaction with Practice." *Archives of Family Medicine* 7: 242–47.

Huff, K. L., and D. Fang. 1999. "When Are Students Most at Risk of Encountering Academic Difficulty? A Study of the 1992 Matriculants to U.S. Medical Schools." *Academic Medicine* 74: 454–60.

Hundley, G. 2000. "Male/Female Earnings Differences in Self-Employment: The Effects of Marriage, Children, and the Household Division of Labor." *Industrial and Labor Relations Review* 54 (1): 95–114.

Huston, S., et al. 2001. "Physician Gender and Hormone Replacement Therapy Discussion." *Journal of Women's Health and Gender-Based Medicine* 10 (3): 279–87.

Hymowitz, Carol. 2005. "Women Internalize Stereotypes of Themselves as Weaker Leaders." *Wall Street Journal Online,* October 25. http://www.careerjournal.com/columnists/inthelead/20051025-inthelead.html.

India Central Bureau of Health Intelligence. 2005. Health Information of India. http://cbhidghs.nic.in/hia2005/6.02.htm.

Institute of Medicine. 2004. *Improving Medical Education: Enhancing the Behavioral and Social Science Content of Medical School Curricula.* Washington, D.C.: National Academy Press.

Iqbal, Yasmine. 2005. "Focusing on Near Misses Can Bring Major Improvements." *ACP Observer.* http://www.acponline.org/clinical_information/journals_publications/acp_internist/sep05/nearmiss.htm.

Iverson, Kenneth. 1996. *Getting into a Residency: A Guide for Medical Students.* Tucson: Galen Press.

Ivins, J., and Gerry Kent. 1993. "Women's Preferences for Male and Female Gynaecologists." *Journal of Reproductive and Infant Psychology* 11 (4): 209–14.

Jacobs, Jerry A. 1996. "Gender Inequality and Higher Education." *Annual Review of Sociology* 22: 153–85.

Jacobs, Jerry A., and Kathleen Gerson. 2004. *The Time Divide: Work, Family, and Gender Inequality.* Cambridge: Harvard University Press.

Jacobs, Jerry A., and Teresa Labov. 2002. "Gender Differentials in Intermarriage among Sixteen Race and Ethnic Groups." *Sociological Forum* 17 (4): 621–46.

Jacobson, Christine, Jack Resneck, and Alexa Boer Kimball. 2004. "Generational Differences in Practice Patterns of Dermatologists in the United States." *Archives of Dermatology* 140: 1477–82.

Jagsi, Reshma, Elizabeth A. Guancial et al. 2006. "The 'Gender Gap' in Authorship of Academic Medical Literature: A 35-Year Perspective." *New England Journal of Medicine* 355: 281–87.

Jancin, Bruce. 2002. "Gender Differences in Ob.Gyn. Resident Attrition: Most Men Leave to Change Career." *OB/GYN News,* June 1. http://www.findarticles.com/p/articles/mi_m0CYD/is_11_37/ai_87078818.

Jarman, B. T., et al. 2004. "The 80-Hour Work Week: Will We Have Less-Experienced Graduating Surgeons?" *Current Surgery* 61: 612–15.

Jarnberg, Per-Olof, James S. Hicks, and Brenda A. Quint Gaebel. 2001. "Scheduling of Call and Operating Room Staffing: A Nationwide Survey of Academic Anesthesiology Centers." *Anesthesiology* 95: A1110.

Jefferson Medical College Alumni Bulletin. 2007. "We Are Family." Spring: 19–23.

Jenkins, Brian. 1997. "More Doctors Join Unions to Fight HMOs." *CNN Interactive,* December 25. http://www.cnn.com/HEALTH/9712/25/docs.unions/index.html.

Jonas, H. S., S. L. Etzel, and B. Barzansky. 1991. "Educational Programs in U.S. Medical Schools." *JAMA: Journal of the American Medical Association* 266: 913–20.

Jones, A. M., and K. B. Jones. 2007. "The 88-Hour Family: Effects of The 80-Hour Work Week on Marriage and Childbirth in a Surgical Residency." *Iowa Orthopaedic Journal* 27: 128–33.

Kahn, G. S., B. Cohen, and H. Jason. 1979. "The Teaching of Interpersonal Skills in U.S. Medical Schools." *Journal of Medical Education* 54: 29–35.

Kaiser, Jocelyn. 2005. "Gender in the Pharmacy: Does It Matter?" *Science* 308 (5728): 1572.

Kalet, Adina, Michele P. Pugnaire et al. 2004. "Teaching Communication in Clinical Clerkships: Models from the Macy Initiative in Health Communications." *Academic Medicine* 79: 511–20.

Kanter, Rosabeth Moss. 1977. *Men and Women of the Corporation.* New York: Basic Books.

Kantor, Jodi. 2006. "On the Job, Nursing Mothers Are Finding a 2-Class System." *New York Times,* September 1. http://news.blogs.nytimes.com/2006/08/31/on-the-job-nursing-mothers-are-finding-a-2-class-system/.

Kassebaum, D. G., and P. L. Szenas. 1995. "Medical students' Career Indecision and Specialty Rejection: Roads Not Taken." *Academic Medicine* 70: 937–43.

Kassebaum, D. G., P. L. Szenas, and M. K. Schuchert. 1996. "Determinants of the Generalist Career Intentions of 1995 Graduating Medical Students." *Academic Medicine* 71 (2): 198–209.

Katz, Pearl. 1999. *The Scalpel's Edge: The Culture of Surgeons.* Boston: Allyn and Bacon.

Keil, L. 1998. *Community Tracking Study Physician Survey: Round 1, General Distribution Survey Methodology Report* (Technical Publication 9). Washington, D.C.: Center for Studying Health System Change.

Kelly, John, and Margaret Toepp. 1994. "Practice Parameters: More than 1,500 Have Been Developed since 1989 and More Are in the Works." *Michigan Medicine* 93: 36–40.

Kemper, P. 1996. "The Design of the Community Tracking Study: A Longitudinal Study of Health System Change and Its Effects on People." *Inquiry* 33 (Summer): 195–206.

Kennedy, R. 2006. "At Some Medical Schools, Humanities Join the Curriculum." *New York Times,* April 17.

Kenney, G. M., and Allison Cook. 2007. "Coverage Patterns among SCHIP-Eligible Children and Their Parents." *Health Policy Online,* February 9. http://www.urban.org/url.cfm?ID=311420

Kikano, G. E., M. A. Goodwin, and K. C. Stange. 1998. "Physician Employment Status and Practice Patterns." *Journal of Family Practice* 46: 499–505.

Kilborn, Peter T. 1998. "H.M.O. Fiscal Incentives Linked to Doctors' Discontent." *New York Times,* November 19.

Kim, C., L. McEwen et al. 2005. "Is Physician Gender Associated with the Quality of Diabetes Care?" *Diabetes Care* 28 (7): 1594–98.

Kirk, Lynne M. 2006. "Who Will Take Care of You and Me? Facing the Crisis in Primary Care." *ACP Observer,* July–August. http://news.acponline.org/journals/news/jul06/toc.htm.

Klass, P. 1988. "Are Women Better Doctors?" *New York Times Magazine,* April 10.

Klebanoff, M. A., P. H. Shiono, and G. G. Rhoads. 1990. "Outcomes of Pregnancy in a National Sample of Resident Physicians." *New England Journal of Medicine* 323: 1040–45.

Kletke, P. R., D. W. Emmons, and K. D. Gillis. 1996. "Current Trends in Physicians' Practice Arrangements: From Owners to Employees." *JAMA: Journal of the American Medical Association* 276: 555–60.

Klingensmith, Mary. 2003. "Current Data on the Impact of Duty Hours on Hospitals, Patients, Faculty, and Resident: Review of Published Studies Relating to the Issue." Power point presentation. American College of Surgeons. http://www.facs.org/edu cation/gs2003/gs43klingensmith.pdf.

Koehn, Nerissa, George Fryer et al. 2002. "The Increase in International Medical Graduates in Family Practice Residency Programs." *Family Medicine* 34: 429–35.

Kohn, Linda T., Janet M. Corrigan, and Molla S. Donaldson. 2000. *To Err Is Human: Building a Safer Health System.* Washington, D.C.: National Academy Press.

Kolata, Gina. 2007. "Sharp Drop in Rates of Breast Cancer Holds." *New York Times,* April 19.

Kongar, Ebru. 2006. "Importing Equality or Exporting Jobs? Competition and Gender Wage and Employment Differentials in U.S. Manufacturing." January. http://ssrn. com/abstract=878123.

Konrad, A. M., J. E. Ritchie Jr., P. Lieb, and E. Corrigall. 2000. "Sex Differences and Similarities in Job Attribute Preferences: A Meta-Analysis." *Psychological Bulletin* 126: 593–641.

Kornstein, S., S. Norris, and S. W. Woodhouse. 1998. "Women in Medicine: Shaping the Future." *Virginia Medical Quarterly* 125 (1): 44–49.

Kotwall, C. A., C. L. Covington et al. 1996. "Patient, Hospital, and Surgeon Factors Associated with Breast Conservation Surgery: A Statewide Analysis in North Carolina." *Annals of Surgery* 224: 426–29.

Kowalczyk, Liz. 2004. "Rejecting Health Insurers: Doctor's Decision Reflects Discontent within Profession." *The Boston Globe,* January 30.

Kunz, Meredith Alexander. 2007. "Flexible Options Help Balance Career, Family Needs." *Stanford News Service,* January 24. http://news-service.stanford.edu/news/2007/ january24/med-flexible-012407.html.

Kupersanin, Eve. 2001. "Recent Changes May Affect IMG Psychiatrists." *Psychiatric News* 36: 28.

Kwan, Rita, and Robert Levy. 2006. *A Primer on Resident Work Hours.* Reston, Va.: American Medical Student Association.

Lambert, Emily, and Eric Holomboe. 2005. "The Relationship between Specialty Choice and Gender of U.S. Medical Students, 1990–2003." *Academic Medicine* 80: 797–802.

Landrigan, Christopher P., Laura K. Barger et al. 2006. "Interns' Compliance with Accreditation Council for Graduate Medical Education Work-Hour Limits." *JAMA: Journal of the American Medical Association* 296: 1063–70.

Ledley, F., and F. Lovejoy. 1993. "Factors Influencing the Interests, Career Paths, and Research Activities of Recent Graduates from an Academic Pediatric Residency Program." *Pediatrics* 92 (3): 436–41.

Leicht, Kevin, and Mary Fennell. 2001. *Professional Work.* Malden, Mass.: Blackwell.

Leppert, P., and R. Artal. 2002. "A Survey of Past Obstetrics and Gynecology Research Fellows." *Journal of the Society for Gynecologic Investigation* 9 (6): 372–78.

Lerner, Barron H. 2002. "TIMELINE: Breast Cancer Activism: Past Lessons, Future Directions." *Nature Reviews Cancer* 2: 225–31.

Levinson, W., R. Gorawara-Bhat, and J. Lamb. 2000. "A Study of Patient Clues and Physician Responses in Primary Care and Surgical Settings." *JAMA: Journal of the American Medical Association* 284: 1021–27.

Levinson W., K. Kaufman, and S. W. Tolle. 1992. "Women in Academic Medicine: Strategies for Balancing Career and Personal Life." *Journal of the American Medical Women's Association* 47: 25–28.

Levinson, Wendy, and Nicole Lurie. 2004. "When Most Doctors Are Women." *Annals of Internal Medicine* 141: 471–75.

Levinson, W., D. L. Roter et al. 1997. "Physician-Patient Communication: The Relationship with Malpractice Claims among Primary Care Physicians and Surgeons." *JAMA: Journal of the American Medical Association* 277: 553–59.

Levy, S., P. Dowling et al. 1992. "The Effect of Physician and Patient Gender on Preventive Medicine Practices in Patients Older Than Fifty." *Family Medicine* 24: 58–61.

Ley, T., and Leon Rosenberg. 2002. "Removing Career Obstacles for Young Physician-Scientists: Loan-Repayment Programs." *New England Journal of Medicine* 346 (5): 368–72.

Light, D., and S. Levine. 1988. "The Changing Character of the Medical Profession: A Theoretical Overview." *Milbank Quarterly* 66: 10–32.

Linzer, Mark, Thomas Konrad et al. 2000. "Managed Care, Time Pressure, and Physician Job Satisfaction: Results from the Physician Worklife Study." *Journal of General Internal Medicine* 15: 441–50.

Lorber, Judith. 1984. *Women Physicians: Careers, Status, and Power.* New York: Tavistock.

——. 2000. "What Impact Have Women Physicians Had on Women's Health?" *Journal of the American Medical Women's Association* 55 (1): 13–15.

Lovecchio, Karen, and Lauren Dundes. 2002. "Premed Survival: Understanding the Culling Process in Premedical Undergraduate Education." *Academic Medicine* 77: 719–24.

Lowe, K. B., G. K. Kroeck, and N. Sivasubramaniam. 1996. "Effectiveness Correlates of Transformational and Transactional Leadership: A Meta-Analytic Review of the MLQ Literature." *Leadership Quarterly* 7: 385–425.

Luft, Harold. 1987. *Health Maintenance Organizations Dimensions of Performance.* New Brunswick, N.J.: Transaction Books.

Lugtenberg, Marjolein, Phil Heiligers, Judith de Jong, and Lammert Hingstman. 2006. "Internal Medicine Specialists' Attitudes towards Working Part-Time: A Comparison between 1996 and 2004." *BMC Health Services Research,* 6: 126.

Lurie, N., K. Margolis et al. 1997. "Why Do Patients of Female Physicians Have Higher Rates of Breast and Cervical Cancer Screening?" *Journal of General Internal Medicine* 12 (1): 34–43.

——. 1998. "Physician Self-Report of Comfort and Skill in Providing Preventive Care to Patients of the Opposite Sex." *Archives of Family Medicine* 7 (2): 134–37.

Lyon, D. S. 2002. "Graduate Education in Women's Health Care: Where Have All the Young Men Gone?" *Current Women's Health Reports* 2: 170–74.

Lyons, M. F. 2001. "Physician Executives Breaking Out of Middle Management." *Physician Executive* 27: 18–21.

Magrane, Diane, Valarie Clark et al. 2004. "Women in U.S. Academic Medicine Statistics and Medical School Benchmarking, 2003–2004." http://www.aamc.org/members/wim/statistics/stats04/start.htm.

Magrane, Diane, Jonathan Lang et al. Medical Students Selected Years 1965–2007. "Women in U.S. Academic Medicine Statistics and Medical School Benchmarking, 2006–2007–2006." Washington, D.C.: Association of American Medical Colleges. Table 1. http://www.aamc.org/members/wim/wimguide/wim6.pdf.

Maguire, Phyllis. 1999. "How Direct-to-Consumer Advertising Is Putting the Squeeze on Physicians." *ACP Internist.* March. http://www.acponline.org/clinical_information/journals_publications/acp_internist/mar99/squeeze.htm.

Makary, M. A., J. B. Sexton et al. 2006. "Operating Room Teamwork among Physicians and Nurses: Teamwork in the Eye of the Beholder." *Journal of the American College of Surgery* 202: 746–52.

Mandelblatt, J. S., C. D. Berg et al. 2001. "Measuring and Predicting Surgeons' Practice Styles for Breast Cancer Treatment in Older Women." *Medical Care* 39 (3): 288–42.

Mannheim, Karl. 1952. "The Problem of Generations." In *Essays on the Sociology of Knowledge*, ed. Paul Kecskemeti, 276–322. London: Routledge and Kegan Paul.

Marder, W. D., David Emmons, Philip Kletke, and Richard Willke. 1988. "Physician Employment Patterns: Challenging Conventional Wisdom." *Health Affairs* 7: 137–45.

Mark, Saralyn, and Jhumka Gupta. 2002. "Reentry into Clinical Practice." *JAMA: Journal of the American Medical Association* 288: 1091–96.

Marshall, Eliot. 2005. "From Dearth to Deluge." *Science* 308: 1570.

Marsteller, Jill, and Randall Bovbjerg. 1999. *Federalism and Patient Protection: Changing Roles for State and Federal Government.* Urban Institute: Washington, D.C. August 11.

Mathias, J. M. 1997. "Surgeons Decry OR Layoffs of Nurse Managers." *OR Manager* 13: 1.

Matorin, A., et al. 1997. "Women's Advancement in Medicine and Academia: Barriers and Future Perspectives." *Texas Medicine* 93 (11): 60–64.

Matteson, M. T., and S. V. Smith. 1977. "Selection of Medical Specialties: Preferences vs. Choices." *Journal of Medical Education* 52: 548–54.

Mattila-Lindy, S. H., E. Hemminki et al. 1998. "Physicians' Gender and Clinical Opinions of Reproductive Health Matters." *Women and Health* 26 (3): 15–26.

Mawardi, B. H. 1977. "Styles of Practice of Female Physicians." *Annual Conference on Research in Medical Education* 16: 227–30.

Mayer, K. L., H. S. Ho, and J. E. Goodnight. 2001. "Childbearing and Child Care in Surgery." *Archives of Surgery* 136: 649–55.

Mayer, K. L., R. V. Perez, and H. S. Ho. 2001. "Factors Affecting Choice of Surgical Residency Training Program." *Journal of Surgical Research* 98: 71–75.

Mazzuca, Josephine. 2003. "Teen Career Picks: The More Things Change . . ." In GALLUP *Brain.* Washington, D.C.: Gallup Organization.

McCann, J. L., R. S. Phillips et al. 2005. "Physician Assistant and Nurse Practitioner Workforce Trends." *American Family Physician* 72 (7): 1176.

McDonald, L. 1988. "Women Physicians and Organized Medicine." *Western Journal of Medicine* 149 (7): 777–78.

McFarland, K. F., and D. R. Rhoades. 1998. "Gender-Related Values and Medical Specialty Choice." *Academic Psychiatry* 22: 236–39.

McGuire, L., et al. 2004. "Career Advancement for Women Faculty in a U.S. School of Medicine: Perceived Needs." *Academic Medicine* 79 (4): 319–25.

McKinlay, J. B. 1977. "The Business of Good Doctoring or Doctoring as Good Business: Reflections on Freidson's View of the Medical Game." *International Journal of Health Services* 15: 161–95.

McMahon, G. T. 2004. "Coming to America: International Medical Graduates in the United States." *New England Journal of Medicine* 350: 2435–37.

McMurray, Julia, P. J. M. Heiligers et al. 2005. "Part-Time Medical Practice: Where Is It Headed?" *American Journal of Medicine* 118: 87–92.

McMurray, J., M. Linzer et al. 2000. "The Work Lives of Women Physicians: Results from the Physician Work Life Study." *Journal of General Internal Medicine* 15 (6): 372–80.

McNeil, Donald G. 2004. "Real Men Don't Clean Bathrooms." *New York Times*, September 19.

Mechanic, David. 1991. "Sources of Countervailing Power in Medicine." *Journal of Health Politics, Policy, and Law* 16: 485–91.

———. 2003. "Physician Discontent: Challenges and Opportunities." *JAMA: Journal of the American Medical Association* 290: 941–46.

Mechanic, David, D. D. McAlpine, and M. Rosenthal. 2001. "Are Patients' Office Visits with Physicians Getting Shorter?" *New England Journal of Medicine* 344: 198–204.

Medical News Today. 2007. "Lack of Control over Work Hours Leads to Physician Burnout." *Medical News Today,* April 15. http://www.medicalnewstoday.com/articles/67795.php.

Migliore, M., C. K. Choong et al. 2007. "A Surgeon's Case Volume of Oesophagectomy for Cancer Strongly Influences the Operative Mortality Rate." *European Journal of Cardiothorac Surgery* 32: 375–80.

Miles, S. H., L. W. Lane et al. 1989. "Medical Ethics Education: Coming of Age." *Academic Medicine* 64: 705–14.

Miller, H. I., and G. Conko. 2001. "Precaution without Principle." *Nature Biotechnology* 19: 302–3.

Miller, N. H., D. J. Miller, and M. Chism. 1996. "Breastfeeding Practices among Resident Physicians." *Pediatrics* 98: 434–37.

Miller, R. H., H. S. Luft et al. 1993. *Managed Care: Performance and Prospects,* ed. D. Margaret F. Schulte. Vol. 9. Washington, D.C.: American Foundation of Health Care Executives.

Miller, S. H. 1998. "Competitive Forces and Academic Plastic Surgery." *Plastic and Reconstructive Surgery* 101: 1389–99.

Moen, Phyllis. 2003. *It's About Time: Couples and Careers.* Ithaca: Cornell University Press.

Morantz-Sanchez, R. M. 1985. *Sympathy and Science: Women Physicians in American Medicine.* New York: Oxford University Press.

More, Ellen. 1999. *Restoring the Balance: Women Physicians and the Profession of Medicine.* Cambridge: Harvard University Press.

Morrell, D. C., M. E. Evans, R. W. Morris, and M. O. Roland. 1986. "The 'Five Minute' Consultation: Effect of Time Constraint on Clinical Content and Patient Satisfaction." *British Medical Journal (Clinical Research and Education)* 292 (6524): 870–73.

Morris, M., and B. Western. 1999. "Inequality in Earnings at the Close of the Twentieth Century." *Annual Review of Sociology* 25: 623–57.

Mullan, F. 2005. "The Metrics of the Physician Brain Drain." *New England Journal of Medicine* 353: 1810–18.

———. 2006. "Doctors for the World: Indian Physician Emigration." *Health Affairs* 25: 380–93.

Murray, Alison, Jana Montgomery et al. 2001. "Doctor Discontent: A Comparison of Physician Satisfaction in Different Delivery System." *Journal of General Internal Medicine* 16: 451–59.

Murray, Alison, Dana G. Safran et al. 2000. "Part-Time Physicians: Physician Workload and Patient-Based Assessments of Primary Care Performance." *Archives of Family Medicine* 9: 327–32.

Myers, J. S., L. M. Bellini et al. 2006. "Internal Medicine and General Surgery Residents' Attitudes about the ACGME Duty Hours Regulations: A Multicenter Study." *Academic Medicine* 81: 1052–58.

Nabel, E. G. 2006. "The Women's Health Initiative." *Science* 313: 1703.

National Center for Education Statistics. 2004. "Trends in the Educational Equity of Girls and Women." http://nces.ed.gov/pubs2005/equity/Section4.asp.

———. 2006a. "Degrees in the Biological and Biomedical Sciences Conferred by Degree-Granting Institutions, by Level of Degree and Sex of Student: Selected Years, 1951–52 through 2004–05." *Digest of Education Statistics.* Table 281.

———. 2006b. "Total Fall Enrollment in Degree-Granting Institutions, by Attendance Status, Age, and Sex: Selected Years, 1970 through 2015." *Digest of Education Statistics.* Table 177.

———. 2006c. "Total Fall Enrollment in Degree-Granting Institutions, by Level, Sex, Age, and Attendance Status of Student: 2005." *Digest of Education Statistics.* Table 178.

National Association of Legal Professionals. 2006. "Few Lawyers Work Part-Time, Most Who Do Are Women." http://www.nalp.org/press/details.php?id=65.

National Research Council. 1998. *Trends in the Early Careers of Life Scientists.* Washington, D.C.: National Academy Press.

National Resident Matching Program. 2007a. "Charting Outcomes in the Match." Washington, D.C.: Association of American Medical Colleges.

———. 2007b. "Results and Data 2007 Main Residency Match." Washington, D.C.: Association of American Medical Colleges.

Neittaanmaeki, Lisa, R. Luhtala, I. Virjo, and E. E. Kumpusalo. 1993. "More Women Enter Medicine: Young Doctors' Family Origin and Career Choice." *Medical Education* 27: 440–45.

Newton, D. A., M. S. Grayson, and L. F. Thompson. 2005. "The Variable Influence of Lifestyle and Income on Medical Students' Career Specialty Choices: Data from Two U.S. Medical Schools, 1998–2004." *Academic Medicine* 80: 809–14.

Nickerson, K. G., N. M. Bennett, D. Estes, and S. Shea. 1990. "The Status of Women at One Academic Medical Center: Breaking through the Glass Ceiling." *JAMA: Journal of the American Medical Association* 264: 1813–17.

Nonnemaker, L. 2000. "Women Physicians in Academic Medicine: New Insights from Cohort Studies." *New England Journal of Medicine* 642: 399–405.

Nora, L. M., M. A. McLaughlin et al. 1996. "Does Exposure to Gender Discrimination and Sexual Harassment Impact Medical Students' Specialty Choices and Residency Program Selections?" *Academic Medicine* 71 (10 Suppl.): S22–24.

———. 2002. "Gender Discrimination and Sexual Harassment in Medical Education: Perspectives Gained by a Fourteen-School Study." *Academic Medicine* 77: 1226–34.

Novack, Lesley L., and David R. Novack. 1996. "Being Female in the Eighties and Nineties: Conflicts between New Opportunities and Traditional Expectations among White, Middle-Class, Heterosexual College Women." *Sex Roles: A Journal of Research* 35: 57–77.

O'Connell, Virginia Adams. 2001. "Attrition in Surgical Residency Programs." Ph.D. dissertation, Department of Sociology, University of Pennsylvania.

O'Connor, Karen G., Avrum Katcher, Hannah Sherman, and William L. Cull. 2004. "Balancing Work and Personal Life: Perceptions of Part-Time and Full-Time Pediatricians." Paper presented at the Pediatric Academic Societies Meetings, San Francisco, May.

Office of Extramural Research, National Institutes of Health. 2005. "Sex/Gender in the Biomedical Science Workforce." U.S. Department of Health and Human Services. October 7. http://grants.nih.gov/grants/policy/sex_gender/q_a.htm#q3.

Office of Women's Health Research. 2004. "Comprehensive 1991–2004 Report on Women's Health Research Funded or Co-funded by the Office of Research on Women's Health," October. http://orwh.od.nih.gov/CompReport91-04.pdf.

O'Rand, A., and J. Farkas. 2002. "Couples' Retirement Timing in the United States in the 1990s." *International Journal of Sociology* 32 (2): 11–29.

Organization for Economic Cooperation and Development (OECD). 2007. "OECD Health Data (2007)." University of Edinburgh.

Orzano, A., and R. Cody. 1995. "Gender Concordance between Family Practice Residents and Diagnoses in an Ambulatory Setting." *Family Medicine* 27 (7): 440–43.

Pai, C. W., Y. A. Ozcan et al. 2000. "Regional Variation in Physician Practice Pattern: An Examination of Technical and Cost Efficiency for Treating Sinusitis." *Journal of Medical Systems* 24 (2): 103–17.

Parkerton, P. H., E. H. Wagner, D. G. Smith, and H. L. Straley. 2003. "Effect of Part-Time Practice on Patient Outcomes." *Journal of General Internal Medicine* 18: 717–24.

Pasko, T., et al. 2000. *Physician Characteristics and Distribution in the U.S.* 2000–2001 edition, 18–19. Chicago: American Medical Association.

Pescosolido, B. A., S. A. Tuch, and J. K. Martin. 2001. "The Profession of Medicine and the Public: Examining Americans' Changing Confidence in Physician Authority from the Beginning of the 'Health Care Crisis' to the Era of Health Care Reform." *Journal of Health and Social Behavior* 42: 1–16.

Phelps, Charles. 2003. *Health Economics.* Boston: Addison Wesley Group.

Philibert, I., and J. Bickel. 1995. "Maternity and Parental Leave Policies at COTH Teaching Hospitals." *Academic Medicine* 70: 1056–58.

Phillips, Robert, Doreen Harper et al. 2002. "Can Nurse Practitioners and Physicians Beat Parochialism into Plowshares?" *Health Affairs* 21: 133–42.

Phillips, Robert L., and Barbara Starfield. 2003. "Why Does a U.S. Primary Care Physician Workforce Crisis Matter?" *American Family Physician* 68 (8): 1494.

Pinn, V. W., and M. T. Chunko. 1999. "The National Institutes of Health Office of Research on Women's Health and Its DHHS Partners: Meeting Challenges in Women's Health." *Journal of the American Medical Women's Association* 54 (1): 15–19.

Plante, Lauren. 2004. "Obstetricians Wanted: No Mothers Need Apply." *Annals of Internal Medicine* 140: 840–41.

Potee, R. A., A. J. Gerber, and J. R. Ickovics. 1999. "Medicine and Motherhood: Shifting Trends among Female Physicians from 1922 to 1999." *Academic Medicine* 74: 911–19.

Powell, H. S., J. Bridge et al. 2006. "Medical Students' Self-Reported Experiences Performing Pelvic, Breast, and Male Genital Examinations and the Influence of Student Gender and Physician Supervision." *Academic Medicine* 81 (3): 286–89.

Preston, Jo Anne. 1995. "Gender and the Formation of a Women's Profession: The Case of Public School Teaching." In *Gender Inequality at Work,* ed. Jerry A. Jacobs, 378–407. Thousand Oaks, Calif.: Sage.

Price, Joyce. 1997. "Doctors Increasingly Treat Sexes Differently: Practice 'Gender-Specific Medicine.'" *Washington Post,* May 1.

Pringle, Rosemary. 1998. *Sex and Medicine: Gender, Power, and Authority in the Medical Profession.* Cambridge: Cambridge University Press.

Purnell, Beverly, Leslie Roberts, and Orla Smith. 2005. "Vive la Diference: Introduction to Special Issue." *Science* 308: 1569.

Quadagno, Jill. 1976. "Occupational Sex Typing and Internal Labor Market Distribution: An Assessment of Medical Specialties." *Social Problems* 23 (4): 442–53.

Rabin, Roni. 2006. "Breast-Feed or Else." *New York Times,* June 13.

Rathore, S., J. Chen et al. 2001. "Sex Differences in Cardiac Catheterization: The Role of Physician Gender." *JAMA: Journal of the American Medical Association* 286: 2849–56.

Redman, S., D. Saltman, J. Straton, B. Young, and C. Paul. 1994. "Determinants of Career Choices among Women and Men Medical Students and Interns." *Medical Education* 28 (5): 361–71.

Reed, Marie, and Paul Ginsburg. 2003. "Behind the Times: Physician Income, 1995–99." Data Bulletin 24. Center for Studying Health System Change. http://www.hschange.com/.

Reed, Marie, and Sally Trude. 2002. "Who Do You Trust? Americans' Perspectives on Health Care, 1997–2001." Tracking report 3. Center for Studying Health System Change. http://www.hschange.com/.

Regan, H. B., and G. J. Brooks. 1995. *Out of Women's Experience: Creating Relational Leadership.* Thousand Oaks, Calif.: Corwin Press.

Reinhardt, Uwe. 1997. "The Impending Physician Surplus: Is It Time to Quit?" *JAMA: Journal of the American Medical Association* 277: 69.

Reskin, Barbara F., and Patricia A. Roos. 1990. *Job Queues, Gender Queues: Explaining Women's Inroads into Male Occupations*. Philadelphia: Temple University Press.

Riska, Elianne. 2001. *Medical Careers and Feminist Agendas*. New York: Aldine De Gruyter.

RNSA. 2002. "Physician Shortage Predicted in All Specialties." http://www.rsna.org/publications/rsnanews/jun02/physhortage-1.html.

Robinson, John P., and Geoffrey Godbey. 1997. *Time for Life: The Surprising Ways Americans Use Their Time*. State College: Pennsylvania State University Press.

Rodriguez, H. P., W. H. Rogers, R. E. Marshall, and D. G. Safran. 2007. "The Effects of Primary Care Physician Visit Continuity on Patients' Experiences with Care." *Journal of General Internal Medicine* 22: 787–93.

Romano, M. 2002. "The Doctor-Exec Is In: To Quell Physician Unrest, Some Hospitals Are Dumping Lay Executives and Replacing Them with Doctors." *Modern Healthcare* 32 (September): 6–7, 12, 1.

Rosenberg, L. E. 1999. "Physician-Scientists: Endangered and Essential." *Science* 283 (January 15): 331–32.

Ross, Shelly M. 2003. "The Feminization of Medicine." *Medicine and Society* 5 (9). http://virtualmentor.ama-assn.org/2003/09/msoc1-0309.html.

Roter, D. L., J. A. Hall et al. 1995. "Improving Physicians' Interviewing Skills and Reducing Patients' Emotional Distress: A Randomized Clinical Trial." *Archives of Internal Medicine* 155: 1877–84.

Roter, D., G. Geller et al. 1999. "Effects of Obstetrician Gender on Communication and Patient Satisfaction." *Obstetrics and Gynecology* 93 (5 pt. 1): 635–41.

Roter, D. L., and J. A. Hall. 1992. *Doctors Talking with Patients/Patients Talking with Doctors: Improving Communication in Medical Visits*. Westport, Conn.: Auburn House.

———. 1998. "Why Physician Gender Matters in Shaping the Physician-Patient Relationship." *Journal of Women's Health* 7 (9): 1093–97.

———. 2004. "Physician Gender and Patient-Centered Communication: A Critical Review of Empirical Research." *Annual Review of Public Health* 25: 497–519.

Roter, D., M. Lipkin, and A. Korsgaard. 1991. "Sex Differences in Patients' and Physicians' Communication during Primary Care Medical Visits." *Medical Care* 29 (11): 1083–93.

Roth, C. S., K. V. Watson, and I. B. Harris. 2002. "A Communication Assessment and Skill-Building Exercise (CASE) for First-Year Residents." *Academic Medicine* 77: 746–47.

Rubin, W. 1988. "Survey Shows Increasing Unhappiness of Internists." *Internal Medicine News* 21 (1): 11, 19, 28.

Rutherford, Sarah. 2001. "Any Difference? An Analysis of Gender and Divisional Management Styles in a Large Airline." *Gender, Work, and Organization* 8: 326–45.

Saad, Lydia. 2005. "Be a Doctor Is the Most Common Career Advice: Nursing Still Perceived as a Woman's Job." Vol. 2005. Gallup Poll News Service.

Safran, D. G. 2003. "Defining the Future of Primary Care: What Can We Learn from Patients." *Annals of Internal Medicine* 138 (3): 248–55.

Sage, William M. 2004. "The Forgotten Third: Liability Insurance and the Medical Malpractice Crisis." *Health Affairs* 23: 10.

Samuels, M. E., L. Shi et al. 1999. "A Profile of Women CEOs/Administrators in Community and Migrant Health Centers." *Journal of Health Administration and Education* 17: 111–27.

Sandvik, H., and S. Hunskaar. 1990. "Doctors' Characteristics and Practice Patterns in General Practice: An Analysis Based on Management of Urinary Incontinence." *Scandinavian Journal of Primary Health Care* 8 (3): 179–92.

Santana, Suria. 2003. "Step 2 Clinical Skills Exam Set for June 2004." *AAMC Reporter* (September). http://www.aamc.org/newsroom/reporter/sept03/exam.htm.

Sasser, Alicia. 2005. "Gender Differences in Physician Pay: Tradeoffs between Career and Family." *Journal of Human Resources* 40: 477–504.

Savickas, M. L., D. E. Alexander, A. P. Jonas, and F. M. Wolf. 1986. "Difficulties Experienced by Medical Students in Choosing a Specialty." *Journal of Medical Education* 61: 467–69.

Sax, Linda J. 1992. "Predicting Persistence of Science Career Aspirations: A Comparative Study of Male and Female College Students." Paper presented at the American Educational Research Association Conference, San Francisco, April 24.

Sax, Linda, Alexander Astin, William Korn, and Kathryn Mahoney. 2006. *National Norms for Entering College Freshmen*. Washington, D.C.: Office of Research, American Council on Education.

Schafermeyer, Robert, and Brent Asplin. 2003. "Hospital and Emergency Department Crowding in the United States." *Emergency Medicine Australasia* 15: 22–27.

Scherzer, Eric, and Janet Freedman. 2000. "Physician Unions: Organizing Women in the Year 2000." *Journal of the American Medical Women's Association* 55 (1): 16–19.

Schmittdiel, J., et al. 2000. "Effect of Physician and Patient Gender Concordance on Patient Satisfaction and Preventive Care Practices." *Journal of General Internal Medicine* 15 (11): 761–69.

Scholle, S. H., W. Gardner, J. Harman, D. Madlon-Kay, J. Pascoe, and K. Kelleher. 2001. "Physician Gender and Psychosocial Care for Children." *Medical Care* 39 (1): 26–38.

Schubot, D. B., W. Cayley Jr., and B. C. Eliason. 1996. "Personal Values Related to Primary Care Specialty Aspirations." *Family Medicine* 28 (10): 726–31.

Schwartz, R. W., R. K. Jarecky et al. 1989. "Controllable Lifestyle: A New Factor in Career Choice by Medical Students." *Academic Medicine* 64: 606–69.

Schwartz, W. B., and D. N. Mendelson. 1990. "No Evidence of an Emerging Physician Surplus: An Analysis of Change in Physicians' Work Load and Income." *JAMA: Journal of the American Medical Association* 263: 557–60.

Scott, C. S., H. S. Barrows, D. M. Brock, and D. D. Hunt. 1991. "Clinical Behaviors and Skills That Faculty from Twelve Institutions Judged Were Essential for Medical Students to Acquire." *Academic Medicine* 66: 106–11.

Scott-Coombes, David. 2002. "Reduction in Juniors' Hours Abolishes Concept of Continuity of Care." *British Medical Journal* 324: 736. http://www.bmj.com/cgi/content/full/324/7339/736#art.

Seltzer, V. L. 1999. "Changes and Challenges for Women in Academic Obstetrics and Gynecology." *American Journal of Obstetrics and Gynecology* 180 (4): 837–48.

Shapiro, J., and D. Schiermer. 1990. "Resident Psychosocial Performance: A Brief Report." *Family Practice* 8 (1): 10–13.

Silliman, R., S. Demissie et al. 1999. "The Care of Older Women with Early-Stage Breast Cancer: What Is the Role of Surgeon Gender?" *Medical Care* 37 (10): 1057–67.

Silver, B., and C. S. Hodgson. 1997. "Evaluating GPAs and MCAT Scores as Predictors of NBME I and Clerkship Performances Based on Students' Data from One Undergraduate Institution." *Academic Medicine* 72: 394–96.

Simon, Rita J., and Jean M. Landis. 1989. "The Polls—A Report: Women's and Men's Attitudes about a Woman's Place and Role." *Public Opinion Quarterly* 53: 265–76.

Simon, Vivian. 2005. "Wanted: Women in Clinical Trials." *Science* 308: 1517.

Smith, R. C., J. S. Lyle, J. A. Mettler, and A. A. Marshall. 2000. "Evidence-Based Guidelines for Teaching Patient-Centered Interviewing." *Patient Education and Counseling* 39: 27–36.

Sobecks, N. W., A. C. Justice, 1999. "When Doctors Marry Doctors: A Survey Exploring the Professional and Family Lives of Young Physicians." *Annals of Internal Medicine* 130: 312–19.

Stanton, B. 2007. "Family-Friendly Workplaces as a Foundation for the Future of Pediatrics." *Archives of Pediatrics and Adolescent Medicine* 161: 511–14.

Starr, Paul. 1982. *The Social Transformation of American Medicine*. New York: Basic Books.

Stein, L. 1967. "The Doctor-Nurse Game." *Archives of General Psychiatry* 16: 699–703.

Steinbrook, Robert. 2002. "The Debate over Residents' Work Hours." *New England Journal of Medicine* 347: 1296–1302.

Steinhauer, Jennifer. 1999. "For Women in Medicine, a Road to Compromise, Not Perks." *New York Times,* March 1.

Stevens, Rosemary. 1989. *In Sickness and in Wealth: American Hospitals in the Twentieth Century.* New York: Basic Books.

Stoddard, J. J., J. D. Reschovsky, and J. L. Hargraves. 2001. "Managed Care in the Doctor's Office: Has the Revolution Stalled?" *American Journal of Managed Care* 7: 1061–67.

Stoeckle, John. 1988. "Reflections on Modern Doctoring." *Milbank Quarterly* 66: 76–91.

Stone, Pamela. 2007. *Opting Out?* Berkeley: University of California Press.

Stone, Pamela, and Meg Lovejoy. 2004. "Fast-Track Women and the 'Choice' to Stay Home." *Annals of the American Academy of Political and Social Science* 596: 62–86.

Stratton, T. D., M. A. McLaughlin et al. 2005. "Does Students' Exposure to Gender Discrimination and Sexual Harassment in Medical School Affect Specialty Choice and Residency Program Selection?" *Academic Medicine* 80: 400–408.

Street, R. L. 2002. "Gender Differences in Health Care Provider-Patient Communication: Are They Due to Style, Stereotypes, or Accommodation?" *Patient Education and Counseling* 48: 201–6.

Street, R. L., H. S. Gordon et al. 2005. "Patient Participation in Medical Consultations: Why Some Patients Are More Involved Than Others." *Medical Care* 43: 960–69.

Strober, Myra. H. 1984. "A Theory of Sex Segregation." In *Sex Segregation in the Workplace: Trends, Explanations, Remedies,* ed. Barbara Reskin, 144–56. Washington, D.C.: National Academy of Sciences Press.

Strober, Myra H., and Carolyn Arnold. 1987. "The Dynamics of Occupational Segregation among Bank Tellers." In *Gender in the Workplace,* ed. Clair Brown and Joseph Pechman, 107–57. Wasington, D.C.: Brookings Institution.

Strunk, B. C., and J. D. Reschovsky. 2002. "Kinder and Gentler: Physicians and Managed Care, 1997–2001." Tracking report 5. Center for Studying Health System Change. http://www.hschange.com/.

Sturm, Ronald. 2002. "Effect of Managed Care and Financing on Practice Constraints and Career Satisfaction in Primary Care." *Journal of the American Board of Family Practice* 15: 367–77.

Taljanovic, M. S., T. B. Hunter et al. 2003. "Academic Radiology: The Reasons to Stay or Leave." *Academic Radiology* 10: 1461–68.

Tarlov, A. R. 1983. "Shattuck Lecture: The Increasing Supply of Physicians, the Changing Structure of the Health-Services System, and the Future Practice of Medicine." *New England Journal of Medicine* 308: 1235–44.

Tesch, B., H. Wood, A. L. Helwig, and A. B. Nattinger. 1995. "Promotion of Women Physicians in Academic Medicine: Glass Ceiling or Sticky Floor?" *JAMA: Journal of the American Medical Association* 273 (13): 1022–25.

Thomas, E. J., J. B. Sexton, and R. L. Helmreich. 2003. "Discrepant Attitudes about Teamwork among Critical Care Nurses and Physicians." *Critical Care Medicine* 31: 956–59.

Tierney, A. E., and A. B. Kimball. 2006. "Median Dermatology Base Incomes in Senior Academia and Practice Are Comparable, but a Significant Income Gap Exists at Junior Levels." *Journal of American Academy of Dermatology* 55: 213–19.

Toner, Robin. 1999. "Doctors Say HMO Patients Denied Care." *Cleveland Plain Dealer,* July 29.

Tran, D., H. Frankel, and R. Rabinovici. 2002. "The Profile of Level I Trauma Center Directors." *Journal of Trauma-Injury Infection and Critical Care.* 52: 835–38.

Trix, Frances, and Carolyn Psenka. 2003. "Exploring the Color of Glass: Letters of Recommendation for Male and Female Medical Faculty." *Discourse and Society* 14. http://www.faculty.diversity.ucla.edu/03recruit/committee/stk/docs/SrchBrfngs/Exploring_the_color_of_glass.pdf.

Tu, H. T., and J. L. Hargraves. 2003. "Seeking Health Care Information: Most Consumers Still on the Sidelines." Washington, D.C.: Center for Studying Health System Change. March. Issue Brief 61.

Uchitelle, Louis. 2006. "Lure of Great Wealth Affects Career Choices." *New York Times,* November 27.

Uhlenberg, P., and T. Cooney. 1990. "Male and Female Physicians: Family and Career Comparisons." *Social Science and Medicine* 30 (3): 373–78.

Unger, Mike. 2007. "Study Suggests Shorter Hours for Residents Are Safer." *Penn Current,* October 4.

U.S. Department of Health, Bureau of Women's Health. 2001. "Compendium on Physician Retraining Initiatives." http://www.4women.gov/owh/retrain/.

U.S. Department of Labor, Women's Bureau. 2004. "Women in the Labor Force in 2004." Vol. 2007. Washington, D.C.: U.S. Department of Labor, Bureau of Labor Statistics.

Vaglum, P., J. Wiers-Jenssen, and O. Ekeberg. 1999. "Motivation for Medical School: The Relationship to Gender and Specialty Preferences in a Nationwide Sample." *Medical Education* 33 (4): 236–42.

Van Dis, Jane. 2004. "Residency Training and Pregnancy." *Student JAMA: Journal of the American Medical Association* 291: 636.

Van Eaton, Erik G., Karen D. Horvath, and Carlos A. Pellegrini. 2005. "Professionalism and the Shift Mentality." *Archives of Surgery* 140: 230–335.

Varki, A., and Rosenberg, L. E. 2002. "Emerging Opportunities and Career Paths for the Young Physician-Scientist." *Nature Medicine* 8: 437–39.

Vaughn, Katie. 2006. "Top Docs: The Other Primary Care Provider Nurse Practitioners Combine the Skills of Physicians and Nurses." *Madison Magazine.* http://www.madisonmagazine.com/article.php?section_id=918&xstate=view_story&story_id=224208.

Veloski, J. J., C. A. Callahan, et al. 2000. "Prediction of Students' Performances on Licensing Examinations using Age, Race, Sex, Undergraduate GPA, and MCAT Scores." *Academic Medicine* 75.

Vickers, A. J., F. J. Bianco et al. 2007. "The Surgical Learning Curve for Prostate Cancer Control after Radical Prostatectomy." *Journal National Cancer Institute* 99: 1171–77.

Wajcman, Judy. 1998. *Managing Like a Man: Women and Men in Corporate Management.* University Park: Pennsylvania State University Press.

Walpert, Bryan. 2002. "Working Part Time: Can It Fit into Your Practice?" *American College of Physicians Observer.* http://www.acponline.org/journals/news/jul-aug02/part_time.htm.

Walsh, M. R. 1977. *Doctors Wanted, No Women Need Apply: Sexual Barriers in the Medical Profession.* New Haven: Yale University Press.

Warde, Carole. 2001. "Work–Family Balance." *Annals of Internal Medicine* 134: 343.

Wardrop, Tina. 2004. "As More Women Enter Medicine, Cultures Will Change." *Managed Healthcare Executive.* http://managedhealthcareexecutive.modernmedicine.com/mhe/Managed+Care+Outlook/As-more-women-enter-medicine-cultures-will-change/ArticleStandard/Article/detail/85876.

Warren, M. G., R. Weitz, and S. Kulis. 1999. "The Impact of Managed Care on Physicians." *Health Care Management Review* 24: 44–56.

Wear, D., and C. Keck-McNulty. 2004. "Attitudes of Female Nurses and Female Residents toward Each Other: A Qualitative Study in One U.S. Teaching Hospital." *Academic Medicine* 79: 291–301.

Weeks, W. B., and A. E. Wallace. 2002. "The More Things Change: Revisiting a Comparison of Educational Costs and Incomes of Physicians and Other Professionals." *Academic Medicine* 77: 312–19.

———. 2006. "The Influence of Race and Gender on Family Physicians' Annual Incomes." *Journal of the American Board of Family Medicine* 19: 548–56.

Weinberg Daniel. 2004. "Evidence from Census 2000 about Earnings by Detailed Occupation for Men and Women." *Census 2000 Special Reports* (May).

Weinstein, M. 1988. "Policing the Profession." *American College of Physician Observer* 1: 10–11.

Weisman, Carol. 1984. "Gender Composition of Medical Schools and Specialty Choices of Graduates." *Journal of Medical Education* 59 (4): 347–49.

Wethington, Elaine, Joy Pixley, and Allison Kavey. 2003. "Turning Points in Work Careers." In *It's About Time: Couples and Careers,* ed. P. Moen, 168–82. Ithaca: Cornell University Press.

Whelan, Gerald P., Nancy E. Gary et al. 2002. "The Changing Pool of International Medical Graduates Seeking Certification Training in U.S. Graduate Medical Education Programs." *JAMA: Journal of the American Medical Association* 288: 1079–84.

White, C. B., H. M. Haftel et al. 2006. "Multidimensional Effects of the Eighty-Hour Work Week at the University of Michigan Medical School: Duty Hours." *Academic Medicine* 81: 57–62.

Williams, B. 1999. "Women in Medicine: Still a Long Way to Go, Baby." *Tennessee Medicine* 92: 327–30.

Wissow, Lawrence S., Susan Larson et al. 2005. "Pediatric Residents' Responses that Discourage Discussion of Psychosocial Problems in Primary Care." *Journal of the American Academy of Child and Adolescent Psychiatry* 44: 1127.

Witte, F. M., T. D. Stratton, and L. M. Nora. 2006. "Stories from the Field: Students' Descriptions of Gender Discrimination and Sexual Harassment during Medical School." *Academic Medicine* 81: 648–54.

Wolinsky, F. D. 1988. "The Professional Dominance Perspective, Revisited." *Milbank Memorial Quarterly* 66: 33–47.

Woodrow, Sarah I., Christopher Segouin et al. 2006. "Duty Hours Reforms in the United States, France, and Canada: Is It Time to Refocus Our Attention on Education?" *Academic Medicine* 81: 1045–51.

Woodward, C. A. 2005. "When a Physician Marries a Physician: Effect of Physician-Physician Marriages on Professional Activities." *Canadian Family Physician* 51: 850–51.

Woodward, C., B. Hutchison, J. Abelson, and G. Norman. 1996. "Do Female Primary Care Physicians Practice Preventive Care Differently from Their Male Colleagues?" *Canadian Family Physician* 42: 2370–79.

Wozniak, Gregory. 2001. "The Impact of HMO Penetration on Physician Retirement." *AMA Center for Health Policy Research Policy Research Perspective* (March): 1–3.

Wright, A., L. Schwindt et al. 2003. "Gender Differences in Academic Advancement: Patterns, Causes, and Potential Solutions in One U.S. College of Medicine." *Academic Medicine* 78 (5): 500–508.

Wright, Rosemary, and Jerry A. Jacobs. 1994. "Male Flight from Computer Work: A New Look at Occupational Resegregation and Ghettoization." *American Sociological Review* 59: 511–36.

Wright, S., A. Wong, and C. Newill. 1997. "The Impact of Role Models on Medical Students." *Journal of General Internal Medicine* 12: 53-56.

Xu, G., L. E. Paddock et al. 2001. "Physician Executives Report High Job Satisfaction: Summary of Findings from a Survey of Senior Physician Executives." *Physician Executive* 27: 46–47.

Xu, G., S. L. Rattner et al. 1995. "A National Study of the Factors Influencing Men and Women Physicians' Choices of Primary Care Specialties." *Academic Medicine* 70 (5): 398–404.

Yamagata, Hisashi, Mark Haviland, Leonard Werner, and Rajeev Sabharwal. 2006. "Recent Trends in the Reporting of Medical Student Mistreatment." *AAMC Analysis in Brief:* 6.

Yellin, Jessica. 2004. "How Gender-Specific Medicine Could Change Health Care." *ABC World News*, December 4. http://abcnews.go.com/WNT/story?id=301044.

Young, J., and J. Ward. 1998. "Influence of Physician and Patient Gender on Provision of Smoking Cessation Advice in General Practice." *Tobacco Control* 7: 360–63.

Yutzie, J. D., J. L. Shellito et al. 2005. "Gender Differences in General Surgical Careers: Results of a Post-residency Survey." *American Journal of Surgery* 190 (6): 955–59.

Zelek, Barbara, and Susan P. Phillips. 2003. "Gender and Power: Nurses and Doctors in Canada." *International Journal of Equity Health* 2 (1): 1.

Index